T0184626

"I am extremely excited about the opportunities that Dr. Constantian's innovative, courageous pursuit offers. I have told my colleagues about how we found each other, and how his open-minded response to my books led to his own; I experienced a similar epiphany with Peter Levine's writings. This is a golden chance to enlighten the lay and medical communities and pave the way for a dramatic break-through in the role of trauma in body dysmorphic disorder."

—**Robert Scaer, MD**, author of *The Body Bears the Burden, The Trauma Spectrum*, and *8 Keys to Brain-Body Balance*

"Dr. Constantian writes extremely well and gives the patient a voice that will be chillingly familiar to those who have dealt with these unfortunate individuals. His extensive literature and clinical research establishes the influence of childhood trauma on someone with BDD. We all know these people, and most physicians will ultimately face a BDD patient. His book should be required reading for all lay and professional people who care for the BDD patient."

—**Jack H. Sheen, MD**, author of *Aesthetic Rhinoplasty*

"Dr. Constantian is, in my opinion, spot on in his observations on re-visioning body dysmorphia, which are excellent and long overdue. They are particularly exceptional from the point of view of a reconstructive surgeon."

—**Dr. Peter Levine**, author of *Waking the Tiger: Healing Trauma, In an Unspoken Voice: How the Body Releases Trauma and Restores Goodness, and Trauma and Memory: Brain and Body in a Search for the Living Past: A Practical Guide for Understanding and Working with Traumatic Memory*

"Dr. Constantian introduces a new perspective into the challenging existence of those struggling with body dysmorphia. As a plastic surgeon, he brings a fresh set of insights to the therapeutic world that can free up those chains of shame, trauma and hopelessness that too often define the world of anorexia, bulimia or binge eating disorder, and provides an antidote to such pain and suffering. This is a must book for anyone interested in body distortion."

—**Ralph E. Carson, LD, RD, PhD**, senior clinical and research advisor, Eating Recovery Center and BETR program, and author of *The Brain Fix: What's the Matter with Your Grey Matter*

"Dr. Constantian's unique career focus on revision rhinoplasty patients combined with his intellectual curiosity enabled him to associate childhood trauma with patient satisfaction. This concept is transformational and has broad impact throughout medicine. His book will establish a new paradigm by which plastic surgeons and other health care providers practice medicine. Screening for childhood trauma should become a routine part of the patient's history."

—**Arin K. Greene, MD**, professor of surgery, Harvard Medical School

"In this good read, Dr. Constantian's powerful contribution extensively researches the surgical and mental health literatures to expose the underworld of adverse childhood events. We visualize the toxic trajectory of childhood trauma and its devastating impact on self-worth, distorting reality and body image and driving the desire for excessive plastic surgery. Dr. Constantian shows that resilience is the antidote to childhood trauma. After all, when there is recognition and treatment, optimism follows."

—**Eugene B. Kern, MD**, Endicott Professor of Medicine, Mayo Foundation; professor of rhinology and facial plastic surgery emeritus, Mayo Clinic School of Medicine; and clinical professor of rhinology and facial plastic surgery, State University of New York (SUNY) at Buffalo

CHILDHOOD ABUSE, BODY SHAME, AND ADDICTIVE PLASTIC SURGERY

Childhood Abuse, Body Shame, and Addictive Plastic Surgery explores the psychopathology that plastic surgeons can encounter when seemingly excellent surgical candidates develop body dysmorphic disorder postoperatively. By examining how developmental abuse and neglect influence body image, personality, addictions, resilience, and adult health, this highly readable book uncovers the childhood sources of body dysmorphic disorder. Written from the unique perspective of a leading plastic surgeon with extensive experience in this area and featuring many poignant clinical vignettes and groundbreaking trauma research, this heavily referenced text offers a new explanation for body dysmorphic disorder that provides help for therapists and surgeons and hope for patients.

Mark B. Constantian, MD, FACS, has practiced plastic surgery in Nashua, New Hampshire, since 1978 and has faculty appointments at the University of Wisconsin and the University of Virginia. He is the author of more than 100 professional journal articles and book chapters and two previous textbooks, including *Rhinoplasty: Craft and Magic.*

CHILDHOOD ABUSE, BODY SHAME, AND ADDICTIVE PLASTIC SURGERY

The Face of Trauma

Mark B. Constantian, MD

ILLUSTRATIONS BY RUSTON J. SANCHEZ, MD
FOREWORD BY DAVID L. CORWIN, MD

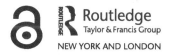
Routledge
Taylor & Francis Group
NEW YORK AND LONDON

First published 2019
by Routledge
52 Vanderbilt Avenue, New York, NY 10017

and by Routledge
2 Park Square, Milton Park, Abingdon, Oxon, OX14 4RN

Routledge is an imprint of the Taylor & Francis Group, an informa business

Library of Congress Cataloging-in-Publication Data
Names: Constantian, Mark B., author. | Sanchez, Ruston (Ruston J.),
    illustrator. | Corwin, David L., writer of foreword.
Title: Childhood abuse, body shame, and addictive plastic surgery :
    the face of trauma / Mark B. Constantian; illustrations by Ruston J.
    Sanchez; foreword by David L. Corwin.
Description: New York, NY : Routledge, 2019. | Includes bibliographical
    references and index.
Identifiers: LCCN 2018039392 (print) | LCCN 2018051905 (ebook) |
    ISBN 9781315657721 (eBook) | ISBN 9781138100305 | ISBN
    9781138100305 (hardback) | ISBN 9781138100312 (paperback) |
    ISBN 9781315657721 (ebk)
Subjects: LCSH: Body dysmorphic disorder. | Body image disturbance. |
    Surgery, Plastic. | Psychic trauma in children.
Classification: LCC RC569.5.B64 (ebook) | LCC RC569.5.B64 C66
    2019 (print) | DDC 616.85/2—dc23
LC record available at https://lccn.loc.gov/2018039392

ISBN: 978-1-138-10030-5 (hbk)
ISBN: 978-1-138-10031-2 (pbk)
ISBN: 978-1-315-65772-1 (ebk)

DOI: 10.4324/9781315657721

For my patients,
Whose behavior I have tried to explain,
whose suffering I have tried to relieve,
and whose resilience has inspired me

And Always for Charlotte
Dès lors et à jamais

CONTENTS

FOREWORD

Mark B. Constantian, MD, has devoted much of his career over the past 40 years caring for patients who are referred to him because of his reputation and skill performing revision rhinoplasties. As an academically oriented plastic surgeon, this area of specialization within the field of plastic surgery has given him a unique opportunity to better inform our understanding of Body Dysmorphic Disorder (BDD). BDD is a frustrating and perplexing condition where individuals with often relatively minor or even no discernable facial abnormalities seek out seemingly endless plastic surgical procedures like repeated rhinoplasties and are often disappointed with the results. The disappointment in BDD patients is usually contrary to their surgeon's and other observers' impression that the plastic surgery accomplished what the patients said they wanted to achieve. Dr. Constantian's description of these patients' obsessive, often negative, and accusatory post-surgical communications, begging for revisions and other additional plastic surgery, sometimes even threatening legal and more rarely physical violence toward their surgeons leads me to believe that this book should become required reading for all practicing and plastic surgeons in training. He acknowledges that BDD patients' suffering is real but that he has come to believe that it has more to do with their childhood adversity than actual physical deformity. Treating these perceived facial deformities with plastic surgery may too often be treating the patients' symptoms of distress and often results in negative consequences and feelings in these patients and accusatory accusations against the surgeons. Dr. Constantian and others who have done research on BDD suggest that the actual cause of BDD is likely associated with childhood abuse, neglect, and other severe childhood adversity.

Dr. Constantian references the paradigm changing Adverse Childhood Experiences Study (ACE Study) by Drs. Vincent J. Felitti and Robert Anda, who first published their findings, with their collaborators, in 1998. He also presents the findings from his clinical case series that used the same questions as the original ACE Study and yielded similar findings.

I worked with both Felitti and Anda to produce two DVDs, the second of which includes videos of their lectures and individual interviews with each of them designed to help educate professionals and the public about their study and findings. In reading some of the chapters from *The Face of Trauma*, Dr. Constantian's description of the insatiable nature of BDD patients reminded me of Dr. Felitti's statement, shared with me and others attending his presentations, that it is "hard to get enough of something that almost works." That the observations and insights in this book come from a plastic surgeon and not a mental health researcher or professional makes total sense. Few mental health professionals see enough of these patients to discern the patterns in their presentation, histories, and discouraging outcomes. Plastic surgeons are the front line caring for BDD patients. Dr. Constantian's lack of preconceptions, rooted in the ideological schools and conventional wisdom of psychiatry and psychology, helped him think and observe "outside the box." He recognized the relationship between childhood abuse and neglect and addictive plastic surgery. Drs. Felitti and Anda are both internists, not psychiatrists. That fact may have also freed them to make the paradigm shifting observations and discoveries of the ACE Study. Major shifts in science and other areas, in some case even disruptive innovations, often come from outside the close circle of individuals viewed as authoritative in those particular fields or topics.*

Hopefully, this book is the beginning of a journey that will lead to better recognition and more effective care for BDD patients. Dr. Constantian describes his great frustration and the bewilderment that he shares with other plastic surgeons treating these unhappy and often disruptive patients. Fortunately, he has not just described how to identify and to avoid these challenging patients. Rather, he seeks to understand the roots of their misery. This is a book of hope and belief in the resilience of human beings to overcome their travail and suffering. It is also a book very much rooted in the tradition of medicine that effective treatment begins with accurate diagnosis and understanding of the pathogenesis of disease. Treating symptoms rather than their root causes is still too common, particularly in the most complex areas of psychiatry and psychology where the pathways, complexity of the brain, and the multiple systems interacting makes the determination of proven pathogenesis much more difficult than infectious disease, metabolic illness, or orthopedic injuries.

This book serves as a bridge between the worlds of plastic surgery and the inter-disciplinary fields focusing on childhood and later life trauma. If read and understood, it may help BDD patients by assisting the plastic surgeons who treat them to better understand the source of these patients' unhappiness and how to better care for them. With time and development of more effective ways of caring for these patients, this knowledge can also diminish the suffering of plastic surgeons who treat BDD patients. As Dr. Constantian reaffirms, effective treatment begins with accurate diagnosis and understanding. At the conclusion of his book,

Dr. Constantian suggests this may begin with asking these patients what happened to them during their childhoods. Dr. Felitti once commented that it took him many years to realize that listening closely to his patients talk about their lives is a most powerful form of doing!

Understanding the associations and connections between adverse childhood experiences and the many later diseases and dysfunctions, including BDD, that afflict so many of those who experience these kinds of adversities, as so eloquently described by Dr. Constantian, is an important foundation for understanding and caring for patients with BDD. It is an important first step for addressing the "Face of Trauma."

David L. Corwin, MD
President, American Professional Society on the
Abuse of Children, 2018–2020
Professor and Director of Forensic Services,
Department of Pediatrics
University of Utah School of Medicine
Salt Lake City, Utah
March 24, 2018

Note

* Kuhn, Thomas, *The Structure of Scientific Revolutions*, Chicago: University of Chicago Press, 1962.

PREFACE

This re-breathing of argon atoms of past breaths . . . has some picturesque implications . . . [and] associate[s] us with the past and the future. . . . If you are more than 20 years old you have inhaled more than 100 million breaths. . . . You contribute so many argon atoms to the atmospheric bank . . . that the first gasp of every baby born on earth a year ago contained argon atoms that you have since breathed. . . . Our next breaths . . . will sample the snorts, sighs, bellows, shrieks, cheers, and spoken prayers of the prehistoric and historic past. Thus we are all linked to the past and to each other.*

★★★★★

These words from an essay by Harlow Shapley, former head of the Harvard College Observatory, is a metaphor for our interconnections as humans. Nowhere is that connection more intimately formed and more easily disturbed than between patient and physician.

From the beginning of this adventure I simply took hold of the free end of a ball of yarn and pulled.

In the mid-1980's, as a young plastic surgeon not yet 10 years in practice, I performed reconstructive nasal surgery on three patients who had good surgical outcomes but extremely stormy postoperative courses. All became recluses. One gave up her university professorship. One became unable to care for her family. One tried to amputate his nose.

At the time, I had heard only a little about body dysmorphic disorder, but these disturbing events drove me to learn more. A disorder that was not contagious or life-threatening nevertheless disrupted patient and family happiness, altered patients' life trajectories and productivity, and in the worst cases ended in suicide. Its apparent cause was a sudden and inexplicable obsession with some physical feature. That's all anyone knew.

From the plastic surgeon's perspective, there were still two gaps. Most of the patients described in the literature were not ones that we saw; that was to be expected. Our patients were not depressed, delusional, or housebound: they were high-performing individuals requesting aesthetic plastic surgery. Most had undergone other cosmetic operations but were not satisfied. Even when the surgical result was good—sometimes exceptional—they became irrationally distraught.

These patients were different. They hadn't had complications. They didn't have bad results. Yet I couldn't comfort them. I couldn't establish relationships of mutual trust: instead, they railed: "What you have done to me borders on the criminal. . . . I trusted you but you deformed me. . . . You experimented on me. . . . You have robbed me of my family, my friends, and my joy in living." None of it made sense.

★★★★★

There was another missing piece: What causes body dysmorphic disorder? For a problem so common and devastating, with so many florid, uniting clinical features, why wasn't the cause more obvious?

The answers came one at a time. I noticed that the behavior of these unhappy postoperative patients was immature. Whatever shroud of normalcy had existed during the preoperative consultation vanished after surgery in a baffling cloud of inexplicable complaints, dramatic swelling, depression, and excessively demanding or disempowered behavior that could overwhelm my staff and me for months.

Then I met a patient who told me that he had been body dysmorphic but recovered. He tells his story in Chapter 1—a disturbing melodrama of significant childhood abuse and neglect. This was my first clue that the chaotic family patterns that I had observed in other patients might have a common root. Perhaps body dysmorphic disorder began in the family.

There is already ample evidence in the mental health literature that childhood abuse and neglect cause shame—the sense of being defective in some way—and that the most common type of shame resulting from childhood trauma is body shame. If traumatized people connect their sense of shame to the way they look, plastic surgery, even unconsciously, seems like an easy pathway to self-esteem. But surgery cannot create self-esteem, and so the dissatisfaction rate among these patients ought to be very high—and it is. Couldn't childhood trauma be one provocative element for body dysmorphic disorder?

The next piece floated down like a message from the spheres. I recognized that I was seeing patients who had undergone multiple unsuccessful rhinoplasties and wanted more surgery. Most had also undergone cosmetic procedures on their faces and bodies. Many were demanding or depressed. What was most unusual was one common thread: 80% originally had noses that they knew were normal—but they had undergone surgery anyway. Why?

Data collected on 100 revision rhinoplasty patients indicated that those who had undergone more than three cosmetic operations, were demanding or depressed, and whose original rhinoplasties were performed on noses that the patients knew were normal had a childhood trauma prevalence of 90%, and the likelihood of total satisfaction after my operation was only 3%. We had identified patients who had body dysmorphic disorder and linked them to histories of childhood abuse or neglect.

★★★★★

The Kaiser Permanente/CDC study had already documented an astounding developmental trauma prevalence of 64% in a middle-class general medical population. What were the prevalences and trauma types in plastic surgery patients? The headline is that, in an elective plastic surgery practice, the overall prevalence of childhood abuse or neglect was 80%—most commonly emotional abuse—significantly higher than the Kaiser/CDC study; and among revision rhinoplasty and BDD patients, it was over 90%.

Perhaps the most inspiring piece was the mediating factor of human resilience. Resilience allows us to conquer ourselves, that makes us, not cisterns, but artesian wells, from which we can draw at will. Resilience appears to be the antidote to developmental trauma.

I needed to know more about what had already been established and so spent four years reading more than 110 textbooks and 750 peer-reviewed manuscripts in the developmental trauma, posttraumatic stress disorder, body image, body shame, eating disorder, self-injury, childhood development, and addiction literature. It became evident to me that there were interconnections—many of them—and that the questions raised by one subspecialty had often been answered others. But the information was sequestered in silos.

Few argue that the vestiges of childhood trauma can propagate into adulthood as shame, addictions, and other self-harming behaviors. Working backward, it is also possible to connect the personality traits, health, and behavior of plastic surgical patients, particularly those with body dysmorphic disorder, to histories of childhood neglect and abuse. It doesn't matter where we start—from childhood or adulthood—the connections between body shame and addictive plastic surgery to developmental trauma are hard to miss. It is important for the readers—especially mental health professionals who have done the heavy lifting—to realize that none of the components that support the link between childhood trauma and body dysmorphic disorder are my conjectures. Each one is found in the established peer-reviewed literature. Developmental trauma causes shame, most commonly body shame. With all this reported evidence, body dysmorphic disorder should not still be an unexplained oddity in which some unlucky people for unknown reasons become obsessively and disablingly self-conscious about their appearances. Body dysmorphic disorder therefore becomes only one more poisonous blossom that grows out of a disruptive and destructive early life, no different than obesity, eating disorders, drug or alcohol addiction, or deliberate self-injury. Trauma-induced shame is the lighter fluid.

★★★★★

I realize that there will be readers who wonder how a surgeon without mental health training could dare to invade the mental health literature and propose a thesis that differs from much prevailing teaching. To that legitimate reservation there are at least three answers. The first is that there is an advantage to long-range perspective. I did not enter this literature search with preconceived notions. I did not intend to rewrite the mental health literature, and I do not believe that I have. I have made an effort to stay within my ken. I simply assembled the observations that others had made into a portrait of body image-disturbed patients that comported with what I saw as a surgeon and what my clinical research revealed. My very distance from these individual specialties perhaps helped me to see unifying themes that might be obscured from the interior.

Second, plastic surgeons have never been very far from trying to understand body dysmorphic patients and body image disorders. Fifty-eight years ago a collaborative study in 98 plastic surgery patients with "minimal deformity" by a plastic surgeon and two psychiatrists from Johns Hopkins University demonstrated psychopathology, depression, obsessive-compulsive disorder, troubled family relationships, or marital difficulties in 73% of the patients. Fifty-five percent had turbulent postoperative courses, some requesting additional surgery.[†] These data almost exactly duplicate our findings, detailed in Chapters 8 and 9, and predate the first description of body dysmorphic disorder in the DSM-III-R by 27 years.

Last, body image is a complex entity with which plastic surgeons cope in every patient, whether the problem is deformity from cancer, congenital anomaly, accidental trauma, or normal aging. All plastic surgeons see the salutary effects of successful reconstructive surgery on patients' psyches, self-esteem, health, and in their eyes. Plastic surgery is always brain surgery, and plastic surgeons are uniquely positioned to understand body image disorders in their context, beyond the inevitable limitations of psychometrics and within the framework of surgical experience and recovery. In this regard, my specialty can and must add a valuable dimension to the voluminous work already contributed by mental health experts.

All threads have two ends; so far this one doesn't. Much of the research in this book is by definition preliminary: it was a side project contemporaneous with a busy surgical practice and teaching schedule. Researchers and clinicians who have the time to expand pieces of what I may have uncovered can add more, and I hope that they will. Those of us interested in body dysmorphic disorder, like players in a playground pickup baseball game, can still recognize the same phenomena, even if we describe them in different dialects.

★★★★★

Finally, this book is also for those survivors and patients who have too few advocacy voices, and who need a way through and out. In writing it, I have tried to straddle the gap between professional medical writing and popular scientific education. Lay readers are much more informed than they were, thanks to electronic media and their own driving curiosity, and now carry knowledge that provides a sophisticated entrée behind the wizard's curtain. Childhood trauma produces toxic shame, contaminates the early life years, and may re-emerge as body shame that can ruin lives as powerfully as any addictions or other maladaptive behaviors.

If patients who seek self-worth and perfection through repeated aesthetic surgeries recognize aspects of themselves in the vignettes or in my discussion of the literature, I hope that they will consider treating the roots of their developmental trauma before seeking surgical solutions that won't work.

For those reconstructive surgeons who have asked, "How do we know who is a surgical candidate?" I hope that the puzzle pieces that I have spread on the table will help them carry out their mission of understanding body image and the suffering that it causes. Shame-motivated surgery is the key.

Perhaps the most extraordinary part of this yarn-pulling is that it began a struggle to explain why some patients with good surgical results could be so irrationally unhappy, but ended as a story about the buoyancy of human resilience, which is so much more enchanting and inspiring.

Mark B. Constantian, MD, FACS
Nashua, New Hampshire
October 2018

Notes

* Shapley, H., *Beyond the Observatory,* New York, Charles Scribner's Sons, 1967, pp. 47–48.
† Edgerton MT, Jacobson WE, Meyer E. Surgical-Psychiatric Study of Patients Seeking Plastic (Cosmetic) Surgery: Ninety-Eight Consecutive Patients With Minimal Deformity. *Br J Plast Surg* 1960; 13:136–145.

ACKNOWLEDGMENTS

During the past five years I have sometimes wondered if I might be assembling a pterodactyl from puzzle pieces that were meant to construct a horse instead, but many steady friends and colleagues have assured me that it really is a horse.

As a third-year medical student at the University of Virginia, my interest in the psychological aspects of plastic surgery was piqued by Dr. Milton Edgerton, chairman of the Department of Plastic Surgery. His seminal papers first identified the problem that we call body dysmorphic disorder, 27 years before it appeared in the DSM-3-R. Though he did not specifically make the etiologic trauma connection, Dr. Edgerton presciently identified each of the personal and family traits of these patients; his 1960 paper reads like a modern publication. We maintained a friendship over the years, and as I began to hatch my new ideas I share them with him. He allowed me to read an unpublished manuscript detailing 20 of his most psychologically disturbed patients, which I have covered in Chapter 1. In many ways, I am simply confirming and extending some of his original observations 58 years later.

Before I began writing, I shared my nascent theories with Doctors Robert Scaer, Bessel van der Kolk, Thomas Pruzinsky, Beatrice Andrews, Thomas Cash, Vincent Felitti, and Peter Levine, who believed that I was facing in the right direction. Their encouragement at that critical time and as the book took shape was critically valuable. Dr. David L. Corwin willingly read chapter drafts and graciously contributed the Foreword.

At The Meadows workshops from 2004 to 2012 and at a postgraduate course for therapists in early 2016, Pia Mellody taught me her model and expanded my earlier concepts. Hers was just the counsel and reinforcement that I needed.

Dr. Mark Albert patiently tracked down and sent many hundreds of journal articles that enlarged my source materials.

Drs. Jenny Chen and Harry Nayar helped assemble and then present our first childhood trauma data to an international audience of plastic surgeons.

Dr. Deepak Narayan graciously proofed my section on Epigenetics.

Robert Aicher, J.D., served as a valued adviser throughout the creative process.

At the Flying E Ranch in Arizona, where I wrote and revised much of the book, Norman Lilley, Ande Taylor, and Debbie Spirito were the first non-medical readers to review early drafts and reassure me that they were actually comprehensible to lay readers.

Nick Zaborek, MA, Assistant Researcher at the University of Wisconsin Department of Surgery, prepared mountains of statistics and answered my endless questions. Together we navigated 10,500 patient data points, and he contributed significantly to the preparation and writing of Chapters 9 and 10.

Dr. Ruston J. Sanchez found time during his busy plastic surgery residency to prepare the cover and artwork and exposed me to concepts of facial analysis that have become our next project.

I am particularly grateful to Dr. Michael Bentz, chairman of the Division of Plastic Surgery at the University of Wisconsin, who gave his residents time to work with me and provided access to the Department of Surgery statisticians, without whom the current product would not have had so much depth.

Between 1958 and 1961, Mary Halkyard taught me Latin, English History, and how to write. I maintained grateful contact with her through all of her 102 years. Without Mary Halkyard, this book would not have been as clear.

Editorial Assistant Jamie Magyar at Routledge (Taylor and Francis) and Editor Amanda Devine advised us in manuscript preparation and handling over 800 endnotes and more than 1,000 text citations. I am grateful for the help of Production Editor Katherine Hemmings and especially for the patient assistance of Project Manager Kate Fornadel. This is the group that finalized the book you hold.

My practice would never run so well without my long-time operating room and office nurse Donna Morton, a woman with the unusual simultaneous qualities of tenderness and tempered steel needed to practice medicine today and to keep pace with the countless projects that I place before her.

Many writers comment on the loneliness of the creative process, and solitary much of it is. But over the years that this research and writing took shape, many wonderful people listened to my ideas, encouraged them, questioned them, and sometimes nudged me toward newer, better directions, among them my professional mentor and close friend Dr. Jack Sheen and his wife, Anitra. I will always be grateful to both.

In the nearly 32 years that we have worked together, everything meaningful I have accomplished has been a team effort with my wife, Charlotte—her FM to my AM—her better frequencies, clearer signals, and smarter ideas. She claims only to be my "logistics person," but she is so much more—my life coach and my dearest, loving partner. Charlotte typed my 830 some-odd references. In the two weeks before the manuscript was submitted, she worked over 150 hours converting endnotes, adding cross references, and tirelessly checking my edits. She is my silent co-author.

I have tried to write a book that I would like to read myself. I hope that both practitioners and patients will believe that I have succeeded, and that those who are survivors of the disorders described here will benefit from the information and be inspired to find ways out.

Mark B. Constantian, MD, FACS
July 2018

THE FIRST PIECE
The Tip of the Thread

1

WHERE THE THREAD BEGAN

What Surgeons Learn From Patients and Their Families

A Successful Surgery; an Unhappy Patient

"I trusted you, but you betrayed me."

The attractive young woman sat on the edge of my examination table, one foot tucked beneath her.* Her husband slouched on the adjoining chair, holding her hand. She stared at me in poisonous silence. I looked back, trying to stay as friendly as someone running for town council. Finally she continued.

"You've ruined my face."

I felt oxygen leave the room. A therapist would tell me that was some kind of boundary failure, but occasional boundary failures are probably good for surgeons. Nine days ago I had performed a difficult revision rhinoplasty, converting a distorted, obstructed nose with a bizarre appearance into something more normal. It was her fifth nasal surgery, but I thought that I had accomplished precisely what she had asked.

I took a deep breath. "I don't understand," I said. "Three days ago, when we took your cast off, you were tearfully happy. You were hugging everyone."

She jerked her head as if shaking off a fly.

DOI: 10.4324/9781315657721-2

"No. You deceived me. You talked about my trauma just to sucker me into surgery. Then you changed the operation. I told you not to shorten my nose, but you did. You made my nose . . ."
She searched for the word. Her husband studied his knuckles.
"Disgusting."
She paced out each syllable, then pointed to her face.
"I can't go back to work—I won't go anywhere—looking like this."
The room air thickened. Her eyes were direct and defiant. She slowed her words to make sure I could follow along.
"You . . . made . . . me . . . ugly."

★★★★★

When we first met we had indeed talked about her abusive childhood. What prompted it was a photo of her nose before she'd had four rhinoplasties, which was straight, symmetrical, and pretty.

"Your nose looked good."
She paused. "I know."
I watched her as I spoke. "So why did you have surgery?"
Her face pinched and her voice became smaller.
"I had to be prettier for my family."
She thought more about that.
"My mother always said she wished I was as pretty as my sister."
She sighed quietly.
"I always disappointed her."
She held out another photograph. Her sister's features were slightly more delicate, but the differences, even to my eye, were small.

At that time I had just published research indicating that the overwhelming majority of patients who had undergone multiple surgeries on noses that the patients already knew were normal had a 90% likelihood of childhood abuse or neglect, and that the chance of making those patients happy in one operation was only 3%.[1,2] These are the desperate people that the literature calls "body dysmorphic" and whose seemingly unaccountable, insatiable addiction for surgical perfection fascinates the popular media. And so at this woman's consultation I had said, "Many patients who have had multiple operations on normal noses have had rough childhoods." Suddenly her mascara blurred and tears trickled down her cheeks. She told me her story.

I explained what I understood about the effects of childhood trauma on body shame, perfectionism, and the drive to plastic surgery, which at the time was limited. She agreed to have trauma therapy after surgery. Her husband had patted her hand. But her nose was disfigured and blocked. I knew that I could repair the surgical problem. My questions to myself weren't, will this patient be easy to manage, but rather, can I get her successfully through an operation despite her childhood—and will she be happy? It was a Hobson's choice: either I did something to help her or I turned her away.

We discussed the reconstruction in detail. I showed the patient and her husband examples of others with similar deformities that had good, mediocre, and even suboptimal results that needed revisions. No, go ahead, she told me. I have to have it fixed. And so I operated. Now it was nine days later.

"You're lying," she said. "It is shorter. You tipped it up after I told you not to do that. You didn't listen. You took advantage of me."

I tried to be reasonable. I showed current photographs. I did just what you asked, I said. Your nose isn't shorter—you can tell because your nostrils aren't visible. Now you can breathe better.

She rotated the mirror, examining herself from different angles.

"It looks like a snout. Me and Miss Piggy."

"That's pretty rough language to use about yourself," I said. She kept going.

"It's crooked. Look at these grafts. I didn't even need grafts. All my friends in the chat room say so."

She narrowed her stare.

"I can hurt you on the Internet, you know."

I decided to let that go.

"I don't believe you have a problem. Just give it time," I said.

I knew it would help to say something profoundly comforting. So far, nothing was coming to me. But she wasn't finished.

"You're a liar. Once I was asleep, you experimented on me."

She leaned forward for emphasis.

"I was just your guinea pig."

She searched my face as if she were reading a map.

"You know what you did," she said, straightening. "You butchered me."

I paused. My composure was atrophying.

"Try not to worry. Even if the result doesn't heal perfectly, I can revise it," I said. "We had talked about that before surgery."

I should stop talking, I thought. She was listening without hearing, as if my voice were background music. Her eyes darkened. The room grew smaller around us. There was so much I didn't understand. Maybe I should print that on my letterhead.

"In my whole life," she said softly, "every man has betrayed me."

Her voice was stiff and flat, as if she were reciting from memory a story that she had learned about someone else, a very long time ago.

What Might Explain This Irrational Behavior?

As of this writing, I have been in practice 40 years; most of my surgeries are now revision rhinoplasties. Despite everything I have learned and taught over the last two decades about my unhappy patients and all the heartfelt stories I have heard from surgeons about their experiences, I still have occasional incidents like this one.

Why do they occur? Why are patients unhappy with surgical results that are successful, even very good?[3] Why can't I reason with them? And why does their anger seem so irrational and personal—so seemingly out of context? Instead of asking, am I still swollen, this intelligent, productive, successful woman was asking, why did you betray me?

Let's speculate. The thesis of this text, supported widely but diffusely in the literature and by my own clinical research, is that this patient's early trauma had left an unhealed, wounded child. The toxic shame generated by her childhood events manifested as body shame and drove her original surgery and each subsequent one. The cardinal problem was not in my office or operating room; it was in her family of origin. Imagine if she had returned home, happy at six days with her reconstructed nose, and some abusive relative had said, "Look at you. You had all that surgery and spent all that money, and you're still as ugly as you always were. You'll never be as pretty as your sister. You're a born loser." She had expected my revision to give her the self-worth that every human deserves but that surgery alone can never supply. Triggered by some reminder of family trauma, she became a wounded child again. She reacted with the coping skills that she had developed—and that were appropriate—at the time, which explains her immature words and intense anger at someone whom she'd trusted with her appearance only a few days before. I was no longer her surgeon. I had become just another perpetrator.

*****

In a perfect world, the relationship between the plastic surgeon and the aesthetic surgery patient would be even more favorable than in other medical encounters, a nicety that does not apply to the patient frightened by a new cancer diagnosis or intoxicated in a lonely emergency room. In cosmetic cases, everything should be different. But there are always exceptions. Part of the thesis of this book is that, unless the surgery was technically flawed, this patient's seemingly inexplicable behavior—to me, at least—is more intriguing and tells a more revealing and provocative story than it may at first seem.

> "It must be a chain of psychological reactions, unpleasant experiences, lingering remarks, frustrations, disturbing self-consciousness that eventually brings the patient to submit to a cosmetic operation. . . . It is not empty vanity.[4] The chain that plastic surgical pioneer Gustave Aufricht so correctly identified stares at us nowhere more intensely and mysteriously than from the condition that we call "body dysmorphic disorder."
>
> Faulkner was right: "The past is never dead. It's not even past."

Body Image Obsession and the Diagnosis of Body Dysmorphic Disorder

My personal introduction to his body dysmorphic disorder (BDD) and unhappy patients was innocent but direct: in the mid-1980s, when few talked about body dysmorphic disorder, I operated on three such patients in short succession without having made the diagnosis beforehand. Their postoperative courses were so stormy that I determined to understand what I had done wrong and dove into the literature.

At the time, body dysmorphic disorder was grouped with the somatoform disorders (like hysteria and hypochondriasis) and defined in the *Diagnostic and Statistical Manual of Mental Disorders, Fourth Edition* (DSM-IV) by three criteria:

(A) Preoccupation with an imagined or trivial defect in appearance that (B) causes clinically significant distress or impairment in social, occupational or other important areas of functioning and (C) is not better explained by another disorder.

On May 8, 2013, the American Psychiatric Association released its newest Diagnostic and Statistical Manual of Mental Disorders (DSM-5).[5] As anticipated from its subcommittee's work, and of particular interest to surgeons, BDD had been redefined and reclassified for the first time since its inclusion in the DSM-111-R in 1987.

In the DSM-5, BDD was promoted to a new chapter, "Obsessive Compulsive and Related Disorders," which also included Obsessive Compulsive Disorder, Hoarding Disorder, and Hair Pulling and Excoriation Disorder. Here is its current definition:

A. Preoccupation with one or more perceived defects or flaws in physical appearance that are not observable or appear slight to others.

B. At some point during the course of the disorder, the individual has performed repetitive behaviors (e.g., mirror checking, excessive grooming, skin picking, reassurance seeking) or mental acts (e.g., comparing his or her appearance with that of others) in response to the appearance concerns.

C. The preoccupation causes clinically significant distress (for example, depressed mood, anxiety, shame) or impairment in social, occupational, or other important areas of functioning (for example, school, relationships, household).

D. The appearance preoccupations are not restricted to concerns with body fat or weight in an individual whose symptoms meet diagnostic criteria for an eating disorder.[5]

These changes from the DSM-IV criteria describe the patient's flaws as "perceived" instead of "imagined," revised wording that is presumably less pejorative and captures the patient's experience more accurately. The DSM-5 also adds a new criterion requiring that the patient must have performed repetitive behaviors (mirror checking, grooming) or mental acts (comparing appearance to others) in response to his or her "perceived flaw," which supports its reclassification with obsessive compulsive disorders. A modifier has been added to allow the examiner to specify the level of insight: "good" or "fair," "poor," or "delusional," and explicitly excludes eating disorders. Although BDD could also be classified with the anxiety disorders because it shares so many traits with posttraumatic stress disorder, these are thoughtful, good changes.

However, the new criteria have perhaps unavoidable practical limitations for surgeons and physicians. Like an 18th century fever, BDD is still described by its surface manifestations. Surgeons rarely see the tortured, delusional, housebound patients treated by mental health professionals. The latter see patients who (for the most part) have an established or suspected diagnosis and who have agreed to be treated. Surgeons see more functional, more guarded, often highly performing individuals who want surgery. Thus specialty differences in diagnosis and perspective are inevitable. These differences are highlighted by the ironic omission of "surgery" to the repetitive behaviors listed in Criterion B—the very route by which many specialists meet body dysmorphic patients. Clinical summaries of my first three BDD patients illustrate the practical distinctions.

Three Patients That Drove Me to the Literature

My first patient was a 60-year-old university professor who wanted modest changes in her nasal shape and correction of an obstructed airway. She had undergone other cosmetic procedures but was dissatisfied with all her results. That ought to have been a clue. She was so anxious on the day of surgery that she almost canceled, which in my youthful inexperience I attributed to normal jitters. That ought to have been another clue. Surgery proceeded uneventfully. The result was objectively very good. I was pleased.

She wasn't. At two weeks, crying and agitated, she demanded an immediate revision, believing that her nose had been over-shortened and that the tip pointed toward the ceiling. She resigned from her teaching position and became a recluse, refusing to see family and only shopping at night where she would not be recognized. "If I return to teaching," she said, "my students will ask, 'What have you done to your nose?'" Her behavior is not uncommon among BDD patients; in several series, 25% to 30% of patients have become housebound.

One of several letters contained photographs and measurements to reinforce her unhappiness.

> *I told you that I wanted my nose shortened by "a hair"—perhaps 1 / 8 inch, perhaps only 1 / 32 inch or 1 / 64 inch. I never in my wildest imagination expected that my nose would be this pointy, short, and turned up. It is a mockery of my long face. It's like someone else's nose has been plucked off and put on my face. I am brokenhearted and devastated by this sawed-off, turned-up snout. How could you have done this to me—and why? I feel so terribly betrayed. I am barely living for the day when you will make this right. You have robbed me of my work, my family, and my joy of living.*

Notice the catastrophic language ("brokenhearted," "devastated," "I am barely living . . ."), the harsh terms for her surgical result ("pointy . . . turned-up snout") and the personal attacks ("I feel betrayed". . ."You have robbed me . . .") These are not the words of an educated, rational, functioning adult. At the end of a year I discharged her. I couldn't revise invisible deformities. She remained dismally unhappy.

★★★★★

My second patient was a physician's wife who had undergone two unsuccessful rhinoplasties. I performed her reconstruction using a bone graft from her skull and ear cartilage. The result was smooth except for a small bump above her left nostril. Given the number of deformities and her delicate skin, the result was good. I reassured her. The bump could be corrected.

She was only happy for two weeks. Then she confined herself to her bedroom. She refused to see family. Improvements were discounted; the small bump was devastating. Her husband pleaded for an immediate revision.

At every visit, the patient arrived in full battle dress, tougher than a railroad spike, and berated me in churlishly abusive language.
  "You're supposed to be an 'expert.' That's a joke. This," she said, jabbing a finger toward her nose. "Is this the best you can do?"

She sat back and folded her arms. She gave me her steely stare. Something about her body reminded me of a clenched fist.

"Forget it. I withdraw the question." She nodded. She had vindicated herself. Suddenly she looked up as if she had thought of something to add.

"I've talked to other surgeons who say they would never use your techniques. You must be an embarrassment to the profession. This surgery has destroyed my life, you know."

She took a step toward the door and looked over her shoulder.

"I used to think you were modest. You've got a lot to be modest about."

Eventually she began to function again. At 12 months, when the time came for revision, I told her that she was discharged.

"You told me you could fix the bump," she hissed.

I took in some air. "I can," I said. "But I won't."

She stared as if I had lit my hair on fire.

"Your first surgery was too disequilibriating, and I don't completely understand why," I said, which at the time was mostly true.

"We can't chance a similar postoperative course. It's not right for you to take that risk."

She left without saying goodbye. Or even closing the door.

★★★★★

My third patient was a 40-year-old auto body repairman with an uncanny ability to describe his tertiary nasal deformities: a sunken bridge and pointed, knuckled tip. "I look like a leprechaun," he said. "And these light reflexes—they aren't right." Every request was precise and realistic. I liked precise and realistic. I liked him. Nothing troubled me.

When I removed his splint he stared into the mirror. His eyes widened. "You have destroyed my face," he said. The man closed his business, drank excessively, and became a recluse. He lurked in my office building stairwell, startling the staff. While I was away at a surgical meeting, he tried to amputate his nose with a razor. Fortunately he only lacerated the skin and was admitted to the psychiatric service. The patient, his family, and his social worker implored me to reoperate. Trying to cut off his nose wasn't weird, they agreed; it was justified. This was a surgical problem. And I had caused it.

I felt like a sapling in a high wind. What was going on here? Notice the common characteristics in these three patients. All were unhappy with good surgical results that met goals that the patients themselves had set. Their families saw nothing inappropriate in the patients' behavior and considered their distress to be the results of inexpert, thoughtless surgery. Each patient used catastrophic, victim language to describe what had happened. In their eyes I was a betrayer, violating their trust and deliberately causing injury for which I wouldn't take responsibility.

★★★★★

It is worth noting that none of these patients fulfilled the DSM-5 criteria for body dysmorphic disorder.[6] None had delusional requests. Their present-ing deformities were neither trivial nor imagined. Each patient was pleasant and compensated before surgery. Each had seen examples of my treatment for similar deformities during consultation, and each agreed to my surgical plan in detail, which they had also received in writing. None exhibited signs of obsessive behavior or distress in daily functioning; on the contrary, each was productive, highly functioning, and active. The usual BDD screening methods would not have applied. Nevertheless, the patients' postoperative distress was real, significant, and debilitating; and the only treatment they would consider was surgery.

Even the new DSM criteria still beg the question—at what point does a shape become a deformity? Who decides what is "not observable" or "slight"? If the focus of a patient's distress is not visible to the family, primary care physician, or mental health professional, does that make it only "perceived"? Is "subtle" the same as "not observable"? And who decides whether the patient is significantly distressed or impaired—i.e., whether the deformity merits the emotional response?

This is not only a theoretical question. It is not hard to find papers on body dysmorphic disorder in which the deformity was evaluated by "panels of non-medical people," "friends and family," or "objective observers." Many studies report BDD diagnoses based on self-reporting by the patients themselves, using Phillips' Body Dysmorphic Disorder Questionnaire,[7] Cash's Body Image Distur-bance Questionnaire,[8] or other useful tools. As a result, even the best BDD litera-ture contains statements such as this: "With the exception of 6 patients, who had slight physical anomalies about which they were excessively concerned, *all body parts of concern appeared normal to the investigators.*"[9] (Italics mine)

Oncologist Naomi Remen has published a collection of essays entitled Kitchen Table Wisdom. *Speaking to one member of identical twins, both suffering from metastatic cancer, she said, " 'We have our bodies but we are not our bodies,' I told him. He and his brother were each souls. They might share a common biology but they did not share a common destiny."*[10]
So true—yet these patients are their bodies. Why?

Body Dysmorphic Disorder in the Plastic Surgery Literature

I am only one of the recent researchers who has tried to understand the seemingly irrational patient, the patient with the minimal deformity, or the obsessive patient addicted to plastic surgery. How can some patients with good postoperative results be so distraught, so enraged, and why can't their surgeons reason with them?

The plastic surgical and mental health literatures have described body dysmorphic disorder in detail but never given sufficient explanations for its cause. That is what has bothered me most. Each patient gave me a glimpse of the source, yet every time I turned the corner looking for the truth about body dysmorphic disorder, it seemed to have turned the next corner, just beyond my sight.

★★★★★

Dissatisfaction after rhinoplasty is legendary, as is the degree to which some patients will go to obtain flawless results.[11–18] Fifty-eight years ago, Edgerton, Jacobson, and Meyer[19] produced clinical support for my current data in a study of 98 aesthetic surgery patients with "minimal deformity," 46 of whom sought rhinoplasty and 68 of whom underwent surgery. Of the operated group, 73% demonstrated psychopathology, depression, obsessive compulsive disorder, troubled family relationships, or marital difficulties. Fifty-five percent had turbulent postoperative courses, some requesting additional surgery. These data almost exactly duplicate the prevalences of depression, demanding behavior, and trauma in our recent published clinical research.[1, 2] (Chapters 8, 9) Anxiety, depression, obsessive behavior, perfectionism, and the linkage between self-esteem and body image have also been documented in rhinoplasty patients.[20]

A classic survey of 692 plastic surgeons had defined the characteristics of the "insatiable plastic surgery patient": often unmarried with impressively low self-esteem, either grandiose or passive and obsequious, obsessive about appearance, potentially aggressive or highly anxious, vague about surgical goals, and having "minimal deformities" that nevertheless distressed them intensely. Fifty-one percent of the surveyed surgeons would not operate on patients with those characteristics. Of those that did operate, only 7% thought that the patients had benefited, though most of the patients continued to seek more procedures. These patients often had unusual family dynamics—oppressive parents who tried to control the procedure. The patients were obsessive about the details of their surgical goals, often bringing photographs, drawings, or plaster models to show the surgeon, and frequently displayed victim anger, as if they were being persecuted by their physicians. "A review of the literature," the paper concluded, "indicates that this syndrome has not been described previously."†

The authors of this paper were Norman Knorr, John Hoopes, and Milton Edgerton, and the publication year was 1967. What is most remarkable about these observations is not only that they defined a recognized but undescribed surgical entity, but also implied that the family itself might be germane to its pathogenesis. All the ingredients were there: oppressive family, low self-esteem, grandiosity or disempowerment, victim behavior by the patient, and coexisting obsessions and perfectionism. It would be 20 more years before body dysmorphic disorder (BDD) would be formally defined in the DSM-3R.

In 1982, Greenley, Young, and Schoenherr correctly recognized that psychologically disturbed patients have wide varieties of negative outcomes.[21] This was their explanation: psychologically distressed patients are so dissatisfied with their lives that their doctors don't like them, which prompts the patients to become even more unhappy with their lives and doctors, so the positive feedback loop spirals downhill.

The authors also documented perfectionism, low self-esteem, hostility, phobia, paranoia, grandiosity, and "damaged personalities" in rhinoplasty patients.[22, 23] As far back as 1960, Clarkson and Stafford-Clark, discussing the importance of collaboration between plastic surgeons and psychiatrists, presented a patient diagnosed as a paranoid schizophrenic, the most severely disturbed patient in their series. Photographs indicate that, like our most difficult patients and the one who opened this chapter, the patient had a normal nose.[24–26]

Body Image Landmarks in the Plastic Surgical Literature

Plastic surgeon John Goin and his wife, psychiatrist Marcia Goin, were among the first to explain the profound psychological ramifications of cosmetic and reconstructive plastic surgery. Their 1981 text, *Changing the Body: Psychological Effects of Plastic Surgery*, impacted many of us.[27] What the surgeon observes postoperatively, they said, is "the kind of malfunctioning that occurs under stress" and follows a predictable pattern within each personality. They warned about the patient who too easily "leans upon a commanding figure . . . who will guide, nurture, and defend them." This description is prescient of Pia Mellody's "Love Addict," classically the result of childhood abandonment, producing an immature adult who seeks a rescuer (Chapter 3).[28] Goin and Goin also cautioned against the "paranoid personality pattern," patients who constantly project their fear and anger onto the surgeon: "It is not I who am angry with you; quite the contrary, it is you were angry with me."[29] This is the patient in our first vignette: I didn't change; you did. Goin and Goin identified hysterical, obsessive compulsive and "doer" personality patterns, as well as the coping mechanisms they use: regression (which we recognize now as emergence of the wounded child or the adapted wounded child); repression, projection, reaction formation (thoughts experienced as their opposites); denial; and displacement ("killing the messenger").[30, 31]

Body image requires varying degrees of postoperative adjustment and may be complicated by ethnic, racial, or familial factors. The Goins often give examples of patients using disaster or catastrophic language, so evident in the patient examples we have seen. They quote Freud's observation that the ego is "first and foremost a bodily ego," by which he meant that the infant's initial world experience develops from bodily sensations first. In fact, our senses continue to influence our individual realities throughout our lives, generating thoughts, emotions, and actions. When traumatic events occur, they are registered somatically.[32–35]

In particular, the Goins drew appropriate attention to the high prevalence of unhappy rhinoplasty patients, which is perhaps why I am writing this book rather than someone else. They believed that, as a midline structure, the nose is a genital equivalent to the penis, emitting secretions, its mucosa reactive to sexual arousal, and its olfactory sense responsive to the opposite sex. Perhaps, they argue, the nose is a scapegoat for displaced anger toward the parents; and in fact, data at that time indicated that rhinoplasty patients, particularly men, were more psychologically disturbed than the general population.[36] This, however, is 46-year-old data and less applicable today.

Neurologist and trauma researcher Robert Scaer has suggested that the nose may be a target organ for victims of developmental trauma because olfaction is the only sense that bypasses the thalamus and sends unmodified sensory signals straight to the amygdala, the brain's alarm center.[37] For example, violent crime victims may not remember anything about their perpetrators except the smell of cigarettes or alcohol.[38] He may be right.

★★★★★

Aside from the facial centrality of the nose and its ethnic and familial linkage, perhaps the reason that some of our most unhappy patients have had rhinoplasties is not so complicated. If developmental trauma produces body shame and if young abused or neglected patients believe that their self-esteem depends upon changing themselves with surgery, what feature will they select? If a boundaryless parent intends to impose surgery on a teenager, there aren't many better options. The child is too young for blepharoplasty or facelift, and most don't need otoplasties. What is left besides rhinoplasty?

The plastic surgery literature consistently describes the same few characteristics that define what surgeons call "the difficult patient": excessive anxiety and frequent telephone calls requiring extra time from surgeon and staff; patients who dominate and interrupt and indicate they have never been properly informed; imperfect recollection of the surgical consent and discussion of complications; vague surgical objectives; obsessive compulsive or perfectionistic behavior; excessive, manipulative flattery; distress about minimal or imagined deformities; depression, tearfulness, and lack of humor; failure to follow preoperative and postoperative instructions; histories of multiple cosmetic surgeries on different areas; obsession about prior surgical failures; use of catastrophic language to describe the preoperative feature, the surgical result, or the prior surgeon ("hate," "disgusting," "ugly"; "I wish the surgeon were dead").[39]

The Edgerton Contribution

Perhaps the boldest investigator into the impact of plastic surgery on mental health was Dr. Milton Edgerton, chair of the Department of Plastic Surgery at the University of Virginia when I was a medical student and surgical intern there and a defining influence on my own career. Earlier, as a plastic surgeon at The Johns Hopkins Hospital and then at the University of Virginia, Edgerton had integrated psychiatrists and psychologists into his department and generated significant collaborative, ground-breaking research that would have been impossible to duplicate by either discipline alone.

His defining paper for our purposes reported aesthetic surgery results in a series of 100 severely psychologically disturbed patients, treated between 1951 and 1989 in conjunction with the mental health professionals at the University of Virginia or previously at The Johns Hopkins Hospital.[40] Each patient was considered to be so psychologically disturbed that surgery would have been ordinarily contraindicated, but the team treated them anyway. Eighty-seven patients ultimately underwent surgery.

The patients were diagnosed with severe neuroses, personality disorders, or psychoses, and many manifested extreme anxiety, self-consciousness, and depression. The responses to their deformities were exaggerated, and most had been unable to find surgeons who would operate on them. Patients were identified by their adamant desires for surgical correction, major disruptions in psychological or social functioning, exaggerated responses to their perceived physical deformities, requests for "unusual" surgical treatments, or by major difficulties in communicating with the surgeon. In screening, the authors determined that the patients' perceptions of their deformities should take precedence over the surgeon's own aesthetic judgments, a bold and still somewhat unconventional decision that makes the study findings all the more provocative.

★★★★★

This was admittedly a daring study, and the authors knew it. Screening was intense. Patients were stratified and graded on a 1–6 Likert scale according to four psychological criteria: communication ability, compliance, trust in the team, stability, and "internal" motivation (i.e., surgery not compelled by or to please others), and by surgical criteria according to technical difficulty, operative risk, possibility of an unfavorable result, ease of correction, and compatibility with the patient's request. Patients who scored more than 10 on either their psychological or surgical characteristics were not considered surgical candidates.

Table 1.1 compares the characteristics and risk assessments in the three groups of patients as stratified in the text. Experienced clinicians will readily see how accurate they still are.

Psychological functioning was graded at three levels. "Significant" dysfunction defined patients whose self-consciousness or anxiety markedly impacted their lives and was accompanied by occupational and marital problems. "Moderate" disturbance defined patients whose lives were dominated by their senses of deformity; most had limited work and social lives. "Severe" dysfunction defined those patients whose entire lives were dominated by their delusions; these patients had few friends and no consistent employment. Many had undergone repeated inpatient psychiatric treatment. Any of these patients would today be defined as body dysmorphic, and it is safe to say that few plastic surgeons would operate on them. In fact, the inclusion criteria that Edgerton and his co-authors set defines

TABLE 1.1 Comparisons of the Three Groups of Plastic Surgery Patients

	Groups		
	I *Emotionally* *Stable*	*II* *Stable* *with* *Support*	*III* *Unstable* *even with* *Support*
Patient Characteristics			
1. Overall psychological strength	High	Average	Low
2. Appropriateness of psychological reaction to deformity	High	Average	Low
3. Patient's willingness to describe the deformity in great detail	Average	Low	High
4. Patient's degree of consistency regarding their impressions and descriptions of their deformity	Average	Average	High
Nature of Surgeon-Patient Relationship			
5. Surgeon's likelihood of empathizing with patient's perception of deformity	High	Average	Low
6. Responsiveness to surgeon's suggestions regarding change	High	Average	Low
7. Ability of patient to place trust in the surgeon	High	Average	Low
8. Surgeon's degree of comfort offering treatment	High	Average	Low
Differences in Potential Gains and Risks of Surgery			
9. Possibilities of favorable impact of surgery on psychological health	Average	High	Very High
10. Possibilities for unfavorable post-operative psychological repercussions	Low	Average	High
11. Likelihood for litigation against surgeon	Low	Average	Low

Adapted from Edgerton MT, Langman MW, Pruzinsky T. "Plastic Surgery and Psychotherapy in the Treatment of 100 Psychologically Disturbed Patients." 1994, unpublished, used with permission

those patients whom most surgeons and mental health professionals believe should never have plastic surgery. That is part of what makes this study so extraordinary.

★★★★★

All patients were treated with intensive preoperative psychotherapy, some over extended periods and under constant reevaluation. Group consensus was required before surgery could be undertaken, which meant that some patients waited more than two years before being cleared.

Surgical deformities cited by the patients were ranked "mild," "moderate," or "marked," but investigators noted that there was little correlation between the magnitude of the anatomical deformity and the degree of preoperative distress or the significance of the *postoperative* improvement. This lack of correlation between the magnitude of the preoperative deformity and the distress that it provokes is cited repeatedly as an unexplained phenomenon in the body image literature, and has been flagged by plastic surgeons as a critical determinant in the decision to operate.

Seven patients were rejected for noncompliance, unrealistic objectives, or inability to describe their surgical goals; distrust of the team; geographic restrictions; or requests for operations that were too complex or unrealistic, e.g., "Can you thin both my lips without reducing sensation?"

★★★★★

Eighty-seven patients were ultimately selected for surgery and had a total of 318 operations performed by the same surgeon; therefore many had several surgeries. Thirty-two percent of these operations were rhinoplasties. Seventeen percent of the patients had personality disorders and 13% were psychotic, most of the latter troubled by delusions rather than hallucinations. Sixty percent of the patients had undergone previous unsuccessful surgeries. This is important because it also indicates that 40% were requesting their first cosmetic surgeries, a concept that is counterintuitive to most surgeons, who may assume that only revision patients are the most difficult.[41] Even primary patients can be body dysmorphic. In a review of 1,000 consecutive rhinoplasty patients in my own practice 18 years ago, 11.5% of the body dysmorphic patients had never undergone nasal surgery.[42]

Women underwent more operations than men (4.1 vs. 2.7), which seems to contradict the axiom that men are harder to please than women. Forty-three percent were unmarried. Thirty-four percent had nasal surgery. Body dysmorphic disorder was the most common psychiatric diagnosis and was treated before surgery when recognized. Associated other diagnoses were somatoform and anxiety disorders, obsessive-compulsive disorder, eating disorders, or personality disorders. Only 5% of the patients were considered to be psychotic.

Results of the Edgerton Study

What was the outcome of this intrepid work? Patients were followed for an average of 6.2 years, some as long as 25 years. Patients' self-image and social functioning were rated, and 82.8% had either marked (50.6%) or modest (32.2%) psychological improvement. All patients said that they would undergo the surgery again. Only 13.8% had no discernible subjective or objective emotional improvement; however, none sought further surgery elsewhere. Most importantly, no patients exhibited the types of negative outcomes predicted when significantly psychologically disturbed patients undergo surgery: no attempted suicides, no psychotic decompensations, no threats of litigation, and only one patient expressed unhappiness about the surgical result. Given their patient cohort, the outcomes are rather extraordinary.

Three patients, however, were psychologically worse postoperatively. One was a 61-year-old woman who was unhappy after her rhinoplasty, which she believed had made her nose larger. Postoperatively, the team elicited a history of early childhood trauma (specifics not given). The second patient was distraught by a minor postoperative asymmetry after a browlift. The third patient underwent a rhinoplasty without having specified her surgical goals and without complying with the postoperative regime. The team recognized that these patients' psychological disturbances were not identified early enough, a problem that all plastic surgeons sometimes face. The patient seeking surgery, intent on making a good impression on the surgeon, may be an equilibrated, "adult adapted wounded child" (Chapter 3). Postoperatively, when the patient realizes that surgery has not created self-esteem, he or she regresses to an earlier age, and the illusion of functional adulthood disappears like a genie returning to the bottle.

★★★★★

The cases illustrated in this paper demonstrate the breadth of the surgical challenge in a plastic surgery population. The team judged most of the preoperative deformities to be negligible but highly distressing—therefore fulfilling BDD criteria. One-third of the patients requested changes that the team considered to be anti-aesthetic. One patient underwent 17 operations in order to look like television personality Johnny Carson. One patient was successfully treated with small cartilage grafts to restore a loss of personal identity that was altered by a prior rhinoplasty. This latter motivation is not uncommon: In my review of 150 consecutive revision rhinoplasty patients, 15% were motivated to undergo other operations because of perceived losses in personal, familial, or ethnic identity.[43] Thus a surgical outcome congruent with the patient's body image is not only appropriate for so-called ethnic patients, but rather for anyone seeking aesthetic surgery.

The authors conclude that the majority of significantly psychologically disturbed patients could still benefit from aesthetic surgery performed by a team with established methodologies for screening and coordinated management. They even argue that such patients might even be more tolerant of imperfect results simply out of gratitude that someone finally took them seriously.

That is perhaps the most optimistic color that can be painted on their conclusions, and will not be every surgeon's experience. However, the Edgerton, Langman, and Pruzinsky paper makes critical points not often found in the literature. The authors' completed but unpublished text, which Dr. Edgerton permitted me to study, contains complete histories for 21 of these patients.[40]

Emerging Themes

Already new themes begin to emerge from the case studies. Many patients used "catastrophic" language to describe themselves ("ugly," "crushed," "shattered," "caustic and angry," "bitter," "disgusting," and "devastated"). This is childlike thinking—everything bad lasts forever and can never be corrected. A sizable number reported facial feature criticism and teasing by family members. Some wanted to change features that resembled those of despised family members. Some sought surgery for perceived losses of personal identity from prior operations. Some patients were excessively controlling and demanded enormous amounts of time from surgeon and staff. Patients were often described as having "low self-esteem" and would ignore any surgical improvements. Most were emotionally vulnerable and required careful handling by the staff. In one patient, PTSD from an automobile accident ten years previously resurfaced along with significant marital instability. This same phenomenon has been verified recently.[44] The patients were often solitary, untrusting, perfectionistic, and guarded. Many adults still lived with their parents. Some were discovered to have occult eating disorders; in other cases adult patients were accompanied by parents who dominated the consultation. Of particular importance was the nasal configuration of the rhinoplasty patients: most had straight, symmetrical noses without dorsal humps, a key indicator to a childhood trauma history.[1,2]

Edgerton Study Conclusions

Discussing these cases, the authors make several critical points.

1. Personal identity is unique and individual. Patients respond to internal standards of beauty that may not be obvious to the physician; therefore the degree of postoperative happiness may seem disproportionate to the preoperative deformity *if the surgeon does not understand its significance.*[45]
2. Many patients had "minimal deformities," but even patients with significant deformities could be emotionally unstable. Therefore the correlation between degree of deformity, psychological health, and degree of postoperative patient satisfaction was not always reliable.[46] This last observation flies in the face of the current criteria for BDD that characterize the disorder by its incongruity: minimal or imagined deformity, large patient response, and low postoperative satisfaction.
3. Those patients requiring the most time from the team lived in extremes: disempowered ("hand-holders") or demanding, falsely empowered "hot potatoes."
4. Many patients, even those who were deemed "severely psychologically disturbed" could be satisfactorily screened for surgery by the surgeon's assessment of the patient's communication ability, trust in the team, motivation, emotional stability, and compliance.
5. Although surgeons consider the healthiest surgical motivation to be "internal," in practice almost no patients were motivated entirely without considerations of how others would react. However, patients without any internal motivation were not suitable candidates.

6. The risk to any patient's mental health if surgery failed depended significantly upon his or her innate "psychological health."
7. Despite the group characteristics, malpractice suits were uncommon.
8. There were 7 absolute contraindications to surgery:

- Any patient who was withdrawn or uncommunicative
- Any untrusting patient
- Any angry or noncompliant patient
- Any deformity beyond the surgeon's technical skill
- Any patient in poor physical health
- Any patient with unrealistic expectations
- Any patient whose geographic or economic constraints made sufficient postoperative care and follow-up unlikely

★★★★★

Most fascinating was the outcome: 82.8% of the patients had decreases in their depression and anxiety and significant improvements in social functioning. Only 3.4% were unhappy with their outcomes. Even in cases where the surgeon performed procedures that were against his surgical judgment but in concert with the patient's aesthetic, the outcome was still successful. Today, most surgeons would consider that practice prohibitively risky.

Finally, this study refutes the assumption that a deformity must be "substantial enough" to merit treatment, even in a psychologically difficult population. The patient measures the real magnitude of the surgical problem. Even patients with minimal or "imagined" deformities could undergo technically skilled surgery with successful outcomes. The size of the problem, by itself, should not be a contraindication for surgery. "Almost every patient of ours has had—at least to some small degree—the defect they described. . . . It is very important, in understanding . . . these patients, that we recognize the *validity* of the deformity, even when it is very minor."[40]

Insights From the Edgerton Research

What emerges from the published paper and unpublished text are several themes: (1) *"Psychopathology" in surgical patients runs a continuum, but these patients live at the extremes*: grandiosity or disempowerment; uncontained emotions or excessive sensitivity to others' opinions; distorted realities; inability to moderate behavior; or inability to self-care and comply with postoperative instructions. (2) *The severity of a patient's perceived deformity does not always correlate with the distress that it creates or the satisfaction that the patient will achieve postoperatively*, which in this series was often significantly greater than had been predicted by the treating physicians and mental health team. (3) *Careful diagnosis, detailed planning, the specifics of the patient's aesthetic goals, and a knowledge of the patient's personality and resilience are critical to satisfactory surgical outcomes in all patients*, regardless of where they fall within the spectrum of mental health.[47] (4) *The surgeon must make the patient's requested changes precisely, without variations.* (5) *The majority of psychologically disturbed patients in the Edgerton series had family histories that indicated significant abuse or neglect, a point on which Dr. Edgerton and I have discussed and agreed* (Edgerton, personal communication, 2014). (6) *The current DSM-5 diagnosis of body dysmorphic disorder therefore has more practical use in mental health than in plastic surgery* because its criteria depend upon establishing the degree of deformity and the distress and compensatory behavior that it produces, all of which are subjective.

> *Some doctors, just because of their personality [sic] are able to manage certain types of patients with which other doctors, equally learned, face certain failure. The personality of each doctor differs. It certainly cannot be taught, and it is a question of how far it can be learned.*
>
> *So wrote Arthur Hertzler, MD,[48] a wise country physician who practiced in Kansas from the late 1800's until 1946. He recognized that physicians have their histories, too, which determines which specialties they choose, which patients they like, and which patients like them.*

Body Image and BDD: Demographics and Diagnostic Tools

Across all cultures, body dysmorphic patients focus on their noses more than any other body part.[49] As a result, rhinoplasty patients with BDD symptoms are easy to find and test. Picavet, Prokopakis, Gabriels, et al. studied 226 patients seeking rhinoplasty.[50] Each patient was given three self-evaluation questionnaires that measured the patient's opinion of his or her nasal shape, the severity of body dysmorphic disorder symptoms, and quality of life. Patients requesting aesthetic changes were more likely to have BDD symptoms than those requesting functional (airway correction) changes, as were revision rhinoplasty patients and those with psychiatric histories. The more rhinoplasties any patient had undergone, the more severe the BDD symptoms. As found in so many other studies, there was also no correlation between the patients' opinions of their deformities and the researchers' opinions. Further, there was an inverse correlation between the patients' subjective deformities and their psychological distress: those patients with the smallest deformities were the most upset (suggesting that nasal shape alone was not driving the desire for surgery). Depression, substance abuse, social phobia, obsessive compulsive disorder, and personality disorders were the most common co-morbidities. The authors report that 33% of the patients in this entire cohort showed at least moderate symptoms of body dysmorphic disorder (43% among their aesthetic rhinoplasty patients). However, only 2% met the full diagnostic criteria. The rest scored "moderate preoccupation" with a defect that the authors judged was minimal. The headline is that 33% to 43% of rhinoplasty patients in this study had body dysmorphic disorder, though a precise diagnosis could only be made in 2%.

✦✦✦✦✦

In a 2013 study of 166 rhinoplasty patients, the same authors confirmed that body dysmorphic disorder symptoms as measured by the Yale-Brown Obsessive Compulsive Scale Modified for Body Dysmorphic Disorder provided prospective evidence of unhappiness following rhinoplasty.[51] In this group also, only 2% met full criteria for moderate or severe BDD symptoms. However, one-third of another group not considered to have BDD (because they had visible deformities) still had moderate to severe psychological distress, adding evidence to the observation that even patients with obvious deformities can be distressed and difficult to manage after surgery.[52]

What are we to make of these studies? In the unhappy postoperative patients, what was the quality of the surgical results? Did the unhappy patients behave like functional adults, or did they act immature, demanding, grandiose, disempowered, or needy? All surgeons have patients who are happy though they have reasons not to be, as well as those who seek endless, trivial revisions despite good—or even excellent—results.[53] Why?

Specific psychometric tests that assess "global" body image dissatisfaction, body dimensions, body appreciation, body shape, body shame, body checking, body image avoidance, body image compulsive actions, drive for leanness, muscle appearance satisfaction, body image avoidance, and questionnaires for men, women, and adolescents (Chapter 4) may be better research than clinical tools. Their practical use in many studies relies on the assumption that any patient's self-tested response to a facial or body feature, if deemed excessive by a psychometric, accurately establishes a mental health disorder. Can patients diagnose themselves? If so, wouldn't the diagnosis of body dysmorphic disorder depend on who is examining the patient?

Body Dysmorphic Disorder Is Ideally a Two-Specialty Diagnosis

What does this data mean? It means that unless the patients being studied have also been evaluated by a surgeon who treats the deformity in question, the diagnosis of BDD must be considered speculative. Even those patients evaluated by structured clinical interviews would benefit from this added information. Imagine, for example, a rhinoplasty patient with postoperative valvular obstruction who has already had septal and turbinate surgery but cannot sleep or exercise, has intercurrent sinus infections, and who has become depressed and obsessed about having corrective surgery. The physical findings may be subtle, but they are real. This is not body dysmorphic disorder, and there are many such patients. Or imagine a patient who has a perfectly acceptable rhinoplasty result but who is distraught because a personal, ethnic, or familial trait was inadvertently destroyed by the surgery: these perceived losses motivate a sizable percentage of patients seeking revision rhinoplasty, many of whom have been diagnosed with BDD, and it is not BDD.

Outcome Studies: The Disjunction Between the Deformity and the Emotion

Cosmetic diagnoses are always in context. In cancer or trauma, the diagnosis is unquestioned and the patient's response can be presumed to be "normal" within his or her cultural norm. It is not so with body image issues, best seen in the interface between mastectomy and breast reconstruction, where the cancer diagnosis and the patient's body image come face to face. Deformities have different meanings to different patients, influenced by the patient's personality, culture, and past. The same intensity of emotion that would be considered appropriate for a patient with a disfiguring facial cancer or burn might be diagnosed as BDD when the deformity is cosmetic.

A key factor is not the size of the defect but the patient's response to it (Gorney, personal communication, 2006).[54] Therapists using cognitive-behavioral therapy to treat patients with BDD note their Manichean, black-and-white, all-or-nothing thought patterns. *The challenge for therapists and surgeons is not necessarily to change the patient's belief but rather its significance.* For better or worse, it is the patient's reality that really counts.

Similarly, the driving motivation for plastic surgery is often more complex than the deformity: not every person with an unattractive nose wants a rhinoplasty. Body image, family and peer influences, especially teasing, gender influences, and childhood sexual abuse[55–62] each shape body image.[63] The comprehensive review by Sarwer, Pruzinsky, Cash, Goldwyn, Persing, and Whitaker summarizes many aspects of our current information about the psychology of aesthetic and reconstructive plastic surgery.[64] Earlier literature from the 1940's and 1950's focused on rhinoplasty patients: the results were sobering. Most rhinoplasty patients were thought to be emotionally disturbed and 53% had personality disorders. This psychopathology was attributed to the genital metaphor that the penis represented unconscious displacement of sexual conflicts to the nose, or to a female patient's attempt to divorce from her father.

★★★★★

So-called second-generation studies in the 1970's and 1980's were not much more sophisticated. Rhinoplasty patients were allegedly more hostile, neurotic, and obsessive than other cosmetic patients, and in one series only half of the patients were considered to be "normal." A subsequent study found increased levels of anxiety, obsessiveness, and paranoia compared to controls.[65]

Studies since 1990 have provided more optimistic results and more accurately reflect the patients that we see today. Until recently, rhinoplasty patients were the most studied group, but now facelift and body contour patients have been added to the mix, with better surgical outcomes reported. Measurements of anxiety, depression, and neuroticism decrease following surgery, except in patients diagnosed with body dysmorphic disorder. Sarwer has proposed that physical and psychological factors create two body attitudes: valence (how important body image is to self-esteem); and value (the degree of body dissatisfaction).[65] He concludes that patients who have high valences, and therefore derive much of their self-worth from their appearances, and who also have negative body images (high-value) are more likely to seek cosmetic surgery and may be less happy afterward.

More recently, Picavet, Gabriels, Grietens, et al. reported a series of 166 patients who were tested preoperatively for body dysmorphic disorder by the Yale-Brown Obsessive Compulsive Scale; postoperative satisfaction was similarly evaluated with a visual analog scale and the Rhinoplasty Outcome Evaluation.[66] Preoperative body dysmorphic disorder symptoms correlated inversely with postoperative satisfaction at three months. Their paper makes another important observation, namely that one-third of the patients who did not fulfill the diagnosis of body dysmorphic disorder because their nasal deformities were observable still showed body dysmorphic symptoms preoperatively. Although the point of the paper was to emphasize the surgical dangers of the disorder, the authors parenthetically make two points that I believe are often overlooked: that the physical deformity itself, large or small, does not define body dysmorphic disorder, nor does it determine a patient's postoperative satisfaction. Others have made the same observation.[21, 67–70]

As a result of cultural changes and greater interest in and acceptance of plastic surgery, surgeons now routinely correct deformities that are less severe than those treated two decades ago. Even minor variations from the "ideal" may be legitimate indications for surgery in the right patients. Therefore the degree of deformity is becoming progressively more irrelevant. Edgerton's series, several decades old, includes many patients with deformities that are modest, even by today's standards.

Letter From an Unhappy Patient

The following letter excerpts from an unhappy patient poignantly illustrate the themes that suffuse this chapter: delusion in assessing the surgical result; abusive family treatment; intense, unjustifiable suspicion and distrust of the surgeon; alternating rebuke and seduction; a belief that if she does enough research, she will get her desired result; and a firm conviction that the surgeon is lying.

"It is now the start of the seventh month. The distress of waiting to heal is more than I can bear. Every day at 3 o'clock my nose swells so much it cracks my makeup and I have to leave work."

"My sister told me that my looks are ruined. I have not heard one positive comment from anyone. It is cruel to leave me like this. Complete

strangers stare at me on the street and ask, 'What have you done to your nose? How can you walk around like that?' Even the postman turns away from me in disgust."

"Doctors on the Internet say that their patients do not swell and are happy right away. I know that you don't consider me an attractive person but I am begging you for compassion and help."

"I just want to thank you for effectively ruining my life. Each plastic surgeon I have seen has admitted that my nose is too wide but that I should go back to you because you are such a 'professional' and would be able to fix it, and you certainly would not want an unhappy patient. No one will operate on me because they are intimidated by you. We know that you don't care if I am happy or not."

"What you did to me, my nose, my face, my life, is unforgivable. It borders on the criminal. I thought I could trust you. I know you left the operation in the middle and never finished it. Another surgeon tells me you gave me a nose like a truck driver. He knew if he didn't do something I would end my life. Now it's worse and I need money."

"You may be a professor and write textbooks; but I know you have disfigured many patients. . . . And don't think that God doesn't know it."

What drives these unhappy patients' pain?

The Tip of the Thread: A Childhood Story of Body Dysmorphic Disorder

The thesis for understanding these tortured individuals unraveled slowly. The first critical piece was provided by a young man who told me that he had once had body dysmorphic disorder but had been cured. I had never heard such a statement, but I liked him immediately. With the approval of his therapist, I performed the surgery he requested. He was a grateful patient. Afterward, I asked if he would answer some questions about his unusual story. The following is his edited answer.[‡] It was the next bit to fall into place.

I was an extremely shy, self-conscious, and unconfident child and adolescent. I could barely get two words out in history class without becoming tongue-tied and my voice becoming quivery. I felt OK about the way I looked. I didn't think about my nose at all.

It was my stepfather who told me that something was wrong. . . . He spent a lot of time trying to convince me that my nose looked weird. I suppose he didn't feel too good about himself—he was a 50-year-old parking lot attendant with . . . a large "Greek" nose.

It took him years. . . . He said, "Your nose droops. I'm going to call you 'droopy nose,'" doing his best imitation of a seven-year-old. I looked in the mirror, turning my head, but everything seemed OK. I was angry that he was trying to upset me. One day, he pointed out my brother's nose. "Look," he said. "It looks chopped off at the end." I looked closely at my brother's nose apart from his face. My stepfather was right.

The harassment continued. "Your nose goes down straight like this," he said, while tracing his finger through the air, "and then . . . it droops. It's getting worse—a family nose." My biological father was mentally ill, so I found this frightening.

Finally, the summer before my senior year in high school, I submitted to photographs taken by my stepfather with the expressed purpose of showing me what was wrong with my nose. He struggled to find the perfect angle. And I let him.

That year I got dumped by my first girlfriend. I would take out the photographs whenever I felt down. I noticed my nose looked flat at the end. With a pen, I drew in my own tip graft to make my nose look average. One day, I got angry and scribbled through my tip. Generalized self-hatred had transferred to my nose. The battle was over.

I started looking in the mirror with a second mirror so I could scrutinize my nose in profile. I'd work myself into a state of agitation. . . . I thought by changing my nose, I would stop thinking about it for even a second, and free my mind. . . . I didn't give too much instruction to the doctor. "Just don't make me look like a pig."

I didn't like the way I looked after surgery but I hoped that I had broken even—my nose still looked weird but at least I had actively tried to change something I didn't like about myself. My stepfather's reaction: "It still looks weird." My brother's reaction: "It still looks Jewish."

I would use two mirrors to look at myself, vacillating back and forth about whether my nose looked OK. My brother committed suicide. I blamed myself for not being more involved in my brother's life. I felt I didn't cry enough. I felt numb. Every day I would wake up and think about my brother. . . . I tried desperately to feel some grief and a connection to him. I went to a psychiatrist to feel less like an evil person who had caused his brother to kill himself. I hated myself so much, and considered myself an uncaring person. I lost my ambition to be a doctor; if I couldn't help or care about my brother, how could I care about strangers.

*****

My life lost meaning. Again I got obsessed with my nose. I felt sure that it looked operated on and strange. I avoided socializing. I asked all my friends whether they had noticed anything weird looking about my nose. No one had.

I remember wanting to drown myself when I went to the beach. I felt my nose looked shapeless, short, and snubby, but I don't remember thinking much about my nostrils.

I had another surgery. I remember catching a glimpse of myself after the bandages were removed and noticing a lot of nostril.

My inheritance ran out. I moved back to my parents' house. I felt like a complete failure. I had no car and practically no friends. I felt a sense of guilt. . . . I had become very sensitive to the fact that there was a huge amount of suffering in the world and I was doing very little to help allevi-ate it. My nose obsession grew to its greatest level ever. My nose looked 'suspended.' I tried to pull it down. I pushed my nostrils up. I wrote to my surgeon. By this time I was looking at my nose for hours at a time, arguing with myself. "If it's so obvious to me, why isn't it obvious to everyone else?"

I would walk around the house looking at my nose in various lighting. I had no money. I begged my brother and my parents for money. I felt totally helpless.

Various medications were tried. I grew suicidal because I couldn't stop thinking about how deformed my nose looked to me and, I imagined, to others. Some medications made me sick; some made me confused. My life was out of control while I looked for a magic pill. I was in and out of hospitals. I remember being so confused that I spent a whole night try-ing to figure out how to put on my T-shirt. I failed. I went into a 10-day coma from serotonin poisoning. I was in the blackest mood of my life, and I stayed in bed sleeping. I went back to the hospital. I got electroshock therapy. I went to a group home to live because my mother couldn't stand the stress anymore. I spent my days in treatment chatting with other nuts. At first the ECT [electroconvulsive therapy used to treat severe depression] made me so confused I didn't know who I was.

A lot of the negative energy was removed from my nose. I started to think that my problem was not my nose, but that I was 36 years old and didn't know how to support myself financially, and that I'd never had a girlfriend, and that I would be in this awful situation for the rest of my life unless I worked to change it [emphasis mine]. . . . *I thought, "My life sucks. . . . I had better do something about helping myself before I can help them." I got a job delivering newspapers. Then I got a job as a substitute teacher. I sold my brother's guitar and moved out of the group home. I got my first real girlfriend at age 37. I got certified as a teacher and got my first real job as a math teacher at 38.* I still didn't like my nose: the nostrils, the idea that I even got that first nose job in the first place, but instead of carrying the obsession with myself all day, the last thing I said to myself as I left the mirror was, "That's not your real problem." [emphasis mine]

*****

Let me answer your specific questions:

Q: *Are there stages to developing BDD?*
A: *In my experience, there are different levels of BDD, but the onset is fairly abrupt.*
Level 0: Lack of nose consciousness.
Level 1: Nose consciousness in private moments; dissatisfaction, mostly forgotten in public.
Level 2: On the brink. Carrying nose consciousness around while in public, fighting it off with varying degrees of success, struggling, wasting time in front of the mirror.
Level 3: Over the edge. Full-blown obsession, spending several hours in front of the mirror, difficulty thinking of anything else.
Q: *Were all my perceptions distorted, or just my body image, or just my nose?*
A: *Just my nose.*
Q: *Did I view my surgery differently when BDD developed? Was it no longer successful in my eyes?*
A: *Since I didn't notice my nostril visibility before the surgery, I wondered whether in fixing my supratip deformity, my surgeon inadvertently created the nostril visibility problem. I knew my surgeon was regarded as the best in the world, so I figured the nostrils were probably a preexisting problem that I had not noticed. I wished that my nose was longer. As far as my profile went, even with BDD, I thought my surgeon did a great job with what he had to work with, but I figured that the material just wasn't there.*
Q: *How did my friends and associates view this period? Did anyone understand?*
A: *My friends were very supportive for long periods, although many gave up on me. I think my friends were more understanding than I would have expected them to be.*
Q: *How easy was it to find a psychiatrist who understood this problem?*

A: I didn't really find anyone whom I felt helped me, but I don't think there is really any way to help someone with BDD, other than hit-or-miss methods. ECT helped me, I guess, but I worry that I may have sustained brain damage in the process, because I am definitely more forgetful than I was in the past.

Q: [What are the] clues for a surgeon to make the diagnosis of BDD?

A: Honest patients will tell you if they have BDD, if they know about BDD. If they answer questions posed to them honestly about how much they think about their appearances, and if they believe their obsession is negatively affecting their lives, the surgeon will be able to determine whether these persons have BDD.

Not surprisingly, when my life is not going well, I have a tendency to develop BDD.

Many People Have Similar Pasts

Other individuals may recognize parts of themselves in this man's story. If I needed evidence that some individuals with BDD come from traumatizing family units, this letter provided it. My patient told the chilling story of systematic child abuse by his stepfather. He describes the early attention that his stepfather brought to his nose, his initial resistance to his stepfather's beliefs, and his growing obsession with a perceived deformity once the stepfather's view prevailed. The patient was tormented by his failure to protect his brother, whose suicide was not coincidental. He was abandoned by his father early in life and his mother later in life. His degree of nasal obsession paralleled his life trajectory: when his life got worse, so did his nose. Therapy was ineffective; but his innate resilience facilitated an epiphany.

What This Information Means

The Edgerton series and the vignettes in this chapter illustrate that, in the absence of independent examination by a surgeon who treats the deformity in question, clinical assessments may reflect not only BDD but rather anxiety, depression, obsessive compulsive disorder, eating disorders, generalized worry disorder, poor insight, social anxiety disorder, or cognitive distortions instead, each of which may co-exist alone or with BDD.[71] The primary dangers here are twofold: the tendency to produce false positives, and the dilution of study conclusions by including patients who do not really have BDD.

As good as the DSM-V criteria for body dysmorphic disorder are, physicians and surgeons not in the mental health field would be helped by criteria that match the characteristics of the patients that they see: apparently functioning adults seeking surgery. There is potentially enormous additive value in the discrete perspectives of different specialties.

Which discipline should make the diagnosis of body dysmorphic disorder? The answer, I believe, is both: BDD must be a two-specialty diagnosis. Though surgeons see a different patient population than mental health experts, their obsessed patients fulfilled the same criteria, as we shall see. Secondly, an accurate assessment of the physical deformity by the surgeons who treat them is the missing piece in much of the BDD literature, and a consensus decision would strengthen the research done by both specialties and decrease the prevalence of false positive diagnoses. I hope that the authors of the next DSM revision will consider these changes.

★★★★★

The surgical question is actually much broader than rhinoplasty—and much broader than plastic surgery. Why do some cancer patients collapse at their diagnoses, fail to heal their wounds, have numerous unexpected complications, and turn favorable-stage diseases into bad prognoses? No one knows. Why are other patients with advanced disease still alive 20 years later? No one knows. Why can one man undergo a severe hand injury and return to work quickly, whereas another with the same injury develops a Complex Regional Pain Syndrome?[72] No one knows. What is the body image of patients who have had multiple cosmetic operations? No one knows. What experiences most impact burn recovery, postoperative pain levels, or cancer treatment? No one knows. What life stories yield the best patients, or the worst?[73] No one knows.

Recurrent themes emerge: poor self-esteem, familial disharmony or childhood abuse, shame, PTSD,[§] body image disorders, and "patient personality," which influence not only plastic surgery but almost every area of medicine—cancer treatment, heart disease, drug or alcohol abuse, obesity management, mental health disorders, autoimmune disease, and many other common, serious conditions. Could childhood experiences contribute to this puzzle?

Patients have histories, as do their physicians and their physicians' physicians.[74] We spend our careers trying to find out what makes patients happy. The answer turns out to be an even simpler question: What makes people happy?

Notes

* All stories are real, but all patients are composites.
† Knorr NJ, Edgerton MT, Hoopes JE. The "Insatiable" Cosmetic Surgery Patient. *Plast Reconstr Surg* 1967; 40:3:285–289.
‡ From Constantian, M.B.,[41] used with permission of publisher and patient.
§ The evidence continues to accumulate. A study in 106,464 patients [Song, Fang, Tomasson, *JAMA* 2018;319:23:2388–2400] indicates that a PTSD history significantly increased the risk of 41 different autoimmune diseases, including rheumatoid arthritis, psoriasis, Crohn's disease, and celiac disease. The use of SSI's seemed protective.

References

1. Constantian MB, Lin CP. Why Some Patients Are Unhappy: Part 1: Relationship of Preoperative Nasal Deformity to Number of Operations and a History of Abuse or Neglect. *Plast Reconstr Surg* 2014; 134:4:823–835.

2. Constantian MB, Lin CP. Why Some Patients Are Unhappy: Part 2. Relationship of Nasal Shape and Trauma History to Surgical Success. *Plast Reconstr Surg* 2014; 134:4:836–851.

3. Picavet VA, Prokoalos EP, Gabriels L, et al. High Prevalence of Body Dysmorphic Disorder Symptoms in Patients Seeking Rhinoplasty. *Plast Reconstr Surg* 2011; 128:2:509–519.

4. Aufricht G. *Philosophy of Cosmetic Surgery*. Read at the meeting of the American Association of Plastic Surgeons, Skytop, PA, May 8, 1957.

5. American Psychiatric Association. *Desk Reference to the Diagnostic Criteria from DSM-5*. Washington, DC: American Psychiatric Publishing; 2013:131, 325–326.

6. American Psychiatric Association. *Desk Reference to the Diagnostic Criteria from DSM-5*. Arlington [VA]: American Psychiatric Publishing; 2013:93–114, 143–149.

7. Phillips KA. Appendix: Measures and Resources. In: Phillips KA, ed. *Body Dysmorphic Disorder: Advances in Research and Clinical Practice*. New York: Oxford University Press; 2017, 522–525.

8. Cash TF, Smolak, eds. *Body Image: A Handbook of Science, Practice, and Prevention*. New York: The Guilford Press; 2011, 135.

9. McElroy SL, Phillips KA, Keck PE, et al. Body Dysmorphic Disorder: Does It Have a Psychotic Subtype? *J Clin Psychiatry* 1993; 54:10:389–395.

10. Remen RN. *Kitchen Table Wisdom: Stories That Heal*. New York: Riverhead Books; 1996.

11. Chauhan N, Alexander AJ, Sepehr A, et al. Patient Complaints with Primary Versus Revision Rhinoplasty: Analysis and Practice Implications. *Aesth Surg Jl* 2011; 31:7:775–780.

12. Ercolani M, Baldaro B, Rossi N, et al. Five-Year Followup of Cosmetic Rhinoplasty. *J Psychosom Res* 1999; 47:283–286.

13. Ercolani M, Baldaro B, Rossi N, et al. Short-Term Outcome of Rhinoplasty For Medical or Cosmetic Indication. *J Psychsom Res* 1999; 47:277–281.

14. McKinney P, Cook JQ. A Critical Evaluation of 200 Rhinoplasties. *Ann Plast Surg* 1981; 7:357–361.

15. Meningaud JP, Benadiba L, Servant JM, et al. Depression, Anxiety, and Quality of Life: Outcome 9 Months After Facial Cosmetic Surgery. *J Craniomaxillofac Surg* 2003; 31:46–50.

16. Naraghi M, Atari M. Comparison of Patterns of Psychopathology in Aesthetic Rhinoplasty Patients Versus Functional Rhinoplasty Patients. *Otolaryngol Head Neck Surg* 2015; 152:2:244–249.

17. Sinno H, Izadpanah A, Thibaudeau C, et al. The Impact of Living with a Functional and Aesthetic Nasal Deformity After Primary Rhinoplasty: A Utility Outcomes Score Assessment. *Ann Plast Surg* 2012; 69:431–434.

18. Wright MR. Management of Patient Dissatisfaction with Results of Cosmetic Procedures. *Arch Otolaryngol Head Neck Surg* 1980; 106:466–471.

19. Edgerton MT, Jacobson WE, Meyer E. Surgical-Psychiatric Study of Patients Seeking Plastic (Cosmetic) Surgery: Ninety-Eight Consecutive Patients with Minimal Deformity. *Br J Plast Surg* 1960; 13:136–145.

20. Veale D, De Haro L, Lambrou C. Cosmetic Rhinoplasty in Body Dysmorphic Disorder. *Brit J Plast Surg* 2003; 56:6:546–551.

21. Greenley JR, Young TB, Schoenherr RA. Psychological Distress and Patient Satisfaction. *Medical Care* 1982; XX:373–385.

22. Fitzpatrick S, Sherry S, Hartling N, et al. Cosmetic Surgery. *Plast Reconstr Surg* 2001; 127:6:177e.

23. Hewitt PL, Sherry SB, Flett GL, et al. Perfectionism and Cosmetic Surgery. *Plast Reconstr Surg* 2003; 1:112:346.

24. Clarkson P, Stafford-Clark D. Role of the Plastic Surgeon and Psychiatrist in the Surgery of Appearance. *Brit Med J* 1960; 2:5215:1768–1771.

25. Klewchuk EM, McKusker CG, Mulholland C, et al. Cognitive Biases for Trauma Stimuli in People with Schizophrenia. *Br J Clin Psychol* 2007; 46:3:333–345.

26. Yu K, Kim A, Pearlman SJ. Functional and Aesthetic Concerns of Patients Seeking Revision Rhinoplasty. *Arch Facial Plast Surg* 2010; 12:291–297.

27. Goin JM, Goin MK. *Changing the Body: Psychological Effects of Plastic Surgery.* Baltimore: Williams & Wilkins; 1981.

28. Mellody P. How the Symptoms Sabotage. In: *Facing Codependence.* New York: Harper Collins; 2003:51–60.

29. Goin JM, Goin MK. *Changing the Body: Psychological Effects of Plastic Surgery: Rhinoplasty: The "Minimal Defect."* Baltimore: Williams & Wilkins; 1981:133.

30. Goin MK, Rees TD. A Prospective Study of Patients' Psychological Reactions to Rhinoplasty. *Ann Plast Surg* 1991; 27:210–215.

31. Goin MK. Psychological Understanding and Management of Rhinoplasty Patients. *Clinics in Plastic Surgery* 1977; 4:1:3–7.

32. Morrison J. Childhood Sexual Histories of Women with Somatization Disorder. *Am J Psychiatr* 1989; 146:2:239–241.

33. Phillips KA, Siniscalchi JM, McElroy, SL. Depression, Anxiety, Anger, and Somatic Symptoms in Patients with Body Dysmorphic Disorder. *Psychiatric Quarterly* 2004; 75:4:309–320.

34. Sack M, Henniger S, Lamprecht F. Changes of Body Image and Body Awareness in Eating-Disorder and Non Eating-Disorder Patients After Inpatient-Therapy. *Psychotherapie, Psychosomatik, medizinische Psychologie.* 2002 Feb;52:2:64–9.

35. van der Kolk BA, Perry LC, Herman JL. Childhood Origins of Self-Destructive Behavior. *Am J Psychiatry* 1991; 148:12:1665–1671.

36. Goin JM, Goin MK. *Changing the Body: Psychological Effects of Plastic Surgery: Psychological Screening of the Rhinoplasty Patient: The Male Patient.* Baltimore: Williams & Wilkins; 1981:137.

37. Scaer RC. *8 Keys to Brain-Body Balance.* New York: W W Norton & Company; 2012.

38. Rose S, Brewin CR, Andrews B, et al. A Randomized Controlled Trial of Individual Psychological Debriefing for Victims of Violent Crime. *Psychological Medicine* 1999; 29:793–799.

39. Connell BF, Gunter J, Mayer T, et al. Roundtable: Discussion of "The Difficult Patient." *Facial Plastic Surgery Clinics of North America* 2008; 16:2:249–258.

40. Edgerton MT, Langman MW, Pruzinsky T. Plastic Surgery and Psychotherapy in the Treatment of 100 Psychologically Disturbed Patients. *Plast Reconstr Surg* 1991; 88:4:594–608.

41. Ambro BT, Wright RJ. Psychological Considerations in Revision Rhinoplasty. *Facial Plast Surg* 2008; 24:288–292.

42. Constantian MB. Unhappy Patients and Those with Body Dysmorphic Disorder. In: Constantian MB, ed. *Rhinoplasty: Craft and Magic.* St. Louis: Quality Medical Publishing; 2009:1401–1448.

43. Constantian MB. What Motivates Secondary Rhinoplasty? A Study of 150 Consecutive Patients. *Plast Reconstr Surg* 2012; 130:667–678.

44. Kilpatrick DG, Resnick HS, Milanak ME, et al. National Estimates of Exposure to Traumatic Events and PTSD Using DSM-IV and DSM-5 Criteria. *J Traumatic Stress,* 2013; 26:5:537–547.

45. Adamson PA, Zavod MB. Changing Perceptions of Beauty: A Surgeon's Perspective. *Facial Plast Surg* 2006; 22:3:188–193.
46. Ong J, Clarke A, White P, et al. Does Severity Predict Distress? The Relationship Between Subjective and Objective Measure of Appearance and Psychological Adjustment During Treatment for Facial Lipoatrophy. *Science Direct* 2007; 4:239–248.
47. Thurston A. The Unreasonable Patient. *JAMA* 2016; 315:7:657–658.
48. Hertzler AE. *The Horse And Buggy Doctor*. New York: Harper & Brothers; 1938:155, 291.
49. Phillips KA. *The Broken Mirror: Understanding and Treating Body Dysmorphic Disorder*. Revised and expanded edition. New York: Oxford University Press; 2005.
50. Plomin R, Owen MJ, McGuffin P. The Genetic Basis of Complex Human Behaviors. *Science* 1994; 264:1733–1739.
51. Picavet VA, Gabriels L, Grietens J, et al. Preoperative Symptoms of Body Dysmorphic Disorder Determine Postoperative Satisfaction and Quality of Life in Aesthetic Rhinoplasty. *Plast Reconstr Surg* 2013; 131:4:861–868.
52. Adamson PA, Chen T. The Dangerous Dozen: Avoiding Potential Problem Patients in Cosmetic Surgery. *Facial Plastic Surgery Clinics of North America* 2008; 16:2:195–202.
53. Cordeiro CN, Clarke A, White P, et al. A Quantitative Comparison of Psychological and Emotional Health Measures in 360 Plastic Surgery Candidates: Is There a Difference Between Aesthetic and Reconstructive Patients? *Annals of Plast Surg* 2010; 65:3:349–353.
54. Gorney M. Mirror, Mirror on the Wall: The Interface Between Illusion and Reality in Aesthetic Surgery. *Plast Reconstr Surg* 2010; 125:411.
55. Byram V, Wagner HL, Waller G. Sexual Abuse and Body Image Distortion. *Child Abuse Negl* 1995; 19:507–510.
56. Dyer A, Borgmann E, Kleindienst N, et al. Body Image in Patients with Posttraumatic Stress Disorder after Childhood Sexual Abuse and Co-Occurring Eating Disorder. *Psychopathology* 2013; 46:186–191.
57. Felitti VJ, Anda RF. The Lifelong Effects of Adverse Childhood Experiences, Chapter 10. In *Chadwick's Child Maltreatment: Sexual Abuse and Psychological Maltreatment*, 4th edition. Florissant [MO]: STM Learning; 2014.
58. Copeland WE, Wolke D, Angold A, et al. Adult Psychiatric and Suicide Outcomes of Bullying and Being Bullied by Peers in Childhood and Adolescence. *JAMA Psychiatry* 2013; 70:4:419–426.
59. Troop NA, Redshaw C. General Shame and Bodily Shame in Eating Disorders: A 2.5-Year Longitudinal Study. *Eur Eat Disorders* 2012; 20:373–378.
60. Wertheim EH, Paxton SJ. Body Image Development in Adolescent Girls. In: Cash TF, Smolak L, eds. *Body Image*. 2nd edition. New York: The Guilford Press; 2011:76–84.
61. Wolf N. *The Beauty Myth: How Images of Beauty Are Used Against Women*. New York: Anchor Books (Doubleday); 1991.
62. Youssef NA, Green KT, Dedert EA, et al. Exploration of the Influence of Childhood Trauma, Combat Exposure, and the Resilience Construct on Depression and Suicidal Ideation among U.S. Iraq/Afghanistan Era Military Personnel and Veterans. *Arch Suicide Res* 2013; 17:2:106–122.
63. Cash TF. Body Image and Plastic Surgery. In: Sarwer DB, Pruzinsky T, Cash TF, Goldwyn RM, Persing JA, Whitaker LB, eds. *Psychological Aspects of Reconstructive and Cosmetic Plastic Surgery*. Philadelphia: Lippincott Williams & Wilkins; 2006:37–59.
64. Goldwyn RM. Psychological Aspects of Plastic Surgery: A Surgeon's Observations and Reflections. In: Sarwer DB, Pruzinsky T, Cash TF, et al. eds. *Psychological Aspects of Reconstructive and Cosmetic Plastic Surgery: Clinical, Empirical, and Ethical Perspectives*. Philadelphia: Lippincott Williams & Wilkins; 2006:13–22.

65. Sarwer DB, Wadden TA, Pertschuk MJ, et al. The Psychology of Cosmetic Surgery: A Review and Reconceptualization. *Clin Psychol* Rev 1998; 18:1–22.

66. Phillips KA. Appendix: Measures and Resources. In: Phillips KA, ed. *Body Dysmorphic Disorder: Advances in Research and Clinical Practice.* New York: Oxford University Press; 2017.

67. Cash TF, Smolak, eds. *Body Image: A Handbook of Science, Practice, and Prevention.* New York: The Guilford Press; 2011.

68. de Brito MJA, Nahas FX, Cordas TA. Body Dysmorphic Disorder in Patients Seeking Abdominoplasty, Rhinoplasty, and Rhytidectomy. *Plast Reconstr Surg* 2016; 137:2: 462–471.

69. de Brito MJA, Nahas FX, Ferreira LM. Should Plastic Surgeons Operate on Patients Diagnosed with Body Dysmorphic Disorder? *Plast Reconstr Surg* 2012; 129:2:406e–407e.

70. Rumsey N, Harcourt D. Who Is Affected by Appearance Concerns, in What Way, and Why? Summary and Synthesis. In: Rumsey N, Harcourt D, eds. *The Psychology of Appearance.* Oxford [UK]: Oxford University Press; 2012:439–448.

71. Buhlmann U, Hartmann AS. Cognitive and Emotional Processing in Body Dysmorphic Disorder. In: Phillips KA, ed. *Body Dysmorphic Disorder: Advances in Research and Clinical Practice.* New York: Oxford University Press; 2017:285–298.

72. Dilek B, Yemez B, Kizil R, et al. Anxious Personality Is a Risk Factor for Developing Complex Regional Pain Syndrome Type I. *Rheumatol Int* 2012; 32:915–920.

73. Levis DJ, Carrera R. Effects of Ten Hours of Implosive Therapy in the Treatment of Out-Patients: A Preliminary Report. *J Abnorm Psychol* 1967; 72:504–508.

74. Humikowski CA. For What It's Worth. *JAMA* 2015; 313:8:799–800.

2

WHAT THE MENTAL HEALTH LITERATURE SAYS ABOUT BODY DYSMORPHIC DISORDER

Body preoccupations are not 20th and 21st century inventions, even among wartime generals:

> [Stonewall] Jackson was obsessive about anything that involved his health. . . . During his early military service . . . "Jackson became convinced that one of his legs was bigger than the other, and that one of his arms was likewise unduly heavy. He had acquired the habit of raising the heavy arm straight up so that, as he said, 'the blood would run back into his body and lighten it." . . . The major believed that one side of him was smaller than the other, and to correct this he would exercise the smaller side more frequently.[1]

It is when the body implies worth that we suffer.

★★★★★

The florid, burly man sat on my examination table. His eyes were opaque and expressionless. I looked at his history, which said that this would be his sixth rhinoplasty.

"Why did you have your first surgery, Harvey?"

Sigh. "I was sixteen. It was terrible. I had this beautiful nose that was long and had a nice high bridge with a bump, like this." He curled his index finger to show me.

"Do you have a photograph?"

DOI: 10.4324/9781315657721-3

He opened a large manila envelope and peered inside.

Sigh. "I have lots."

He selected one and handed it across to me slowly and soberly, as if it were the most important thing he would do all day. His hands were soft and damp.

"See? It was beautiful. And I had surgery and my nose became small and low and short and I didn't look like myself. Then I had another surgery that made it worse, and my nostrils changed, and I couldn't breathe." His voice had the timbre of a child who didn't want to go to bed.

"Can I have a Kleenex?" He mopped heavy sweat from his forehead and continued.

"I hate it. Every time I look in the mirror all I see is my nose."

He slumped in front of me as if he were waiting outside the headmaster's office.

"I want you to put it back like this." He pointed at a yellowed photograph of a blond and smiling young man with wide, compassionate eyes, ready to live the dream.

"If you liked your nose, why did you have surgery?"

"I had surgery . . ." His voice got smaller. He looked around the room, empty except for us. He nodded to himself, reassured that no one else was there.

"I had the surgery so people would love Harvey."

He mopped his forehead again. I thought of rubbing mine. I had never heard someone refer to himself in the third person. His eyes widened and defocused. Maybe it would help to change the subject.

"What type of work do you do?" He had perspired so heavily that his body left a moist imprint on my examination room paper, like the chalk tracing that the police draw on the floor to show where the body had lain. I silently hoped that he had inherited lots of money and wasn't working at all.

"Me? Oh, I pilot private charters down the Amazon River, right to the Roosevelt branch."

Indeed this man led divers hundreds of feet into the depths of the Amazon to dangerous underwater lakes and caves. We will see personalities like this again: vigorously competent in one area and paralyzed by trauma triggers in another.

I operated to lengthen his nose and restoring his bridge height and tip to simulate the original. A year later he returned.

"My nose—it's a little better." He paused and shifted his weight, but remained tight as a guitar string.

"But I need a little more tip projection. Like this." He squeezed his nose between his thumb and index finger. "Forward 2 mm. Then it will be perfect." He turned toward me, a drowning man looking for a lifeguard.

"Please do it. That's all I need to be happy."

With hesitation, I performed a second surgery. The surgical risk was low and the procedure would be easy for him. Maybe this man, clearly competent in other areas, would move on. The observable difference was real but subtle, exactly what he wanted.

Four months later he returned. Disheveled, he was hard and soft at the same time, limp with defeat. His clothes fit poorly. His flowered shirttails hung over his belt. Since I'd seen him he'd eaten a lot of food marinated in cholesterol. He wore a small bandage across his nasal tip.

"You made my tip too big." His eyes darted to see that we were alone, then quickly lifted the edge of the bandage and replaced it.

"See? It's awful. People stare. Yesterday I passed two women and one laughed. They were laughing at my nose. You have to put the tip back." His eyes widened.

I would have liked to add something professorial but didn't know what it was, so I waited.

"You can do that right now, OK?" His voice constricted so that it was barely audible.

"The last change was a two millimeter difference," I said.

"No, it's much bigger now. It's huge. And my teeth don't fit. My jaw moved."

"That's impossible," I said. *"I only operated on your nasal tip."*

"No, my jaw moved." He nodded decisively and pressed it to show me. He really believed what he was saying.

"I can't stand it. Please fix my tip."

He had grown a little Victorian stage villain's mustache and played with it absently.

"It's too soon to operate safely," I said. *"I don't understand what happened. You were happy when you left."*

His eyes got wider.

"I just want you to put the tip back the way it was. Can you operate now?"

He paused for emphasis. The energy in his body seemed to compress.

"It has to be perfect."

"I can't operate yet. Do you remember what I said?"

He looked into his shoes. Almost imperceptibly he shook his head. I felt like I was trying to speak over a fire alarm that only he could hear. His composure was tumbling. He took a deep breath, and his voice got louder.

"Look, I've sold my guitar and quit my job. I moved in with my father."

I straightened.

"I thought he beat you."

He shook his head.

"The guy is sick and nobody else is willing."

"Maybe that's why you're unhappy," I said. He didn't react. The alarm was too overpowering. I decided to add something.

"If you carry his fear, you will end up living his life, you know."

His focus didn't move.

"Look, if I hold the mirror just here, my nostrils look funny."

He squinted at the ceiling. "And there's something wrong with your lights. I can see it much better in my bathroom mirror."

He sighed and his shoulders fell.

"You have to help me. Forget what I told you. It wasn't me talking before the last operation. Now this is the real me."

Nosology and Diagnostic Criteria of Body Dysmorphic Disorder

Even through this distressed man's Byzantine logic, he fulfills all textbook components for body dysmorphic disorder: a modest aesthetic deformity that would be imperceptible except to surgeons; significant distress; and compensatory behavior (multiple surgeries).[2–5] So did General Jackson. Yet the deformities were real and improvable, both aesthetically and functionally. When I first saw him, the patient was high-functioning in a risky occupation. I empathized with his desire to restore his lost sense of personal identity after making a teenager's decision. But there are other elements: Why did he feel so desperately unloved that surgery was the solution? What role did his father's constant abuse play? Why did he care what others decided were his deficiencies? What was the connection between caring for a parent whom he disliked and his sudden dissatisfaction with the surgical result? What else did I never uncover that influenced his body image and search for perfection? Did he have a genetic abnormality, family disposition, sensitive ego, or neurotransmitter defect? Or was this just a disorder that had appeared without reason?

★★★★★

Except for collaboration by surgeons and mental health professionals, plastic surgeons might be just complaining to each other about their eccentric patients without understanding what they saw. The work done by Edgerton, starting in the 1950's, and the early writings of Goin and Goin in 1970's and 1980's described the clinical pathology; but the inclusion of body dysmorphic disorder in the DSM-111-R in 1987 was an important step that allowed researchers to begin to systematically characterize the disorder and its associated pathology. Voluminous research done by mental health professionals dedicated to understanding body dysmorphic disorder has given us a precise description of these patients' lives and behavior, and clues to their treatment. But it also raises new questions.

BDD is not a new disorder, but rather the current term for a disease that was previously called dysmorphophobia in the eastern European, German, and Russian psychiatric literature. Freud described a patient he called "the Wolf Man," whose behavior included the obsessive and mirror-checking traits of the disease. Having previously treated this patient for "compulsive neurosis," Freud later commented that he still "neglected his daily life and work because he was engrossed, to the exclusion of all else, in the state of his nose. . . . His life was centered on the little mirror in his pocket, and his fate depended on what it revealed or was about to reveal."[6]

The DSM-III first classified BDD as "dysmorphophobia," categorized as an atypical somatoform disorder.[7] In the DSM-III-R, BDD became a somatoform disorder, "characterized by preoccupation with an imagined defect *in a normal-appearing person* [italics mine] accompanied by excessive concern by the patient, without delusional intensity, and not accompanied by anorexia nervosa or transsexualism."[7] Anorexia nervosa and BDD may, however, coexist, and in one study of 41 patients with both disorders, 69% had sought plastic surgery.[8] In 93.8% of those patients, BDD preceded the anorexia symptoms. Both disorders exist in milieux of body shame, abuse, neglect, and disordered family life, so that their association makes sense.

DSM-IV added a delusional variant, characterizing patients completely convinced that their physical deformities were real.[7, 9] But who decides what is real? At what point does body image become abnormal? How much distress is justified when the patient has an unexpected, unacceptable surgical change in body image? These are not easy questions because the answers depend a great deal upon who is examining the patient.

The committee charged with making recommendations for the DSM-V examined each of these issues thoroughly.[10] It determined that the word "preoccupation" was adequate because many BDD patients reported obsessing (or "worrying," the cognitive component of anxiety) about their appearance flaws for three to eight hours a day, a third for more than eight hours.[11] Based on its similarity to obsessive compulsive disorder (OCD), BDD was previously characterized as part of that spectrum.[12–16] Nevertheless, there were ways in which BDD did and did not fit that conceptualization. The primary similarities between BDD and OCD were their compulsive actions such as mirror checking or excessive grooming and their responses to pharmacotherapy and cognitive-behavioral therapy. Patients with BDD are notorious for their poor insight; between 35% and 40% are delusional.[17, 18] The intensity with which BDD patients experience their perceived flaws is similarly uncharacteristic of OCD. The Committee recommended substituting the word "imagined" with "perceived," even though it agreed that most deformities were only visible to the patients. Would that still be true if the examining physician were trained to treat the patient's alleged deformity? We do not know.

A new criterion added compulsive behaviors to the diagnosis. The authors emphasized the resemblance to OCD compulsions and specifically cited BDD patients' compensatory behaviors (mirror checking, excessive grooming, skin picking, reassurance seeking, or comparing his or her appearance to others'). Surgery is not included.

Although "distress or impairment in functioning" became an added criterion, the Committee correctly recognized that many non-BDD individuals are distressed or preoccupied by some physical feature: 46% in one study of college students, and 87.4% in a nationwide survey.[7] As a result, the Committee required that the distress (depression, anxiety, shame) and the type of impairment in social, occupational, or household functioning be specified.[19] Finally, the Committee recommended a distinction between BDD appearance obsessions and those characterized relating to body fat or weight.

*****

The Committee also considered whether body dysmorphic disorder shared similarities with hypochondriasis, and decided that it did not. Its reasoning was based on the inapplicability of the ICD-10 criterion C for hypochondriasis: "Persistent refusal to accept medical advice that there is no adequate physical cause for the symptoms for physical abnormality, except for short periods . . ." This criterion assumes that all physical diagnosis is accurate and that the physician is right but the patient is wrong, which is not always true. Another limitation is that patients who have undergone surgery know what actually happened; subsequent providers don't. BDD diagnosis has been held back by this schism.

Another distinction between BDD and somatization disorders was evidence that women with BDD were less aware of being ill than unaffected individuals.[20] There is a reasonable explanation for this finding: patients who survive developmental trauma never learn appropriate self-care and suffer trauma-derived illnesses and symptoms (Chapter 9).[21–25] I see evidence of poor self-care in my own patients, who willfully disregard preoperative and postoperative instructions even though they know the dangers. This behavior is fundamentally paradoxical.[22] Abuse and neglect contribute to body dissociation and poor body care, reflecting changes encoded in the right cerebral hemisphere.[26]

Finally, the Committee eliminated the separation between delusional and nondelusional BDD, recognizing that the distinction is often difficult. "Insight" is a more appropriate measure. Delusionality has to be based on whether the treating clinician sees what the patient sees: if he or she doesn't, the patient is, in theory, delusional—another assumption that is not always true. However, "insight" does not always take into account the degree of deformity, whether the patient's distress is appropriate, whether the cost/benefit analysis of surgery is to the patient's advantage; and whether the patient recognizes that his or her compensatory actions were merited. These fine points are not always clear in actual practice.

My comments are not meant to be criticisms of the Committee's work or the final version in the DSM-V.[27] But there is a great deal to be gained in the future by more collaboration between treating physicians and mental health experts. BDD is ideally a two-specialty diagnosis without which there can be too many false positives and negatives, and where patients with legitimate surgical problems can be saddled forever with diagnoses that they do not deserve. This already happens. On the other hand, too many surgeons and physicians, particularly from my specialty, have been missing in action in contributing information and new research on BDD. Their perspectives are uniquely contextual and would provide an important service.

Etiology, Prevalence, Demographic Characteristics, Phenomenology, and Comorbidity

In the population at large, representative samples have given a body dysmorphic disorder prevalence of about 2%. However, the prevalence for patients who seek dermatologic or surgical treatment is estimated at 7% to 25%.[28–30]

A number of good self-administered questionnaires have been constructed by various researchers to diagnose body dysmorphic disorder and associated body dissatisfaction.[31] Among the more commonly used scales, the Derriford Appearance Scale, Short Form,[32] the Centre for Appearance Research Salience Scale and the Center for Research Valence Scale,[33] the Short Form Health Survey, Version 2 (Short Form-36), the Rosenberg Self-Esteem Scale, and the Eating Attitudes Test (referenced in[34]), the Cosmetic Procedure Screening Questionnaire,[35] the FACE-Q,[36] the Objectified Body Uneasiness Test,[37] PreFACE,[38] the Body Dysmorphic Disorder Self questionnaire,[39] and the Brown Assessment of Beliefs Scale.[40] Only the last two are either clinician-administered or followed up.

Self-diagnosis has its limitations: patients may deny or elaborate. Even physician evaluation imposes a margin of error unless the physician is trained to correct the problem that the patient sees. What this may mean is that we have no accurate idea of the real prevalence of body dysmorphic disorder. In fact, because the diagnosis depends so much on subjective decisions, like the severity of the deformity and life disruption, there are bound to be erroneous type I (false positive) or type II (false negative) errors.

Particularly relevant to our discussion is recognition that body dysmorphic disorder usually begins in early adolescence, with a mean onset at age 16.7 years (range 4–43).[2, 3, 28, 41–43] The younger the onset of body dysmorphic disorder, the more severe the symptoms, and the greater the delusionality, substance abuse, associated disorders, and attempted suicide.[39, 42, 44–46] The high prevalence of childhood trauma before age 18 in the Kaiser/Permanente study and in our own patients (Chapter 9) cannot be ignored in this regard. Not surprisingly, BDD in the teen years is alleged to interfere with the development of self-esteem and body image—as do abuse and neglect (Chapter 3).[47–53]

BDD is almost always a chronic disease, with only a 20% chance of full remission within four years, and a high probability of relapse (42%).[54] If one etiologic component is a dysfunctional family inflicting developmental trauma on a growing child unable to escape the toxic environment, these findings get easier to understand.

★★★★★

One day after surgery she took a taxicab from New Haven and charged into my office, head down and breathless.

"I have to ask, I am so worried, a pillow fell on my nose last night and I think it might have ruined my result. What about moving my lips? Can talking affect my nose?" I was in surgery. My staff reassured her that the splint would protect her.

By the day of dressing removal, she was radiant. "This was fun. Let's book my next surgery."

As she left, she looked over her shoulder. "And I think I'll put tape on my tip: I read it on the Internet."

At her next appointment she returned with a bright new helmet of blonde hair, showing what I thought was remarkable expanse of cleavage for a doctor's office.

"I feel so good! I love cosmetic surgery! What else can we do? How about breast surgery; will you examine my breasts?"

I wouldn't. She was 45 and single, the only other lawyer in her father's office.

I examined her nose. "You look great. I'll see you in four months."

Her eyes widened. "Oh, oh, I can't go that long. Can I come back next week?"

We made an appointment in four months. Two weeks later, her desperate phone calls began. Worries popped like corn in a pan. I can't breathe. I think my nose is crooked. My grafts are dissolving. I have bone coming out of my nose. I've had unprotected sex—it's making my surgery fall apart. No doctors in the emergency rooms know what to do. I think I have a hole in my septum. My nose is sinking into my face. I think he disfigured me. I need injections for my forehead creases. I need filler in my nose."

Twenty-three emails later, each of which I answered, the phone rang. She spoke without taking a breath.

"I blew my nose too soon. And my bones are completely curved to the left. I hope you don't get mad. I am hitting a rough patch. I really want a pretty face."

The daily emails continued—wild and free-floating.

"I want you to like me and care about me. It seems that you do, because you are such a remarkably kind person. I don't want to talk about trauma therapy again. It's not psychological."

"My psychiatrist won't see me. I am disfigured. I'm going to another doctor. I've gone ten months hiding without looking at anyone. I'm really plummeting. I can't live like this anymore. My tip looks mushy. Will second-hand smoke affect me?"

"My mother was hospitalized for insanity. She was mentally unbalanced and spoiled, but she was smart and pretty. She said I wasn't as pretty as the other girls. I was bad a lot. She spanked my wet bathing suit when I lost my tricycle."

In the space of 18 months, she sent 151 emails, often two or three in a day.

"I have rights. I demand that you see me. If you won't, I'll hire a lawyer to force you."

She never saw the relevance of trauma therapy. The problem was surgical.

"I have to see him today. I know it's too soon but I'll pay any amount of money."

Consider the attitudes, behaviors, and attributes of the disquieted patients described so far: The intense need to continue or increase their behaviors—in this case operative treatment, despite disappointment—in order to relieve inner tension; a life organized around appearance and surgery; extreme mood changes; passionate—even operatic—emotions; tenuous worlds built on delusion, poor self-care, and underpowered insight.

What word describes this behavior—so irrational, so desperate, so willing to pay anything, so urgent for a fix? Addiction.

Clinical Presentation of Body Dysmorphic Disorder

Samples of treated and untreated body dysmorphic disorder patients cite the most frequent areas of concern as follows: skin (80.0%), hair (57.5%), nose (39.0%), stomach (32.0%), teeth (29.5%), weight (29.0%), breasts (26.0%), buttocks (21.5%), eyes (21.5%), thighs (20.0%), eyebrows (19.5%), overall appearance of face (19.0%), small body build (18.0%), legs (18.0%), face size or shape (16.0%), chin (14.5%), lips (14.5%), arms (13.5%), hips (12.5%), cheeks (10.5%), and ears (10.5%).[20, 29, 55–62] The most common body area for which BDD patients seek surgery is the nose.[28, 41, 63]

Most series find that body dysmorphic disorder is more common in women than men.[64] My own review of 1,000 consecutive rhinoplasty patients in 2007 indicated that 40% of the BDD patients were men, even though men comprised only 22% of the total patient population; thus men were disproportionately represented.

Certainly the plastic surgery literature warns more about the dangers of male compared to female patients even though most series show a gender dominance of affected females. However, when females are traumatized, they are more likely to react with depression ("flight" or "freeze"), whereas men are more likely to become combative ("fight").[51, 65] Thus, although unhappy men seem to be less numerous, they can be more memorable.

More severely affected patients may each average five to seven areas of concern, as we have also documented.[98, 99] Treatment does not decrease the number of areas that affected patients dislike nor resolve compensatory behaviors (e.g., excessive mirror checking, grooming, camouflaging).[66, 67] Reality processing is poor, and untreated patients often have poorer insight than those who have been treated.[12, 18] Many such patients are highly impaired, disabled in their social and work lives, and frequently miss work or school because of the disorder. Some leave school permanently.

Suicidal behavior is 10–25 times higher for ideation and 2–12 times higher for attempt than in the general population.[28] A 2005 report by the same authors noted that the predictors for suicidal ideation or attempts were the presence of comorbid lifetime major depression and PTSD. The odds of prior suicide attempt are more than six times greater for patients with both body dysmorphic disorder and PTSD.[68]

Comorbidities, Information Processing, and Other BDD Characteristics

Comorbidity with mood disorders, bipolar disorder, obsessive-compulsive disorder (OCD), and eating disorders is also high, confirming previous reports indicating that 12% of OCD patients also have BDD; that 33% of BDD patients have OCD, and others that link anxiety, anger, somatic complaints and delusionality with body dysmorphic disorder.[16–18, 30, 58, 69–74] A study of 191 delusional and non-delusional body dysmorphic disorder patients correlated similar features in both groups, including demographic and disease characteristics, degree of functional impairment and life quality, and comorbidities. Both groups had similar remission rates; but delusional subjects were less well educated, more likely to have attempted suicide, less likely to be under adequate treatment, and had worse BDD symptoms.[18] An earlier report on the same patient sample, BDD severity and the likelihood of suicide and substance abuse was also associated with comorbid post-traumatic stress disorder.[68]

Patients with body dysmorphic disorder who also have obsessive compulsive disorder are younger and have an earlier onset of OCD, are more likely to be female, less likely to be married, more severely depressed, more likely to have social phobia or psychotic disorder diagnoses, more likely to be hoarders, need more reassurance, more likely to have suicidal ideation, and more likely to abuse substances.[16, 39]

BDD patients have other comorbidities, including anorexia nervosa (39% in one study) and alexithymia (difficulty identifying and naming feelings).[75] The association between body dysmorphic disorder, alexithymia, and eating disorders may be mediated by a "global emotion-processing deficit": the widespread effect of PTSD on the midbrain and cortex would be an excellent candidate. Other BDD patients have established memory dysfunction, specifically the ability to learn and recall (but not store information).[76]

Altered information processing was found in OCD patients, but BDD participants rated appearance-relevant scenarios even worse than the OCD patients ("I am sure they are judging the way I look"),[77] even though none of the BDD participants met criteria for comorbid social phobia. Thus, as the vignettes illustrate, these patients interpret ambiguous events as threatening, confirming their unflattering opinions of themselves and making them emotionally vulnerable. Even in general conversation; their external boundaries are porous.[52] Other researchers have confirmed these findings.[78] These authors note that social anxiety commonly co-existed with depression and posttraumatic stress disorder (PTSD). The constant tendency to interpret neutral cues as negative and threatening will clearly affect patient trust, often strikingly impaired without justification—a trait also found in childhood trauma and PTSD victims.[65, 79, 80] Not surprisingly, BDD patients perceive much higher degrees of life stress than unaffected controls in self-reported surveys.[81] Who can blame them?

The Brain in Body Dysmorphic Disorder

What happens to the brains of BDD patients? There is some provocative information, especially relevant to the similarity of memory dysfunction in these patients and those with PTSD and childhood trauma. Functional magnetic resonance imaging (fMRI) indicates that BDD patients focus on visual details rather than holistic, global ones.[76] This finding makes intuitive sense because of the way BDD patients can obsess over trivial appearance details or fabricate delusional beliefs about various features. Additional preliminary research in a small number of subjects demonstrated asymmetry of the caudate nucleus, the left side dominating, and greater white matter volume, although gray matter volume was unchanged.[28, 82] The orbitofrontal cortex and anterior cingulate (which inhibits amygdalar fear-conditioning) were smaller, though the thalamus was larger.[83] When stimulated by photographs of their own faces, BDD patients demonstrated hyperactivity in their left orbitofrontal cortices and bilateral caudate nucleus heads compared to controls; these findings were similar to those found in OCD patients, suggesting that the brain circuits in both disorders may be similar, which would not be surprising.[16,84,85] Overactivity has been noted in the orbitofrontal cortex/anterior cingulate cortex/caudate nucleus and thalamus (the so-called "worry circuit") in OCD patients.[86] These same changes occur in patients with PTSD.[80,87,88] Parallel changes in BDD patients would not be surprising based on the association of both childhood trauma[89] and PTSD in BDD patients (9% in one study[28,90]). An important study tested memory characteristics in 18 BDD patients.[91] The authors found increased attention biases in BDD patients (hypersensitivity) and tendencies to avoid situations where their appearances might be evaluated. Eighty-eight percent reported spontaneous, intrusive memories and images, often dating from childhood and associated with particularly stressful events (bullying, and teasing, being told that he or she was ugly, being too tall or short), paralleling PTSD. Teasing was also common, particularly among adolescents. The target side of teasing is the child's coping strategies: boundaryless children will be more susceptible and disturbed by teasing than those who understand their intrinsic value. Cognitive behavior therapy can be helpful.[92,93] Not surprisingly, childhood trauma survivors have intact boundaries to compliments (ignoring them) but penetrable boundaries to criticism, making them perfect victims for bullying and verbal abuse.

The Links From BDD to PTSD, Memory, and Developmental Trauma

Arousal, avoidance, and re-experiencing, which 88% of these patients recount, characterize posttraumatic stress disorder. It is easy to imagine how the tormenting cacophony of these memory and processing disturbances could create the behavior that we clinicians interpret as depressed or demanding conduct, and that gives some plastic surgery patients such unflattering reputations. Some of our own rhinoplasty patients screened positive for PTSD, particularly those with childhood trauma histories (Chapter 8).

"Memory tempered by personal feeling is what allows humans to imagine both individual well-being and the compounded well-being of the whole society. . . . Memory is responsible for ceaselessly placing the self in an evanescent here and now, between a thoroughly lived past and an anticipated future . . . the tomorrows that are nothing but possibilities," Damasio writes.[22]

But traumatic memory is not ordinary memory.[79,94–97] Traumatic memories are stored and accessed without involvement of conscious memory centers (hippocampus and pre-frontal cortex), explaining why abused patients react to stress inappropriately and can display the poor insight or delusional thinking characteristic of BDD. The shadow factor of abuse or neglect and any associated conditions (e.g., obsessive-compulsive disorder, eating disorder, or perfectionism) also help explain why the severity of many patients' deformities does not correspond to the drive for surgery that it provokes. In fact, among the reasons given by BDD patients for not having sought treatment is "shame."[54] A history of emotional abuse and long-standing interpersonal conflict can be elicited from the majority of patients with BDD.[6, 98–100] When traumatized patients perceive that they are powerless and believe that they have been abused or neglected again (e.g., not achieving an expected surgical outcome, feeling abandoned by the surgeon, experiencing a complication), they plunge into a shamed trauma state and begin to behave and respond with the childish maturity and coping skills that may have been appropriate for the original trauma, but are no longer. This is the unconscious conduct that surgeons perceive as immature, irrational, or "crazy." To these patients, however, their childhood abuse is occurring all over again. There is significant evidence that body image disturbances do not often arise without a background milieu of developmental trauma.[101] The patient who has self-worth as a young teen may develop *body dissatisfaction*; the traumatized patient without self-worth develops *body shame*, which is quite different (Chapter 5).[102] These findings suggest that targeting shame during the treatment of BDD patients might significantly increase success.

★★★★★

Patients with BDD appear to have abnormal perceptual and emotional information-processing capabilities and deficits in memory organization.[76] These patients also have deficits in learning and memory, particularly strategic organization and free recall. However, they are, on the whole, unusually intelligent and can recall information once it is learned.

Reinforcing this schema, the brains of patients with BDD emphasize negative words and interfere with the processing of positive words, making these patients more hypersensitive to criticism and therefore less amenable to reassurance by the surgeon.[103, 104] Similarly, patients with BDD are more likely than control subjects or patients with OCD to interpret others' descriptive or neutral comments as criticism—this trait reflects the reality processing and boundary issues that we will discuss in Chapter 3.[77] In a 2008 comparison of 275 OCD patients with and without BDD, Stewart, Stack, and Wilhelm determined that 15.3% were comorbid, but that the patients with both diseases developed them earlier (OCD appearing first), were predominantly female, more depressed, dominantly unmarried, and had a higher rate of illicit drug use.[16] Although family histories did not differ, the authors do not state what those histories comprised. Another study of 195 patients confirmed these findings and added that those with OCD were more likely to be delusional, whereas the BDD patients were more likely to have suicidal ideation, be depressed, and use illicit drugs. Perhaps most important, the authors conclude that BDD and OCD are related conditions, BDD occurring significantly more frequently in first-degree relatives with obsessive compulsive disorder, suggesting a familial spectrum for the diseases. This is a critical speculation.[28, 53, 105] Patients with BDD are therefore much more sensitive than control subjects to teasing and are more likely to misidentify facial and computerized images.[106] This characteristic has encouraging implications for surgeons who may try to screen patients for BDD by using computer-imaging software.

BDD patients' clinical manifestations are characteristic. Many require constant reassurance, manifest great anxiety, and selectively process information, obsessing about imperfections while filtering out successes. Some patients, like the distressed man described at the beginning of this chapter, ask the same questions repeatedly within minutes but are absolutely unable to recall what they have been told.[104] This is not an act. Part of their hyperaroused behavior can be attributed to the anxiety that results when patients cannot fully "engage" (Chapter 7), but there is probably more. Buhlmann and co-authors[77, 104] reported that their BDD patients always attributed hypothetical body-related scenarios negatively ("I must have said something foolish or insulting"), even when there were other reasonable alternatives. "My father blamed me for the breakup [of his marriage]. . . . He said to me, 'You are no longer my son.' I looked in the mirror and I thought I looked different. . . . I have never looked the same since."[58] Shall we blame the patient's own information processing or his father's toxic emotional abuse?

Body Dysmorphic Disorder in Plastic Surgery Populations

A recent paper from Brazil compared body dysmorphic disorder symptoms in 300 patients (90 abdominoplasty, 151 rhinoplasty, and 59 facelift).[107] Prevalence rates in the three groups were 57%, 52%, and 42%, respectively (not statistically different). As noted by other authors, dissatisfaction began in childhood or adolescence in 90% of rhinoplasty patients, at about age 40 in 90% of abdominoplasty patients, and over the age of 40 in 52% of facelift patients; those findings would be expected. Approximately 80% of patients in all three groups spent more than three hours a day obsessing about their appearances. Most patients exaggerated their deformities (abdominoplasty, 82%; rhinoplasty, 92%; facelift, 76%) in the authors' judgment, suggesting a significant emotional component. Sixty-four percent to 84% of patients compared their target body areas to those of others. The majority avoided mirrors, public and social situations, physical activities, physical and sexual contact; 96% to 100% in each group were obsessed with mirror checking, self-inspection, and camouflage.

Of particular importance to our own discussion was a history of childhood emotional abuse (teasing and bullying) in 69% of abdominoplasty patients, 28% of rhytidectomy patients, and 92% of rhinoplasty patients (identical to our results in revision rhinoplasty patients [Chapter 9]). Similarly, 6% of rhinoplasty patients were sexually abused, as were 4% of rhytidectomy patients; the association of sexual abuse with BDD, highest in the rhinoplasty group, was statistically significant. All childhood or adolescent sexually abused patients had severe body image disturbances. A history of sexual abuse also correlated with both suicidal ideation and attempt. In my ongoing Adverse Childhood Events study (currently 175 consecutive patients), 86% of whom had aesthetic surgery, 27% were sexually abused (Chapter 9).

Childhood trauma, particularly sexual trauma, has been suggested as a cause of BDD, confirmed by the Zlotnick,[28, 108, 109] Didie,[100] Baldock and Veale,[110] and my own reports[6, 98, 99] that document childhood abuse, neglect, and PTSD in BDD patients. Phillips also highlights the importance of shame, often explicitly stated by BDD patients.[28, 111] This is an important observation, though not new: Janet described symptoms that would now be called body dysmorphic disorder and referred to them as "*un obsession de la honte du corps*" (a body shame obsession).[112] "Carried" shame, absorbed from an abusive or neglectful parent, as opposed to healthy shame (also called "embarrassment," Chapter 3) is toxic to the developing child.[47-52] A great number of plastic surgery patients, particularly the most distressed and obsessed, will spontaneously cite shame, lack of self-esteem, defectiveness, and desire to please or fit in with the family as motivations for surgery. Bodily imperfections are seen as impairments to love, companionship, and acceptance—even goodness.

Family Prevalence in Body Dysmorphic Disorder

There is an established family incidence of body dysmorphic disorder.[28, 54, 82] Approximately 20% of BDD patients have a first-degree relative with body dysmorphic disorder; 5.8% of all first-degree relatives have BDD (probably an underestimate because of interviewing limitations), but still three to six times higher than the BDD prevalence in the general population.[12, 113]

Socio-environmental research suggests that "early childhood experiences and psychological vulnerabilities" can plant and reinforce children's aversion to their own appearances.[90] Veale and others have suggested that external events and intrusive thoughts might trigger excessive attention to one's appearance, which in turn may create core beliefs linking self-esteem to appearance; hence the obsession with perceived "ugliness."[36, 67, 97, 111] Once established, it is easy to see how maladaptive thoughts may multiply and initiate ritualistic behavior, camouflaging, social avoidance, reassurance seeking, or other obsessive behavior. Where, however, do these "intrusive thoughts" and "external events," coupled with histories of emotional and sexual abuse, originate? It is hard to imagine a scenario in which the family is never at fault when young children are emotionally abused or neglected. The family of origin is the milieu in which the sense of self, and the attitude toward self, are generated.

Genetics and Neurotransmitters in Body Dysmorphic Disorder

Genetic studies supply provocative information, though they are still inconclusive about etiology. Many genetic studies compare "alleles," the result of genetic mutations that create gene variants, looking for morphologic or visible differences (phenotypes) in the alleles. Alleles can be dominant or recessive, and several may be needed to determine one characteristic; for example, three alleles determine ABO blood type; at least two alleles determine eye color.

Alleles typically have short and long variants. "Serotonin transporter" is a genetically—determined protein that removes serotonin from the spaces between nerve cells in the brain, and so becomes the primary target of serotonin reuptake inhibitor antidepressants (SRI's). The more serotonin remains, the longer its effect lasts. In one study, a higher percentage of people with body dysmorphic disorder have the short allele of serotonin transporter.[41, 82] This is interesting, because the short allele for serotonin transporter has also been associated with alcoholism, depression, PTSD, obsessive-compulsive disorder, and social phobia, neuroticism, "impaired agreeableness,"[114] alcoholism,[115, 116] anxiety and depression,[117] and affective disorders.[118] GABA (gamma-aminobutyric acid), a substance available as the drug gabapentin, is an endogenous inhibitory neurotransmitter used to treat chronic neuropathic pain, epilepsy, anxiety, and other disorders. In one preliminary study, the short allele of the GABA gene is also higher in BDD patients.[28, 82]

Telomeres, the protein caps on our chromosomal tips, vary in length based on the environment. Short telomeres are associated with inflammation, depression, anxiety, sleep deprivation and its consequences,[119, 120] eating disorders, stress (maternal violence, bullying, or physical abuse), alcohol abuse, smoking, psychiatric disorders (bipolar disorder, schizophrenia, non-affective psychoses, and anxiety disorders[121, 122]), and cellular aging; but endurance exercise, active lifestyles, vitamins, high-fiber diets, adequate sleep, not smoking, and modest alcohol use can stop or reverse telomere enzymatic (telomerase) erosion and protect telomere length.[123]

Backing away from the genetic information, however, let us re-examine the family studies. The 20% incidence of BDD in first-degree relatives of BDD patients is acknowledged but not, in my opinion, yet given sufficient prominence. Let's change the disease: Suppose 20% of breast cancer patients had mothers or sisters with breast cancer—would we notice then? Only a 5% to 10% first-degree relative incidence in breast cancer prompted the research that identified genetic mutations in the BRCA-1 and BRCA-2 genes. A single first-degree relative (mother, sister, or daughter) with breast cancer doubles a woman's chance of developing the same disease.

Remarkably consistent in the overwhelming majority of case histories are references to shame, low self-esteem, catastrophic thinking, family ridicule, histories of childhood neglect or abuse, associated substance abuse and depression, suicidal ideation, great difficulty with interpersonal relationships, and brain and abnormalities consistent with those found not only in obsessive compulsive disorder but also in PTSD and complex trauma. When added to the 20% first-degree relative prevalence of BDD, it is hard to argue that these identical manifestations are only unfortunate coincidences and that genetic or neurotransmitter causes always operate alone.

There is limited research on the association between childhood trauma or life trauma and BDD, but the findings have always been significant. Zlotnick and Phillips found a 20% prevalence of BDD in a group of 55 women who had been sexually abused.[28] Nine percent of 200 BDD patients had PTSD.[39] These prevalences suggest that there still is room for investigation into the impact of familial factors that produce body shame and other characteristics of body dysmorphic disorder.

Treatment of Body Dysmorphic Disorder

Both pharmacological and nonpharmacological treatments have been heavily researched and tested. Medication trials have primarily included serotonin reuptake inhibitors (SRI) (fluoxetine, fluvoxamine, citalopram, escitalopram, and clomipramine) tested against despiramine.[54] In one study, clomipramine was more effective than despiramine.[28, 71, 124] Experience with SRI's suggests that BDD patients may require higher doses and longer treatment durations. Combination with other medications (buspirone or clomipramine) may help.[56, 71, 124, 125]

Cognitive Behavior Therapy (CBT) is commonly used and effective for BDD.[36, 126, 127] This therapy involves psychoeducation; learning to recognize triggers, maladaptive thoughts, and erroneous core beliefs; understanding the benefits of behavioral change, performing exposure exercises, and learning to better manage thoughts. Several studies have shown decreased symptom severity at three and six month follow-up, but longer term studies are needed.[126, 128]

Other treatments have included electroconvulsive therapy, rarely used, and, in severe cases, anterior cingulotomy or subcaudate tractotomy, the logic being that they are the areas affected in obsessive compulsive disorder. Coincidentally, the same areas are also affected in childhood (complex) trauma and PTSD. Unfortunately, as my own patients' cases and the literature indicate, plastic surgery is almost always ineffective, and many patients with occult disease, apparently compensated before surgery, only begin to exhibit full-blown BDD postoperatively.[19] Most studies show a surgical dissatisfaction rate of 80% to 90%.[28, 57, 128–138] In my recently reported series of 100 consecutive revision rhinoplasty patients, complete satisfaction after a single revision rhinoplasty in patients who knew their original noses were normal but who had surgery anyway (therefore defining BDD) was only 3%. Another 65% were only partially satisfied and requested more surgery. With few exceptions,[139] most aesthetic surgeons have had the same experience.[140, 141]

Not all unhappy patients go away quietly. In a 2002 survey, 40% of plastic surgeons stated that patients with BDD had threatened them physically or with legal action.[130, 133] In one prominent New York case, a patient with BDD sued her plastic surgeon, asserting that, despite undergoing successful previous operations performed by him, she was unable to give informed consent because of the cognitive distortion produced by her disease.[6] Several unhappy plastic surgery patients murdered their physicians; however, it has not been established whether the patients' psychopathology in these cases was BDD.

What the Family Research Suggests

Our patient vignettes replicate the behavioral difficulties common to both BDD and to patients with "complex trauma," the term for patients exposed to protracted abuse and neglect during childhood: impulsivity, aggression, sexual acting out, poor self-care, uncontrolled anxiety, alcohol and drug abuse, self-destructive actions, depression, panic, trouble with interpersonal relationships, and somatization.[51, 65, 73, 80, 87, 88, 142–145] New experiences may reactivate both BDD and PTSD symptoms.[7, 28, 58, 146–151]

In 2006, an unprecedented and remarkable report appeared in which 75 patients with established body dysmorphic disorder completed the Childhood Trauma Questionnaire and were then interviewed.[100, 152, 153, 154] An astonishing 78.7% reported history of adverse childhood events: 68% emotional neglect, 56% emotional abuse, 34.7% physical abuse, 33.3% physical neglect, and 28% sexual abuse. Severity of sexual abuse correlated with the severity of BDD symptoms. A history of childhood abuse was also correlated with attempted suicide and substance disorder. These data resemble the prevalences in our own patients (Chapter 9). Two of my own BDD patients committed suicide 15 and 20 years after surgery, respectively, capping lives of chaos and substance addiction.

Can we use this information to understand the observations that BDD patients have particular personality traits: introversion, social avoidance, perfectionism, shyness, social anxiety, low self-esteem, depression, obsessive compulsive tendencies, associated anorexia nervosa, sensitivity to rejection, and sensitivity to criticism? Where do these characteristics originate? Are the brains of some patients simply sensitive to appearance remarks that later trigger BDD? Is it coincidental that the brains of individuals traumatized in childhood have the same changes in their caudate nuclei, cingulate cortices, and orbitofrontal complexes as BDD patients?[84, 155–162] Are they only random genetic traits?[163] Is family prevalence relevant? If so, why can't excellent researchers document characteristic genetic profiles? Among patients who do not give histories of BDD elsewhere in the family, are they new mutations? Is there some neurotransmitter abnormality, yet unidentified? Is the neurotransmitter search in BDD patients like trying to understand love by measuring estrogen and testosterone levels?

What This Information Means

If the BDD patient is simply a victim of societal pressures to be thin and beautiful, why aren't all men and women similarly affected?[5] Are these patients simply dupes of dominating male plastic surgeons, as some writers believe,[164, 165] or are they genetically more artistic?[166] In what causative order do we place low self-esteem, PTSD, obsessive compulsive tendencies, family prevalence, adverse childhood events, abnormal memory processing, shame, co-existent eating disorders, addictive behaviors, and patients driven to perfection, even for minor or imperceptible deformities?[167] Which comes first?

These are all valid questions for which we have already had glimpses and for which there is a plausible hypothesis: a model that begins with childhood abuse or neglect, which affects self-esteem, reality, the ability to live in moderation, and self-care; that in turn manifests as body shame (instead of body dissatisfaction); and that then drives these unhappy patients into the personality and behavioral characteristics that we call the unhappy patient, the insatiable patient, or body dysmorphic disorder. Might body dysmorphic disorder only be one of many unhappy—or even addictive—manifestations of the past, an emotional disease before it is physical? Might that theory explain why the size of the deformity is often irrelevant to the personal anguish and behavior it generates? We shall explore these questions in subsequent chapters.

References

1. Gwynne SC. *Rebel Yell: The Violence, Passion and Redemption of Stonewall Jackson.* New York: Scribner; 2014:126.
2. Phillips KA. Body Dysmorphic Disorder: The Distress of Imagined Ugliness. *Am J Psychiatry* 1991; 148:9:1138–1149.
3. Phillips KA. *The Broken Mirror: Understanding and Treating Body Dysmorphic Disorder.* Oxford [UK] / New York: Oxford University Press; 1996.
4. Slaughter JR, Sun AM. In Pursuit of Perfection: A Primary Care Physician's Guide to Body Dysmorphic Disorder. *Am Fam Physician* 1999; 60:6:1738–1742.
5. Slevec J, Tiggemann M. Attitudes Toward Cosmetic Surgery in Middle-Aged Women: Body Image, Aging Anxiety, and the Media. *Psychol Women Quar* 2010; 34:65–74.
6. Constantian MB. Unhappy Patients and Those with Body Dysmorphic Disorder. In: Constantian MB, ed. *Rhinoplasty: Craft and Magic.* St. Louis: Quality Medical Publishing; 2009:1401–1448.
7. Constantian MB. The New Criteria for Body Dysmorphic Disorder: Who Makes the Diagnosis? *Plast Reconstr Surg* 2013; 132:1759–1762.
8. Grant JE, Kim SW, Eckert ED. Body Dysmorphic Disorder in Patients with Anorexia Nervosa: Prevalence, Clinical Features, and Delusionality of Body Image. *Int J Eat Disord* 2002; 32:291–300.
9. Morrison J. *DSM-IV Made Easy: The Clinician's Guide to Diagnosis.* New York: The Guilford Press; 1995.
10. Phillips KA, Wilhelm S, Koran LM, et al. Body Dysmorphic Disorder: Some Key Issues for DSM-V. *Depress Anxiety* 2010; 27:573–591.
11. Phillips KA. Insight and Delusional Beliefs in Body Dysmorphic Disorder. In: Phillips KA, ed. *Body Dysmorphic Disorder: Advances in Research and Clinical Practice.* New York: Oxford University Press; 2017:103–114.
12. Bienvenu OJ, Samuels JF, Riddle MA, et al. The Relationship of Obsessive-Compulsive Disorder to Possible Spectrum Disorders: Results from a Family Study. *Biol Psychiatry* 2000; 48:287–293.

13. Eisen JL, Phillips KA, Coles ME, et al. Insight in Obsessive Compulsive Disorder and Body Dysmorphic Disorder. *Comp Psychiatry* 2004; 45:1:10–15.
14. Halmi KA, Tozzi F, Thornton LM, et al. The Relation among Perfectionism, Obsessive-Compulsive Personality Disorder and Obsessive-Compulsive Disorder in Individuals With Eating Disorders. *Int J Eat Disord* 2005; 38:4:371–374.
15. Phillips KA. Classification of Body Dysmorphic Disorder and Relevance for Patient Care In: Phillips KA, ed. *Body Dysmorphic Disorder: Advances in Research and Clinical Practice*. New York: Oxford University Press; 2017:33–45.
16. Stewart SE, Stack DE, Wilhelm S. Severe Obsessive-Compulsive Disorder with and without Body Dysmorphic Disorder: Clinical Correlates and Implications. *Ann Clin Psychiatry* 2008; 20:1:33–38.
17. Phillips KA, McElroy SL. Brief Reports—Insight, Overvalued Ideation, and Delusional Thinking in Body Dysmorphic Disorder: Theoretical and Treatment Implications. *J Nerv Ment Dis* 1993; 181:11:699–702.
18. Phillips KA, Menard W, Pagano ME, et al. Delusional Versus Nondelusional Body Dysmorphic Disorder: Clinical Features and Course of Illness. *J Psychiatric Res* 2006; 40:95–104.
19. Crerand CE, Sarwer DB, Ryan M. Cosmetic Medical and Surgical Treatments and Body Dysmorphic Disorder. In: Phillips KA, ed. *Body Dysmorphic Disorder: Advances in Research and Clinical Practice*. New York: Oxford University Press; 2017:431–448.
20. Didie ER, Kuniega-Pietrzak T, Phillips KA. Body Image in Patients with Body Dysmorphic Disorder: Evaluations of and Investment in Appearance, Health/Illness, and Fitness. *Body Image* 2010; 7:66–69.
21. Czerwinski SA, Mahaney MC, Williams JR, et al. Genetic Analysis of Personality Traits and Alcoholism Using a Mixed Discrete Continuous Trait Variance Component Model. *Genet Epidemiol* 1999; 17[suppl 1]:S121–S126.
22. Damasio A. *Self Comes to Mind: Constructing the Conscious Brain*. New York: Vintage Books; 2010:315.
23. Daniels JK, Hegadoren KM, Coupland NJ, et al. Neural Correlates and Predictive Power of Trait Resilience in an Acutely Traumatized Sample: A Pilot Investigation. *J Clin Psychiatry* 2012; 73:3:327–332.
24. Das D, Cherbuin N, Tan X, et al. DRD4-exonIII-VNTR Moderates the Effect of Childhood Adversities on Emotional Resilience in Young-Adults. *PLoS One* 2011; 6:5:e20177.
25. Davenport S, Goldberg D, Millar T. How Psychiatric Disorders Are Missed During Medical Consultations. *The Lancet* 1987; August:439–440.
26. Weinberg I. The Prisoners of Despair: Right Hemisphere Deficiency and Suicide. *Neurosci Biobehav Rev* 2000; 24:799–815.
27. American Psychiatric Association. *Desk Reference to the Diagnostic Criteria from DSM-5*. Washington [DC]: American Psychiatric Publishing; 2013.
28. Phillips KA. *The Broken Mirror: Understanding and Treating Body Dysmorphic Disorder*. Revised and expanded edition. New York: Oxford University Press; 2005.
29. Bjornsson AS, Didie ER, Phillips KA. Body Dysmorphic Disorder. *Dialogues Clin Neurosci* 2010; 12:221–232.
30. Grant MM, Cannistraci C, Hollon SD, et al. Childhood Trauma History Differentiates Amygdala Response to Sad Faces Within MDD. *J Psychiatric Res* 2011; 45:7:886–895.
31. Wildgoose P, Scott A, Pusic AL, et al. Psychological Screening Measures for Cosmetic Plastic Surgery Patients: A Systematic Review. *Aesth Surg J* 2013; 33:1:152–159.

32. Carr T, Moss T, Harris D. The DAS24: A Short Form of the Derriford Appearance Scale DAS59 to Measure Individual Responses to Living with Problems of Appearance. *Brit J Health Psychol* 2005; 10:285–298.

33. Moss TP, Rosser BA. The Moderated Relationship of Appearance Valence on Appearance Self Consciousness: Development and Testing of New Measures of Appearance Schema Components. *PLoS One* 2012; 7:11:1–7.

34. Ogden P, Fisher J. *Sensorimotor Psychotherapy: Interventions for Trauma and Attachment.* New York: W W Norton & Company; 2015.

35. Veale D, Ellison N, Werner TG, et al. Development of a Cosmetic Procedure Screening Questionnaire (COPS) for Body Dysmorphic Disorder. *Brit J Plast Surg* 2011; 09:007.

36. Wilhelm S. *Feeling Good about the Way You Look: A Program for Overcoming Body Image Problems.* New York: The Guilford Press; 2006.

37. Cuzzolaro M, Vetrone G, Marano G, et al. The Body Uneasiness Test (BUT): Development and Validation of a New Body Image Assessment Scale. *Eat Weight Disord* 2006; 11:1:1–13.

38. Honigman RJ. A Review of Psychological Outcomes for Patients Seeking Cosmetic Surgery. *Plast Reconstr Surg* 2004; 113:1229–1237.

39. Phillips KA, Gunderson CG, Mallya G, et al. A Comparison Study of Body Dysmorphic Disorder and Obsessive-Compulsive Disorder. *J Clin Psychiatry* 1998; 59:11:568–575.

40. Eisen JL, Phillips KA, Baer L, et al. The Brown Assessment of Beliefs Scale: Reliability and Validity. *Am J Psychiatry* 1998; 155:1:102–108.

41. Picavet VA, Gabriels L, Grietens J, et al. Preoperative Symptoms of Body Dysmorphic Disorder Determine Postoperative Satisfaction and Quality of Life in Aesthetic Rhinoplasty. *Plast Reconstr Surg* 2013; 131:4:861–868.

42. Phillips KA, Pinto A, Jain S. Self-Esteem in Body Dysmorphic Disorder. Body Image 2004; 1:385–390.

43. Bjornsson AS. Comorbidity and Personality in Body Dysmorphic Disorder. In: Phillips KA, ed. *Body Dysmorphic Disorder: Advances in Research and Clinical Practice.* New York: Oxford University Press; 2017:115–124.

44. Phillips KA, McElroy SL, Keck PE, et al. A Comparison of Delusional and Non-delusional Body Dysmorphic Disorder in 100 Cases. *Psychopharmacol Bull* 1994; 30:2:179–186.

45. Sarwer DB, Brown GK, Evans DL. Cosmetic Breast Augmentation and Suicide. *Am J Psychiatry* 2007; 164:7:1006–1013.

46. Sarwer DB, Constantian MB. Psychological Aspects of Cosmetic Surgical and Minimally Invasive Treatments in Plastic Surgery. In: Neligan P, Rubin P, eds. *Plastic Surgery,* 4th edition. New York: Saunders; 2018:24–34.

47. Mellody P. How the Symptoms Sabotage. In: *Facing Codependence.* New York: Harper Collins; 2003:51–60.

48. Mellody P, Freundlich LS. *The Intimacy Factor the Ground Rules for Overcoming the Obstacles to Truth, Respect, and Lasting Love.* San Francisco: Harper Collins; 2003:7–24.

49. Mellody P, Freundlich LS. *The Intimacy Factor the Ground Rules for Overcoming the Obstacles to Truth, Respect, and Lasting Love.* San Francisco: Harper Collins; 2003:11–49.

50. Mellody P, Freundlich LS. *The Intimacy Factor: The Ground Rules for Overcoming the Obstacles to Truth, Respect, and Lasting Love.* New York: Harper Collins; 2003.

51. Mellody P, Miller AW, Miller JK. *Facing Codependence: What It Is, Where It Comes from, How It Sabotages Our Lives.* New York: Harper Collins; 1989.

52. Mellody P, Miller AW, Miller JK. *Facing Love Addiction: Giving Yourself the Power to Change the Way You Love.* New York: Harper Collins; 1992.

53. Phillips KA, Pinto A, Menard W, et al. Obsessive-Compulsive Disorder Versus Body Dysmorphic Disorder: A Comparison Study of Two Possibly Related Disorders. *Depress Anxiety* 2007; 24:6:399–409.

54. Fang A, Matheny NL, Wilhelm S. Body Dysmorphic Disorder. *Psychiatric Clin N Am* 2014; 37:287–300.

55. Phillips KA. Appendix: Measures and Resources. In: Phillips KA, ed. *Body Dysmorphic Disorder: Advances in Research and Clinical Practice.* New York: Oxford University Press; 2017:522–525.

56. Albertini RS, Phillips KA. 33 Cases of Body Dysmorphic Disorder in Children and Adolescents. *J Am Acad Child Adolesc Psychiatry* 1999; 38:453–459.

57. Barone M, Cogliandro A, Persichetti P. Preoperative Symptoms of Body Dysmorphic Disorder Determine Postoperative Satisfaction and Quality of Life in Aesthetic Rhinoplasty. *Plast Reconstr Surg* 2013; 132:6:1078e–1079e.

58. Biby E. The Relationship Between Body Dysmorphic Disorder and Depression, Self-Esteem, Somatization, and Obsessive-Compulsive Disorder. *J Clin Psychology* 1998; 54:4:489–499.

59. Clarke A, Hansen ELE, White E, et al. Low Priority? A Cross Sectional Study of Appearance Anxiety in 500 Consecutive Referrals For Cosmetic Surgery. *Psychol Health Med* 2012; 17:4:440–446.

60. Dyl J, Kittler J, Phillips KA, et al. Body Dysmorphic Disorder and Other Clinically Significant Body Image Concerns in Adolescent Psychiatric Inpatients: Prevalence and Clinical Characteristics. *Child Psychiatry Hum Dev* 2006; 36:369–482.

61. Sarwer DB, Crerand CE. Body Image and Cosmetic Medical Treatments. *Body Image* 2004; 1:99–111.

62. Thomas CS, Goldberg DP. Appearance, Body Image and Distress in Facial Dysmorphophobia. *Acta Psychiatr Scand* 1995; 92:231–236.

63. Jerome L. Body Dysmorphic Disorder: A Controlled Study of Patients Requesting Cosmetic Rhinoplasty. *Am J Psychiatry* 1992; 149:4:577–578.

64. Phillips KA. Body Dysmorphic Disorder: Diagnosis and Treatment of Imagined Ugliness. *J Clin Psychiatry* 1996; 57[suppl 8]:61–65.

65. van der Kolk BA, Pelcovitz D, Roth S, et al. Dissociation, Somatization, and Affect Dysregulation: The Complexity of Adaptation to Trauma. *Am J Psychiatry* 1996; 153:7:83–93.

66. Veale D, Kinderman P, Riley S, et al. Self-Discrepancy in Body Dysmorphic Disorder. *Br J Clin Psychol* 2003; 42:157–169.

67. Veale D, Riley S. Mirror, Mirror on the Wall, Who Is The Ugliest of Them All? The Psychopathology of Mirror Gazing in Body Dysmorphic Disorder. *Behav Res Ther* 2001; 39:1381–1393.

68. Phillips KA, Coles ME, Menard W, et al. Suicidal Ideation and Suicide Attempts in Body Dysmorphic Disorder. *J Clin Psychiatry* 2005; 66:717–725.

69. Josephson SC, Hollander E, Fallon B, et al. Obsessive-Compulsive Disorder, Body Dysmorphic Disorder, and Hypochondriasis: Three Variations on a Theme. *CNS Spectrums* 1996; 1:2:24–31.

70. Keller A, Litzelman K, Wisk LE, et al. Does the Perception that Stress Affects Health Matter? The Association with Health and Mortality. *Health Psychol* 2012; 31:5:677–684.

71. Phillips KA, McElroy SL, Dwight MM, et al. Delusionality and Response to Open-Label Fluvoxamine in Body Dysmorphic Disorder. *J Clin Psychiatry* 2001; 62:2:87–90.

72. Phillips KA, Menard W. Suicidality in Body Dysmorphic Disorder: A Prospective Study. *Am J Psychiatry* 2006; 163:7:1280–1281.

73. Phillips KA, Quinn G, Stout RL. Functional Impairment in Body Dysmorphic Disorder: Prospective, Follow-Up Study. *J Psychiatry Res* 2008; 42:701–707.

74. Hart AS, Niemiec MA. Comorbidity and Personality in Body Dysmorphic Disorder. In: Phillips KA, ed. *Body Dysmorphic Disorder: Advances in Research and Clinical Practice.* New York: Oxford University Press; 2017:125–138.

75. Fenwick AS, Sullivan KA. Potential Link Between Body Dysmorphic Disorder Symptoms and Alexithymia in an Eating-Disordered Treatment-Seeking Sample. *Psychiatry Res* 2011; 189:299–304.

76. Deckersbach T, Savage CR, Phillips KA, et al. Characteristics of Memory Dysfunction in Body Dysmorphic Disorder. *J Int Neuropsychol Soc* 2000; 6:673–681.

77. Buhlmann U, Wilhelm S, McNally RJ, et al. Interpretive Biases for Ambiguous Information in Body Dysmorphic Disorder. *CNS Spectrums* 2002; 7:6:435–443.

78. Kelly MM, Walters C, Phillips KA. Social Anxiety and Its Relationship to Functional Impairment in Body Dysmorphic Disorder. *Behav Ther* 2010; 41:143–153.

79. van der Kolk B. Trauma and Memory. In: van der Kolk B, McFarlane AC, Weisaeth L, eds. *Traumatic Stress.* New York: The Guilford Press; 2007:3289–3296.

80. van der Kolk BA. *The Body Keeps the Score: Brain, Mind, and Body in the Healing of Trauma.* New York: Viking (Penguin Group); 2014.

81 DeMarco LM, Li LC, Phillips KA, et al. Perceived Stress in Body Dysmorphic Disorder. *J Nerv Ment Dis* 1998; 186:11:724–726.

82. McCurdy-McKinnon D, Feusner J. Neurobiology of Body Dysmorphic Disorder: Heritability / Genetics, Brain Circuitry, and Visual Processing. In: Phillips KA, ed. *Body Dysmorphic Disorder: Advances in Research and Clinical Practice.* New York: Oxford University Press; 2017:253–256.

83. Atmaca M, Bingol I, Aydin A, Yildirim H, Okuret I, et. al. Brain Morphology of Patients with Body Dysmorphic Disorder. *J Affect Disord* 2010; 123:1:258–263.

84. Feusner, JD, Hembacher E, Moller, H, Moody, TD. Abnormalities of Object Visual Processing in Body Dysmorphic Disorder. *Psychol Med* 2011; 41:11:2385–2397.

85. Rotge JY, Guehl D, Dilharreguy, B, Tignol, J, Bioulac, B, Allard, M, Aouizerate, B. Meta-Analysis of Brain Volume Changes in Obsessive-Compulsive Disorder. *Biol Psychiatry* 2009; 65:1:75–83.

86. Andrews G, Hobbs MJ, Borkovec TD, et al. Generalized Worry Disorder: A Review of DSM-IV Generalized Anxiety Disorder and Options for DSM-V. *Depress Anxiety* 2010; 27:134–147.

87. Scaer RC. *The Body Bears the Burden: Trauma, Dissociation, and Disease.* 3rd edition. New York: Routledge; 2014.

88. Scaer RC. *The Body Bears the Burden: Trauma, Dissociation, and Disease.* 2nd edition. New York: Routledge; 2007:34, 85,180–181.

89. De Venter M, Smets J, Raes F, et al. Impact of Childhood Trauma on Postpartum Depression: A Prospective Study. *Arch Womens Ment Health* 2016; 19:2:337–342.

90. Phillips KA. Body Dysmorphic Disorder in Children and Adolescents. In: Phillips KA, ed. *Body Dysmorphic Disorder: Advances in Research and Clinical Practice.* New York: Oxford University Press; 2017:173–185.

91. Osman S, Cooper M, Hackmann A, et al. Spontaneously Occurring Images and Early Memories in People with Body Dysmorphic Disorder. *Memory* 2004; 12:4:428–436.

92. Lovegrove E, Rumsey N. Ignoring It Doesn't Make It Stop: Adolescents, Appearance, and Bullying. *Cleft Palate-Craniofac J* 2005; 42:1:33–44.

93. Palacio RJ. *Wonder.* New York: Knopf (Borzoi Books); 2012.

94. McFarlane AC, van der Kolk BA. Trauma and Its Challenge to Society. In: van der Kolk B, McFarlane AC, Weisaeth L, eds. *Traumatic Stress*. New York: The Guilford Press; 2007:27.

95. Saar-Ashkenazy R, Cohen JE, Guez J, et al. Reduced Corpus-Callosum Volume in Posttraumatic Stress Disorder Highlights the Importance of Inter-Hemispheric Connectivity for Associative Memory. *J Traumatic Stress* 2014; 27:1:18–26.

96. van der Kolk B, van der Hart O. The Intrusive Past: The Flexibility of Memory and the Engraving of Trauma. *Am Imago* 1991; 48:425–454.

97. van der Kolk B. The Complexity of Adaptation to Trauma Self-Regulation, Stimulus, Discrimination, and Characterological Development. In: van der Kolk B, McFarlane AC, Weisaeth L, eds. *Traumatic Stress*. New York: The Guilford Press; 2007:182–213.

98. Constantian MB, Lin CP. Why Some Patients Are Unhappy: Part 1: Relationship of Preoperative Nasal Deformity to Number of Operations and a History of Abuse or Neglect. *Plast Reconstr Surg* 2014; 134:4:823–835.

99. Constantian MB, Lin CP. Why Some Patients Are Unhappy: Part 2. Relationship of Nasal Shape and Trauma History to Surgical Success. *Plast Reconstr Surg* 2014; 134:4:836–851.

100. Didie ER, Tortolani CC, Pope CG, et al. Childhood Abuse and Neglect in Body Dysmorphic Disorder. *Child Abuse Negl* 2006; 39:10:1105–1115.

101. Andrews B. Bodily Shame in Relation to Abuse in Childhood and Bulimia: A Preliminary Investigation. *Br J Clin Psychol* 1997; 36:41–49.

102. Franzoni E, Gualandi S, Caretti V, et al. The Relationship Between Alexithymia, Shame, Trauma, and Body Image Disorders: Investigation Over a Large Clinical Sample. *Neuropsychiatr Dis Treat* 2013; 9:185–193.

103. Buhlmann U, Hartmann AS. Cognitive and Emotional Processing in Body Dysmorphic Disorder. In: Phillips KA, ed. *Body Dysmorphic Disorder: Advances in Research and Clinical Practice*. New York: Oxford University Press; 2017:285–298.

104. Buhlmann U, McNally RJ, Wilhelm S, et al. Selective Processing of Emotional Information in Body Dysmorphic Disorder. *Anxiety Disord* 2002; 16:289–298.

105. Simberlund J, Hollander E. The Relationship of Body Dysmorphic Disorder to Obsessive-Compulsive Disorder and the Concept of the Obsessive-Compulsive Spectrum. In: Phillips KA, ed. *Body Dysmorphic Disorder: Advances in Research and Clinical Practice*. New York: Oxford University Press; 2017:481–492.

106. Yaryura-Tobias, José A, et al. Computerized Perceptual Analysis of Patients with Body Dysmorphic Disorder: A Pilot Study. *CNS Spectrums* 2002; 7:6:444–446.

107. de Brito MJA, Nahas FX, Cordas TA. Body Dysmorphic Disorder in Patients Seeking Abdominoplasty, Rhinoplasty, and Rhytidectomy. *Plast Reconstr Surg* 2016; 137:2:462–471.

108. Neziroglu F, Barile N. Environmental Factors in Body Dysmorphic Disorder. In: Phillips KA, ed. *Body Dysmorphic Disorder: Advances in Research and Clinical Practice*. New York: Oxford University Press; 2017:277–284.

109. Zlotnick C, Mattia JI, Zimmerman M. The Relationship Between Posttraumatic Stress Disorder, Childhood Trauma and Alexithymia in an Outpatient Sample. *J Traumatic Stress* 2001; 14:1:177–188.

110. Baldock E, Veale D. The Self as an Aesthetic Object: Body Image, Beliefs about the Self, and Shame in a Cognitive-Behavioral Model of Body Dysmorphic Disorder. In: Phillips KA, ed. *Body Dysmorphic Disorder: Advances in Research and Clinical Practice*. New York: Oxford University Press; 2017:299–312.

111. Simmons RA, Phillips KA. Core Clinical Features of Body Dysmorphic Disorder: Appearance Preoccupations, Negative Emotions, Core Beliefs, and Repetitive and Avoidance Behaviors. In: Phillips KA, ed. *Body Dysmorphic Disorder: Advances in Research and Clinical Practice*. New York: Oxford University Press; 2017:61–80.

112. van der Kolk BA, van der Hart O. Pierre Janet and the Breakdown of Adaptation in Psychological Trauma. *Am J Psychiatry* 1989; 146:12:1530–1540.

113. Grogan S. *Body Image: Understanding Body Dissatisfaction, in Men, Women, and Children*. London: Routledge; 2008.

114. Greenberg BD, Li Q, Lucas FR, et al. Association Between the Serotonin Transporter Promoter Polymorphism and Personality Traits in a Primarily Female Population Sample. *Am J Med Genet Neuropsychiatr Genet* 2000; 96:202–216.

115. Barr CS, Newman TK, Becker ML, et al. Serotonin Transporter Gene Variation Is Associated With Alcohol Sensitivity in Thesus Macaques Exposed to Early-Life Stress. *Alcohol Clin Exp Res* 2003; 27:5:812–817.

116. Barr CS, Newman TK, Lindell S, et al. Interaction Between Serotonin Transporter Gene Variation and Rearing Condition in Alcohol Preference and Consumption in Female Primates. *Arch Gen Psychiatry* 2004; 61:1146–1152.

117. Karg K, Burmeister M, Shedden K, et al. The Serotonin Transporter Promoter Varient (5-HTTLPR), Stress, and Depression Meta-Analysis Revisited: Evidence of Genetic Moderation. *Arch Gen Psychiatry* 2011; 68:5:444–454.

118. Bennett AJ, Lesch KP, Heils A, et al. Early Experience and Serotonin Transporter Gene Variation Interact to Influence Primate CNS Function. *Mol Psychiatry* 2002; 7:118–122.

119. Kobayashi I, Delanhanty DL. Gender Differences in Subjective Sleep After Trauma and Development of Posttraumatic Stress Disorder Symptoms. *J Trauma Stress* 2013; 26:467–474.

120. Xie L, Kang H, Xu Q, et al. Sleep Drives Metabolite Clearance from the Adult Brain. *Science* 2013; 342:6156:1–11.

121. Leon AC, Portera L, Weissman MM. The Social Costs of Anxiety Disorders. *Br J Psychiatry* 1995; 166:27:19–22.

122. Leverich GS, Altshuler LL, Frye MA, et al. Factors Associated with Suicide Attempts in 648 Patients with Bipolar Disorder in the Stanley Foundation Bipolar Network. *J Clin Psychiatry* 2003; 64:5:506–515.

123. Shalev I, Entringer S, Wadhwa PD, et al. Stress and Telomere Biology: A Lifespan Perspective. *Psychoneuroendocrinol* 2013; 38:9:1835–1842.

124. Phillips KA, Simmons RA. Treating a Patient with Body Dysmorphic Disorder Using Medication and Cognitive-Behavioral Therapy: An Illustrative Case Example. In: Phillips KA, ed. *Body Dysmorphic Disorder: Advances in Research and Clinical Practice*. New York: Oxford University Press; 2017:379–396.

125. Rothbaum BO, Davidson JR, Stein DJ, et al. A Pooled Analysis of Gender and Trauma-Type Effects on Responsiveness to Treatment of PTSD with Venlafaxine Extended Release or Placebo. *J Clin Psychiatry* 2008; 69:10:1529–1539.

126. Prazeres AM, Nascimento AL, Fontenelle LF. Cognitive-Behavioral Therapy for Body Dysmorphic Disorder: A Review of Its Efficacy. *Neuropsychiatric Dis Treat* 2013; 9:307.

127. Rasmussen J, Gomez AF, Wilhelm S. Cognitive-Behavioral Therapy for Body Dysmorphic Disorder. In: Phillips KA, ed. *Body Dysmorphic Disorder: Advances in Research and Clinical Practice*. New York: Oxford University Press; 2017:357–378.

128. Clarke A, Thompson AR, Jenkinson E, et al. *CBT for Appearance: Anxiety Psychosocial Interventions for Anxiety Due to Visible Difference.* West Sussex [UK]: John Wiley & Sons, Ltd.; 2014.

129. Goin JM, Goin MK. *Changing the Body: Psychological Effects of Plastic Surgery: Rhinoplasty: The "Minimal Defect."* Baltimore: Williams & Wilkins; 1981:133.

130. Sarwer DB, Wadden TA, Pertschuk MJ, et al. The Psychology of Cosmetic Surgery: A Review and Reconceptualization. *Clin Psychol Rev* 1998; 18:1–22.

131. Crerand CE, Menard W, Phillips KA. Surgical and Minimally Invasive Cosmetic Procedures among Persons with Body Dysmorphic Disorder. *Ann Plast Surg* 2010 Jul; 65:1:11.

132. Moss TP, Harris DL. Psychological Change after Aesthetic Plastic Surgery: A Prospective Controlled Outcome Study. *Psychol Health Med* 2009; 14:5:567–572.

133. Sarwer DB, Crerand CE. Body Dysmorphic Disorder and Appearance Enhancing Medical Treatment. *Body Image* 2008; 5:50–58.

134. Sarwer DB, Magee L, Crerand CE. Cosmetic Surgery and Cosmetic Medical Treatments. In: Thompson JK, ed. *Handbook of Eating Disorders and Obesity.* Hoboken, NJ: Wiley; 2004:718–737.

135. Sarwer DB, Pruzinsky T, Cash TF, et al. *Psychological Aspects of Reconstructive and Cosmetic Plastic Surgery: Clinical, Empirical, and Ethical Perspectives.* Philadelphia: Lippincott Williams & Wilkins; 2006.

136. Schwitzer JA, Albino FP, Mathis RK, et al. Assessing Demographic Differences in Patient-Perceived Improvement in Facial Appearance and Quality of Life Following Rhinoplasty. *Aesth Surg J* 2015; 35:7:784–793.

137. von Soest T, Kvalem IL, Skolleborg KC, et al. Psychosocial Changes after Cosmetic Surgery: A 5-Year Follow-Up Study. *Plast Reconstr Surg* 2011; 128:3:765–775.

138. von Soest T, Kvalem IL, Wichstrom L. Predictors of Cosmetic Surgery and Its Effects on Psychological Factors and Mental Health: A Population-Based Follow-Up Study among Norwegian Females. *Psychol Med* 2012; 42:617–626.

139. Felix GAA, de Brito MJ, Nahas FX, et al. Patients with Mild to Moderate Body Dysmorphic Disorder May Benefit from Rhinoplasty. *J Plas Reconstr Aesth Surg* 2014; May 1:67:5:646–654.

140. Edgerton MT, Langman MW, Pruzinsky T. Plastic Surgery and Psychotherapy in the Treatment of 100 Psychologically Disturbed Patients. *Plast Reconstr Surg* 1991; 88:4:594–608.

141. Knorr NJ, Edgerton MT, Hoopes JE. The "Insatiable" Cosmetic Surgery Patient. *Plast Reconstr Surg* 1967; 40:3:285–289.

142. Kim EY, Park J, Kim B. Type of Childhood Maltreatment and the Risk of Criminal Recidivism in Adult Probationers: A Cross-Sectional Study. *BMC Psychiatry* 2016; 16:294.

143. Lanius RA, Vermette E, Pain C, eds. *The Impact of Early Life Trauma on Health and Disease: The Hidden Epidemic.* Cambridge [UK]: Cambridge University Press; 2010.

144. Scaer RC. Concepts of Trauma: The Role of Boundaries. In: *The Body Bears the Burden: Trauma, Dissociation, and Disease.* 2nd edition. New York: Routledge; 2007:1–7.

145. van Zelst C, van Nierop M, van Dam DS, et al. Associations between Stereotype Awareness, Childhood Trauma and Psychopathology: A Study in People with Psychosis, Their Siblings and Controls. *PLoS One* 2015; 10:2:e0117386.

146. Brady KT. Posttraumatic Stress Disorder and Comorbidity: Recognizing the Many Faces of PTSD. *J Clin Psychiatry* 1997; 58:12–15.

147. Dyck IR, Phillips KA, Warshaw MG, et al. Patterns of Personality Pathology in Patients with Generalized Anxiety Disorder, Panic Disorder with and without Agoraphobia, and Social Phobia. *J Pers Disord* 2001; 15:1:60–71.

148. Powers A, Fani N, Pallos A, et al. Childhood Abuse and the Experience of Pain in Adulthood: The Mediating Effects of PTSD and Emotion Dysregulation on Pain Levels and Pain-related functional impairment. Psychosomatics 2014; 55:5:491–499.

149. Rothbaum BO, Kearns MC, Reiser E, et al. Early Intervention Following Trauma May Mitigate Genetic Risk for PTSD in Civilians: A Pilot Prospective Emergency Department Study. *J Clin Psychiatry* 2014; 75:12:1380–1387.

150. Steenkamp MM, Litz BT, Hoge CW, et al. Psychotherapy for Military-Related PTSD: A Review of Randomized Clinical Trials. *JAMA* 2015; 314:5:489–500.

151. Watkins LE, Han S, Harpaz-Rotem I, et al. FKBP5 Polymorphisms, Childhood Abuse, and PTSD Symptoms: Results from the National Health and Resilience in Veterans Study. *Psychoneuroendocrinol* 2016; 69:98–105.

152. Bernstein DP, Ahluvalia T, Pogge D, et al. Validity of the Childhood Trauma Questionnaire in an Adolescent Psychiatric Population. *J Am Acad Child Adolesc Psychiatry* 1997; 36:3:340–348.

153. Bernstein DP, Fink L, Handelsman L, et al. Initial Reliability and Validity of a New Retrospective Measure of Child Abuse and Neglect. *Am J Psychiatry* 1994; 151:8:1132–1136.

154. Bernstein DP, Stein JA, Newcomb MD, et al. Development and Validation of a Brief Screening Version of the Childhood Trauma Questionnaire. *Child Abuse Neglect* 2003; 169–190.

155. Carballedo A, Lisiecka D, Fagan A, et al. Early Life Adversity Is Associated with Brain Changes in Subjects at Family Risk for Depression. *World J Biol Psychiatry* 2012; 13:569–578.

156. Chugani HT, Behen ME, Muzik O, et al. Brain Functional Activity Following Early Deprivation: A Study of Post-Institutionalized Romanian Orphans. *Neuroimage* 2001; 14:6:1290–1301.

157. Eluvanthingal TJ, Chugani HT, Behen ME, et al. Abnormal Brain Connectivity in Children after Early Severe Socio-Emotional Deprivation: A Diffusion Tensor Imaging Study. *Pediatrics* 2006; 117:6:2093–2100.

158. Lanius R, Lanius U, Fisher J, et al. Psychological Trauma and the Brain: Toward a Neurobiological Treatment Model. In: Ogden P, Minton K, Pain C eds. *Trauma and the Body*. New York: W W Norton & Company; 2006:141–163.

159. Lupien SJ, McEwen BS, Gunnar MR, et al. Effects of Stress Throughout the Lifespan on the Brain, Behaviour and Cognition. *Neuroscience* 2009; 10:434–445.

160. McEwen BS, Morrison JH. The Brain on Stress: Vulnerability and Plasticity of the Prefrontal Cortex Over the Life Course. *Neuron* 2013; 79:16–29.

161. Rauch SL, Phillips KA, Segal E, et al. A Preliminary Morphometric Magnetic Resonance Imaging Study of Regional Brain Volumes in Body Dysmorphic Disorder. *Psychiatry Res: Neuroimaging* 2003; 122:13–19.

162. Reich CG, Taylor ME, McCarthy MM. Differential Effects of Chronic Unpredictable Stress on Hippocampal CB1 Receptors in Male and Female Rats. *Behav Brain Res* 2009; 203:2:264–269.

163. Phillips KA, Zai, G, King NA, et al. A Preliminary Candidate Gene Study in Body Dysmorphic Disorder. *J Obsessive-Compuls Relat Disord* 2015; 6:72–76.

164. Blum VL. *Flesh Wounds: The Culture of Cosmetic Surgery*. Los Angeles: University of California Press; 2003.

165. McLaren L, Kuh D, Hardy R, et al. Positive and Negative Body—Related Comments and Their Relationship with Body Dissatisfaction in Middle—Aged Women. *Psychol Health* 2004; 19:2:261–272.

166. Veale D, Ennis M, Lambrou C. Possible Association of Body Dysmorphic Disorder with an Occupation or Education in Art and Design. *Am J Psychiatry* 2002; 159:10:1788–1790.

167. Sherry SB, Hewitt P, Lee-Baggley D, et al. Perfectionism and Interest in Cosmetic Surgery. *Plast Reconstr Surg* 2005; 115:6:1806–1807.

The Roots

Developmental Trauma and Its Effects

3

THE VALLEY OF THE SHADOW

Core Issues and Parenting

Franz Kafka traces the entire pathway of emotional abuse to toxic shame in *Letter to My Father*—and advances it to bodily obsession and illness.

> I was a fearful child. . . . You would normally admonish me in this way, Can't you do it properly?. . . . And all such questions were accompanied by an evil laugh and an evil face . . . referring to me [in the] third person. . . . I lost my self-respect. . . . I was sick because I was a disinherited son. . . . You would make your reprimands more cutting by referring to me in the third person, as if it wasn't worth talking to me. . . . I feel guilty because of you, my guilt stems uniquely from you.1

Notice that his father referred to him in the third person, a trait that we see in borderline personality disorder. Kafka speaks repeatedly of his father's own shame, and then:

> "I was worried about my hair falling out. . . . I was sick because I was a disinherited son, who needed constant reassurance about his own peculiar existence . . . And who was even insecure about the thing which was next to him: his own body. . . . My back was bent; I could hardly exercise; the road was open to hypochondria."

★★★★★

> It was his eyes that I noticed first: defocused, emotionless, heavy-lidded, impenetrable—what the posttraumatic stress disorder literature calls, "The Thousand Yard Stare."

DOI: 10.4324/9781315657721-5

"So tell me, what don't you like about your nose," I said.

Shrug. "It doesn't look right."

"You already had surgery."

Shrug. He had the slow movements of a third shift custodian. In his hand was the photo of a younger man, just as expressionless.

"What was wrong with your nose?"

His voice was empty and uninterested, its tone uninflected. He looked like he didn't get much exercise. I wondered if I could help.

"I don't know." He hesitated. "It was big." His voice contracted. "I didn't want to look like my father."

The original nose was broad, with a large bump on the bridge and a tip that hung over his upper lip.

"Okay. If you want another operation, what don't you like now?"

He winced at the photograph, which he held like a live grenade.

Shrug. "This thing is too low." He pointed to his columella (the skin between his nostrils).

To my eye, his columella was one of the few areas that didn't need improvement. There were more obvious deformities: his bridge was concave; his nose was short with sunken sidewalls; his tip was shapeless; and there was an odd, irregular lump just below his forehead. I felt it. It was movable.

Shrug. "The last doctor put that in."

"Do you want me to take it out?"

Shrug. Each time the movement got more dramatic. "I don't care. Just push this up." He lifted his columella with a thumb.

Generally men are less analytical about their faces than women, perhaps because they don't change their hair color as often, don't learn about makeup as teenagers, and don't worry about coordinating eyeshadow and lipstick. Maybe that was his problem.

"Let me take photographs. You can show me what you don't like." Perhaps then he would see what I did.

I knew that he wasn't an ordinary patient. Like his father and brothers, he had been a barber. But after his rhinoplasty, he said that his reflection in the barbershop mirror upset him so much that he had stopped working. Ordinarily patients so disabled by one surgery are not good candidates for more surgery, but I understood why he was self-conscious. I would have been.

With permission, I spoke to his psychiatrist. Aside from being depressed, his father had often beaten him.

"Your therapist said that your father was very rough. I am sympathetic. A lot of us didn't have easy childhoods.

"Look at the pictures." I turned them around to face him. "What don't you like?"

He rubbed his eyes with his palms and shrugged just enough to show that he was still listening. Maybe he couldn't collect enough energy to speak.

"This thing is too low."

Patients who can't define surgical goals and are vague and indecisive are famously poor surgical risks and often unhappy postoperatively. Don't operate on patients who don't know what they want. Don't operate on patients who don't smile. None of my choices were comforting.

There are a number of reasonable explanations for why this man might not be able to describe his surgical goals. Perhaps he wasn't insightful or intelligent enough. Perhaps he was too depressed. Perhaps I wasn't interviewing him well.

I have seen other patients like him. Insufficient intelligence and apparent depression are rarely satisfactory explanations for total disempowerment.

What Makes People the Way They Are

"Are people born wicked, or do they have wickedness thrust upon them?" a character asks in the musical *Wicked*. How do we answer this question?

Most of us want to feel important. Not necessarily famous, but to have lived a life that mattered. How we measure that importance varies.

What, then, creates self-worth? Why do some people have it, and others don't? Why do some seem to have too much, and others, none at all? If you don't have self-worth, where do you get it? How, indeed, do we become functional adults?

One of the best models I know to explain these concepts was developed by Pia Mellody, the creative mind behind the trauma treatment program at The Meadows in Wickenburg, Arizona.[2,3,4,5,6] I have also been influenced by John Bradshaw, Judith Herman, Claudia Black, Paul Gilbert, Bernice Andrews, Bessel van der Kolk, Peter Levine, Robert Scaer, and many other fine researchers' interpretations of shame and its fallout.[7–31]

Mellody, a nurse who arrived at The Meadows when it was still a drug and alcohol rehabilitation center, realized that behind many of these addictions lay the footprints of childhood traumas that needed attention and that had become the geneses of coping mechanisms that patients used to medicate their pain. Over twenty-five years she developed an elegant and dense model that explains the effects of childhood trauma in the individual and family. What I find provocative is that the majority of her model organized quickly, within the space of about four years (Mellody, personal communication, 2016), a phenomenon that I have observed in other extremely creative minds: concepts appear rapidly, almost simultaneously, with great energy. What attracts me to this model is not only its clarity and the number of conditions that it explains, but its beautiful simplicity, in my opinion one test of real truth.[32]

★★★★★

I conceptualize the Mellody model into five components:

1. The childhood role that you played in your family of origin
2. Where it came from
3. The developmental age at which you still play it
4. The way in which you relate to others
5. How each of these factors (role, origin, current developmental age, and relational model) influence and impair the five core components that make up a functional adult

The first, second, and third components determine the fourth and fifth. Conversely, individuals who become functional adults through nurturing childhoods or through trauma work and live in moderation, don't play roles, don't act like compensated children, and relate to others in healthy ways that allow appropriate intimacy and self-care. However, these five components do not have linear relationships: they chase each other, strengthening or handicapping us in our lives (See Figure 3.1)

Origins and Core Issues in Relational Trauma

All relational trauma arises from either disempowering abuse or falsely empowering abuse. But first let's examine the characteristics of any functional adult (See Table 3.1).

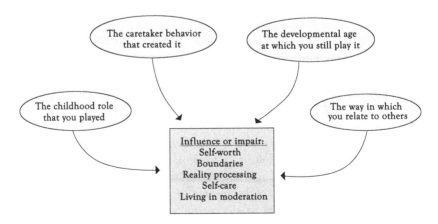

FIGURE 3.1 The Five Core Issues and How They Interrelate

TABLE 3.1 Overview of Developmental Immaturity Issues

Nature of the Child	Core Issues	Secondary Symptoms	Relational Problems	Body Metaphor
Childhood Trauma → Causes	Codependence/ Immaturity → Both Drive	Unmanageability → All Three Create	Problems with Being Intimate	
1. Valuable	1. Self-esteem Issues (Less Than vs. Better Than)	1. Negative Control Issues	1. Relational Esteem Issues	Heart
2. Vulnerable (Protection)	2. Boundary Issues (Too Vulnerable vs. Invulnerable)	2. Resentment Issues/Raging	2. Enmeshment & Avoidance Issues	Skin
3. Imperfect (Reality)	3. Reality Issues (Bad or rebellious vs. Good or Perfect)	3. Spirituality Issues	3. Dishonesty	Brain
4. Dependent (Needs/Wants)	4. Dependency Issues (Too Dependent vs. Anti-dependent or Needless/Wantless)	4. Addiction Issues Mood Disorders Physical Illness	4. Problems with Interdependence	Organs
5. Spontaneous and Open	5. Moderation/Containment Issues (Out of Control vs. Controlling of Others)	5. Intimacy Issues	5. Intensity Issues	Sphincters

Adapted from Mellody, P., 2016, used with permission

The Five Core Issues

1. Self-Esteem (Self-Love, Self-Worth)

Self-esteem is your relationship with yourself. It is the recognition that each of us has individual inherent worth equal to everyone else, not greater or lesser. Unfortunately, life and experience work to destroy the simplicity of that axiom. Parents, families of origin, and culture may teach us to measure our self-worth by comparison to something external: people, success, money, intelligence, or perfection. This is "other esteem," which inevitably fails. Someone else always has more. The pivotal concept is that self-esteem does not have to be earned. Weaknesses do not make us worthless, and strengths do not make us superior. Self-esteem is existential and unfluctuating: "I am enough and I matter, despite my imperfections."

It is easy to imagine how patients who have been devalued or neglected as children and subjected to constant emotional abuse, berating, and criticism might spend their lives trying to achieve perfection through aesthetic surgery. In our current study of adverse childhood events (Chapter 9), the most common trauma type was emotional abuse: "You are worthless." "You are stupid." "You are lazy." "You're ugly." "You will never amount to anything." These statements become the swamp within which the child struggles to survive and grow.

This drive to flawlessness is unconscious—many patients even specify that they are not looking for perfection—but manifest in constant requests for revisions and persistent unhappiness. Problematic for the surgeon is that some of these patients are correct: the surgery should be revised; whether more surgery is justified depends on the deformity, patient motivation, the surgeon's skill and judgment, and the likelihood that the patient will be pleased.

2. Boundaries

Personal boundaries are invisible sleeves that protect and contain us—the skin to the psyche.[33] *External physical boundaries* provide bodily protection and determine physical spaces and physical contacts. *External sexual boundaries* determine when, where, and with whom we will be sexual.

External physical boundaries are breached by any parent who forces surgery on a child or a surgeon who performs procedures not specifically requested by the patient.

Internal listening or talking boundaries protect us from incoming information and contain us when we speak.

Internal listening boundaries fail when someone cannot accurately assess incoming data and therefore becomes excessively sensitive to criticism, teasing, or bullying. Internal speaking boundaries fail when someone cannot contain his or her speech by raging, lying, ridiculing, interrupting, blaming, gossiping, or being sarcastic.

Intact boundaries allow us to detain information long enough to evaluate its truth, then either accept or reject it or get more information. Intact boundaries protect others from our own raging or inappropriate statements. When internal boundaries fail, criticism penetrates like a hot knife. Patients with body dysmorphic disorder are known to be particularly "sensitive" to bullying and teasing (reported by 60% of BDD patients),[34–36] but teasing only hurts when it penetrates porous internal boundaries.

"At twelve, kids at school would remark on the appearance of my nose," one patient wrote. "We moved when I was twelve. I had to reestablish friends and deal with daily harassment. . . . Bullying stays with kids for a lifetime." When we feel "thin-skinned" and over-reactive, we are unprotected; when we are walled-off, we are unconnected. Barricades are not boundaries.

★★★★★

Intact boundaries are critical to personal and professional interactions; boundary failures or violations color our realities. Bullying and teasing are often portrayed as unilateral victimizations when in fact they are bilateral boundary collapses: failure to contain on the bully's part and failure to protect on the victim's. A recent paper has examined the desire for cosmetic surgery in bullies and victims (by self-reporting, with its inherent limitations), and concluded that both groups were more interested in cosmetic surgery than uninvolved adolescents, but for different reasons.[37] Bullies have "good psychological functioning and suffer a few negative long-term consequences" but would like cosmetic surgery to further polish their already high peer group status. Victims, who desire cosmetic surgery even more fervently, have poor self-esteem and seek cosmetic surgery as a way of improving their self-images.

I do not entirely agree. Neither bullies nor their victims have effective boundaries, self-esteem, or reality processing. Both live at the extremes: false empowerment and grandiosity (bullies) or shamed disempowerment (victims)—lashing out or caving in. Both desire aesthetic surgery for the same reason: the imagined result of self-worth. Trauma generates both grandiosity and disempowerment.[38] It is hardly surprising that bullying victims have poor results following aesthetic surgery.[39, 40]

3. Reality

Our realities determine how we bump up against each other—how we assess incoming data—and are rooted in our experiences. Reality has four components: sensory input, which generates thoughts, then creates emotions, and ultimately prompts behavior. Each component must function and contribute accurately or our worlds distort.

When relational trauma is sufficiently serious, children defend themselves by separating from their sensations and detaching from their bodies—as the previous patient illustrates.[10, 21, 41] This response is important to recognize. Separating from one's sensations interferes with the abilities to value and care for oneself, live moderately, maintain intact boundaries, or describe goals to a surgeon. Affected individuals also have impaired capacities to sense their own emotions and to know how they feel. We see these traits in patients who live in the extremes, either overlooking their physical signs and symptoms or exaggerating them in catastrophic language. Schore believes that shame, subjectively experienced as a downward spiral, represents a sudden shift from sympathetic energy—expending hyperarousal to parasympathetic (dorsal vagal) energy—conserving hypoarousal.[40] When traumatic attachment occurs, the developing child interacts with a massively misattuned caregiver who triggers but does not repair—like ringing the doorbell and running away. Relational trauma thus creates prolonged periods of negative affect combined with intense hyperarousal and hypoarousal. When attachment is dysregulated, the child's autoregulation becomes disordered very early, and if untreated can continue throughout life. The infant stores this internal working model in the nonverbal, implicit procedural memory of the right brain, dominantly influenced by the mother during the first year of life, and by the father in the second year. Throughout life, the same right hemispheric attachment model, working unconsciously, appraises, interprets, and regulates interpersonal information and guides future action.[42] The right hemisphere is also responsible for generating self-awareness, self-recognition, and body image.[43, 44] This normal processing is disrupted in PTSD and body dysmorphic disorder, and profoundly affects physician/patient relationships. In PTSD, flashbacks activate the right brain and deactivate the left.[10] Those of us without specific mental health training must remember that patients may reinterpret or process our facial expressions, words, actions, and affect in ways that we do not intend;[45] and that supportive behavior can be critical to managing stressful clinical situations, especially when the patient is deregulating. Patients read the concern on my face before I recognize it myself. Patients may re-interpret—metabolize—what I say into a meaning far from what I meant based on preconditioning or past experience. Ambiguous statements are easily transformed into criticisms, condemnations, or insults. These traits are easily observable in BDD patients.

★★★★★

Early, preverbal conditioning rapidly processes facial expressions, prosody, and eye contact. Fragile patients with impaired abilities to regulate their affects manifest the direct consequences of early relational trauma. At stressful moments, these patients under-regulate or over-regulate their behaviors, dissociating or venting. Patients from abusive or neglectful backgrounds are hypersensitive to trauma and may dissociate or anticipate trauma before it arrives. Patients who clench their fists and jaws before painless dressing changes from physicians whom they already know are examples of such preconditioning. Their behavior only seems irrational to us because we do not recognize their triggers. It is important at these moments to keep patients socially engaged and not let their sympathetic nervous systems control them.

How Disordered Reality Processing Works

Accordingly, what we think or "make up" about incoming sensory information is influenced by our personal histories. A lot of midbrain mischief can happen at this point. If we were raised by caregivers with distorted thinking, their ideas can seep into our own. My mother was untrusting, usually unjustifiably, of her family or acquaintances. She believed that no one was authentic. "If people act nice," she said, "they are just pretending. They don't really like you. They don't know how evil you are." Patients with similar backgrounds may be unjustifiably untrusting of their physicians.

Children who have their realities denied (e.g., not being believed if they were abused) marinate in an environment of shame, overwhelming feelings, and "craziness." Like a post-hypnotic suggestion, the child begins to doubt his or her own sensations and thoughts. Emotionally shaming parents cannot tolerate the child's feelings because they trigger the parents' own feelings. Repressed emotions are always overwhelming. Shame—"the master emotion"[18] —becomes constant, instead of fleeting; hiding it becomes central to life.[10, 46] "Toxic shame is unbearable and always necessitates a cover-up, a false self. . . . Once one becomes a false self, one ceases to exist psychologically . . . what Alice Miller calls 'soul murder'"[47] (quoted by Bradshaw).[18] A child unrelentingly exposed to toxic shaming becomes unable to trust his or her own judgments. Those who cannot judge their own faculties become powerless. Actions that were shamed become hidden. "The people who matter in our lives stay with us, haunting our most ordinary moments. They are with us in the grocery store, as we turn a corner, chat with a friend. They rise up through the pavement; we absorb them through our soles."[48]

The Eight Basic Emotions and Carried Shame

Eight basic emotions (anger, fear, pain, joy, passion, love, shame, and guilt) are generated by the thoughts that we generate from sensory input (Table 3.2). Two of them, shame and guilt, have specific meanings critical to understanding trauma.[49]

Guilt is the sensation provoked by actions that violate one's standards of behavior. Theft or lying produces a gnawing sensation in the gut and emotions of regret, contrition, and remorse are always felt below the diaphragm.

Shame, on the other hand can either be healthy or toxic. *Healthy shame*, or "embarrassment" is the sensation of being exposed. Your face and neck flush. Your head drops. You wish you were invisible. Healthy shame reminds us that we are not gods; it is "permission to be human."[18] When a grateful patient says to her surgeon, "You saved my life," the surgeon feels healthy shame but ideally remains

TABLE 3.2 The Eight Emotions, Your Own and Carried: What They Are and Where They
Are Felt

Basic Emotions		Own	Carried
Anger	Resentment	All Over Body	Gut
	Irritation	Power	Pressure
	Frustration	Energy	Rage
Fear	Apprehension	Tingling in	
	Overwhelmed	Upper Stomach	Extremities
	Threatened	Tightness in	Numbing and/or
		Upper Chest	Tingling
			Panic
Pain	Sad	Lower Chest	Gut
	Lonely	and Heart	Pressure
	Hurt	Hurting	Hopeless
	Pity		
Joy	Hopeful	All Over Body	Uncontrolled
	Elated	Lightness	Laughing
	Happy		
	Excitement		
Passion	Enthusiasm	Excitment	Fanaticism
	or	or	
	Desire	Sexual	Sexual
			Passion
		Arousal	Icky, Slimy, Dirty Feeling
			Nausea
Love	Affection	Warmth &	Warmth &
	Tenderness	Swelling in	Swelling in
	Compassion	Chest Area	Chest Area
	Warmth		
Shame	Embarrassment	Face, Neck,	Gut
	Humble	and/or Upper	Worthless
	Exposed	Chest	
		Hot/Red	
Guilt	Regretful	Gut	Bottom of Feet
	Contrite	Gnawing sensation	Sensation of Being
	Remorseful		Stuck to the Ground

Adapted from Mellody, P., 2016, used with permission

aware of his or her humanity, remembering that he or she was the agent of cure,
not the cause. Healthy shame is felt above the diaphragm.

★★★★★

This anatomical separation of sensations between guilt and healthy shame
correlates nicely with Porges' Polyvagal Theory.[50] Guilt is non-relational and

solitary and in theory should be mediated by the dorsal motor nucleus of the vagus nerve, largely infra-diaphragmatic—our familiar "gut feelings." Conversely, healthy shame is always relational and always connected to those who have seen our frailties. You can't experience healthy shame alone. Because healthy shame is supradiaphragmatic and felt in the face and neck, Porges' model would mediate it by vagus nerve branches from the nucleus ambiguous, which have connections to cranial nerves V, VII, IX, XI, XII and therefore impact the ways in which we engage with each other relationally and socially (Chapter 7).

Carried, or Toxic Shame is never healthy and belongs to the caregiver who sprayed it out. We soak it up. When an abusive or neglectful caregiver has acted shamelessly toward a child without acknowledging his or her behavior, often hiding the abuse behind a wall of anger, *the child picks up the shame as if it were his own or her own* and experiences the sensation of intense worthlessness. The child does not recognize that the shame belongs to the parent, and so this shaming energy does not match the child's thinking. Carried shame can be buried by the child, but recurs when triggered as a "shame attack," characteristically manifested by a patient who suddenly develops a slumped posture, covers his or her mouth, and becomes overwhelmed with feelings of worthlessness. Carried shame can be treated by experiential "chair work," in which trauma survivors can integrate their childhood experiences and return this shame to its perpetrators.

Carried shame is manifested in our vignettes: without adequate provocation, affected patients suddenly become disempowered, collapse, and cannot speak; or conversely assume postures of false empowerment, grandiosity, victimization, or offensive behavior. It is not hard to understand how the emotions felt by the patient, unconsciously triggered by childhood events, or the corresponding emotions felt by the physician, unexpectedly on defense when neither victimization nor rage was appropriate, would confuse both parties and impair their relationship.

Carried shame frequently attaches to one of the five core issues and connects to the part of the self that was injured, creating a "shame bind." "My mother always told me that she wanted an abortion but it was the 1950's, so she was stuck with me," one patient said. This woman has an "existence shame bind," as it appears Kafka did.[1] My mother used to say that her life had been ruined by having children. The effect on a child is strong.

★★★★★

Shame binds can attach to boundaries: if a child has tried to set physical, sexual, talking, or listening boundaries but was not permitted to do so, relevant boundary shame binds occur. When the parents' own sexuality has been shamed, they may shame their children's' sexuality. The greater the abuse and neglect, the greater the shame, the greater the belief in a flawed self, and the more boundaries disappear, leaving the child unprotected. Shame binds can attach to the entire body or to a body part (relevant in body dysmorphic disorder); to an emotion (anger, fear, joy); to intelligence; to behavior (what I do or do not do); to character (what kind of person I am); to any need or want; to appearance, to the need for physical comfort;

or even to spontaneity. Rhinoplasty patients whose original surgeries were forced on them by boundaryless, abusive parents or occurred under the pressures of family ridicule or teasing develop nose shame binds.

Therapist Dan Griffin[51] has written about his own delayed puberty, which required human growth hormone injection treatments. Constantly exposed to a milieu of abuse and neglect by his violent, alcoholic father, Griffin developed a whole body shame bind (personal communication, 2016). "I would stare at my naked body over and over again in the mirror," he wrote, "cursing myself and God. I wouldn't shower for days. I started having night terrors. . . . I became genuinely afraid for my sanity."[51]

How the Parent Manifests in the Child: Shame Binds

As the child begins to mature, each developmental stage reactivates that same stage in the parent. The shame bind or the obsession with an action, need, behavior, personal characteristic, or body part always arises within a milieu of abuse or neglect. Once established, the shame bind develops its own penetrating energy. Complications from parent-forced surgery corrode a patient's boundaries like the original abuse. I have never met a BDD patient who had a nurturing family or who has become a fully functional adult; there is always something missing. By definition, obsession, walls, porous boundaries, shame turned on the self, absent self-worth, suicidal thinking, immoderation, lack of self-care, and distorted reality—the hallmarks of body dysmorphic disorder—are also the manifestations of trauma.

When a shame bind exists, the source can be identified by a therapist who asks the patient what happened just before the shame attack. If, for example, the patient had wanted a boundary to be respected and then suddenly felt shame when it wasn't, the patient has a boundary shame bind. The sensation of worthlessness generated by a shame bind can also generate a protective wall of anger, so the bind may appear and disappear rapidly. It is easy to feel victimized. The sensations of pain and hopelessness can generate anger. The rationale goes like this: I have been victimized, so I am entitled to rage, which gives me the sense of power and thus calms me. The heat of righteous anger is powerful, oddly pleasing, and difficult to control, but always inappropriate and damaging. I have felt it myself. Mellody calls this behavior "offending from the victim position."

Healthy shame is a critical emotion that allows us to balance our humanity and lead abundant, spiritual lives. Toxic shame is a crushingly destructive driver of human behavior that is almost impossible to overestimate and underlies the pain of our most difficult patients and our most unhappy family and friends. It is pointless to argue with someone having a shame attack: pretty soon no one can tell who is really more irrational.

Healthy shame is what I believe Brené Brown means by "humility" and "vulnerability, the recognition that we are imperfect but still 'enough.'"[51] She is also correct that shame interrupts our abilities to connect with others because it requires being seen and being vulnerable, which is dangerous or impossible for shame-based individuals. The sense of abundance that comes from balancing the five core attributes is what I think Brown means by being "wholehearted."

4. Self-Care

Basic to our survival are *needs* for food, clothing, shelter, emotional support, spirituality, education, sufficient money, and medical and dental attention. Our data (Chapter 9) indicate that at least 40% of my own patients were neglected in this way. "*Wants*," on the other hand, are optional, but provide pleasure and the sense of abundance.

Appropriate self-care must be taught. Trauma survivors distort this core issue in the ways that physicians see in their patients. They may ignore their needs and fulfill only their wants like children. They may expect others to care for them—or ignore all needs and become needless, wantless, and anti-dependent. Each strategy is a dead end. We all must learn when to ask for help, when to decline helping others (to avoid being resentfully overextended), and when to enable someone else to learn his or her own independence.

Even the pioneer of neurosurgery built protective walls—characteristic of too many physicians. "Everyone who worked with Cushing knew how he would respond to his son's death. 'Dr. Cushing will hide it all behind a mask,' Elliott Cutler told Madeline Stanton. 'No one will ever see it. Therefore all the worse.'"[52].

Children shamed for their wants never learn what brings them joy, just like children shamed for their dependence never learn to ask for help. Both traits impair lives and make it difficult for patients to be happy, even with successful surgical results.

5. Living in Moderation

The fifth core issue is the product of the interaction between appropriate boundaries (Core Issue 2) and reality (Core Issue 3). Developmental trauma survivors contain their spontaneity behind walls because they don't trust their boundaries. The results are joyless people—rigid, manipulative, controlling, and insufferable—what Mellody calls, "out of control being in control." These traits are characteristic of the "adapted adult wounded child" (See The Age-Dependent Response to Developmental Trauma, below). Alternatively, individuals can become boundaryless and out of control, or "in control being out of control," characteristic of the "wounded child ego state." By comparison, functional adults use personal boundaries to contain their spontaneity and are relational without being abusive.

Equilibrium in the Core

The balance of any functional adult balance is created by an appropriate sense of individual value, power through self-control, and appreciation of life's fullness through appropriate self-care. Imbalances can occur in either direction: when self-value (self-esteem), power (boundaries, reality, and self-care), and abundance (moderation) distort upward, the individual becomes offensively grandiose; when they distort downward, the individual becomes a worthless, hapless, resentful victim who feels entitled to offend others. We all know such people; the vignettes illustrate them. The core issues are so thoroughly interconnected that when one rises or falls, the others move with it.

> *People like Brian and me do not lose contact with our parents because we don't care; we lose contact with them to survive," J.D. Vance writes in* Hillbilly Elegy.[53] *Vance, who escaped familial poverty, alcoholism, violence, and abuse to become a successful attorney recognized the direct connection between childhood trauma and many common adult diseases (Chapter 9). He also understood how childhood had affected his adult behavior: "I began to understand why I used words as weapons . . . I did it to survive. . . . I realized that of all the emotions I felt toward my mother—love, pity, forgiveness, anger, hatred, and dozens of others—I had never tried sympathy.*

The Disequilibrium Caused by Traumatic Parenting

Abusive parenting creates unbalanced children and adults. Such unbalanced behavior is recognizable in personal characteristics. Left untreated, this disequilibriated behavior propagates into adulthood. When life events trigger unconscious memories of original trauma wounds buried deep in their unconscious brains and not accessible to their "thinking" cortices, trauma survivors re-experience the shame of their original wounding *as if it were happening all over again,* and respond dysfunctionally with the immature skills that they had at the time of the wounding.[54] "I don't even know how I got so mad. . . . But then all of a sudden it all kind of just exploded out of me."[55] They behave at the extremes. Disempowered patients operate in a world colored by shame: they can't describe what they want from the doctor, forget appointments and preoperative testing, and arrive late for surgery.

Shame feels bad. On the other hand, grandiosity feels good, at least momentarily, but both are fueled by personal contempt. Whether shame manifests as grandiosity or disempowerment depends upon which way the beam shines: if the contempt shines outwardly, it looks like grandiosity. If the contempt shines inwardly, it looks like disempowerment.[56] Grandiose patients feel both justified and victimized. Even the privileged can feel like victims. It is not an act.

Grandiosity blunts judgment and impairs empathy. Grandiose patients expect surgery on holidays because they are so busy, refuse lab work, dominate conversations, try to impose the surgical plan, expect perfect results, and demand fee discounts. The message is: "I'm going to say what I want because I'm right." Some patients live in each extreme at different times, and under stress others regress to less compensated states where they can be dangerous to themselves or others.

Only functional adults, regulated by their pre-frontal cortices, can be relational, practical, cooperative, realistic, balanced, appreciative, and intimate.

Self-worth affects our ability to be relational. These interactions can be diagrammed on a grid in which relationality is the x-axis and self-esteem is the y-axis (Figure 3.2).

★★★★★

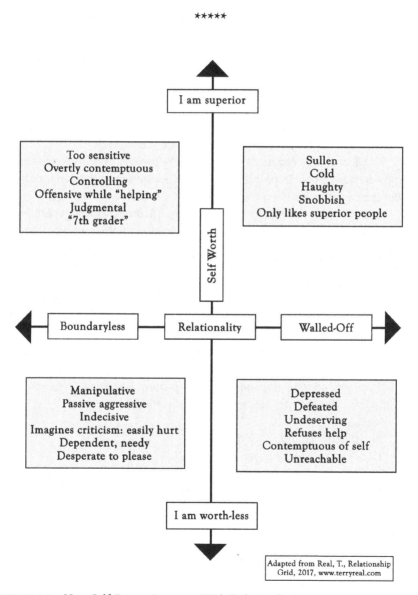

Adapted from Real, T., Relationship Grid, 2017, www.terryreal.com

FIGURE 3.2   How Self-Esteem Intersects With Relationality[33]

If he had stood before I entered the examination room, I wouldn't have fit. About 30 years old, he was an outsized young man, hard muscled, shaped like an oil drum squeezed into a tailored suit. His pocket square puffed exactly above the rim. His haircut was expensive. He seemed to have come straight from the mint.

Every bit of skin I could see, and doubtlessly parts I couldn't, was nicely tanned. He could have been the centerfold for Forbes *Magazine. When I entered he examined me head to foot and offered his hand enthusiastically. I felt like Gulliver.*

"I am so glad to see you, doctor," he said, glowing with self-contentment. "Thank you for taking my case. I know that you're the best in the world."

I tried to smile enigmatically. "Please tell me your story."

"I've flown here because I know that you're the only one who can help me." He slowed the last phrase for emphasis. I knew where this was going, but decided to let him lead me through it.

The patient already had three rhinoplasties. He brought photographs in piles. The first result was very good, but he went to another surgeon hoping for more perfection. He didn't think he got it. A third surgeon operated. I thought the result was excellent.

"No, it has to be better. See, right here, just at my nostrils, see how they go up and then down?" He was staring into the wall mirror, rolling his hands as he searched for the exact words.

"And my middle vault isn't quite right."

He combed his hair back with his fingers. Perhaps he was going to the British embassy later.

"Strangers used to stop and take my picture, you know." His voice trailed off. "But then my mother committed suicide."

He paused.

"I used to get beat up a lot as a kid."

"I'll bet that doesn't happen now," I said.

"That's why I go to the gym."

He turned and settled heavily into a chair.

"It was so bad." He pulled into himself.

"I had to quit my job. Now it's like there are ants crawling and electric shocks in my nostrils. And I have to wear my hair long because they pinned my ears but it came out wrong."

He seemed to have lost his train of thought. I took in some air while he regrouped.

"But my tip—my tip needs more, I don't know, delicacy, right?" He backed away from the mirror, looked himself over, smoothed his eyebrows with both hands

"You can fix it, right?"

I exhaled quietly so it wouldn't sound like a sigh. His observations were subtle but not imaginary. His nostrils were arched. His nasal tip was round. It would be possible to improve both.

"I need to think about it," I said. A few days later a package arrived containing a four page single-spaced letter accompanied by 70 pages of photographs from magazines and my journal publications. Across the bottom of one was written, "The result I want most is on page 69. That's the picture of George Washington."

I liked this man, but his whole life seemed to depend on my surgical outcome. "You've got too much energy invested in another operation," I wrote. "I don't think I can make you happy." Two weeks later he sent six more pages in a poetic, circular scrawl.

"You can do it. I just want a sharply defined angle of rotation with a smooth dorsum that demonstrates the continuity of lines from the supraorbital ridges that you show in your 1984 paper.

"I'm sending you plaster masks of what I want. You'll see how simple it'll be. After all, I'm not looking for perfection.

"And just please burn my photos after you study them."

How Children Adapt to Survive

From the earliest age, children recognize that they need their caregivers to survive. Powerless to feed, clothe, and protect themselves, they learn to adapt to their environments and gradually lose contact with their authentic selves if the environment is traumatic.

For some patients, surviving abuse becomes enough. "My father beat me repeatedly," one man told me. "That broken nose was a badge that I had survived. He didn't win."

The Childhood Role That You Played in Your Family

Children raised in neglectful or abusive households are unconsciously assigned one of three roles by their parents that determine how they manifest the five core issues and how they relate to others (Table 3.3): these are The Hero, the Scapegoat, or the Lost Child. Enmeshment, in which child/parent boundaries

TABLE 3.3 Following the Shame

Enmeshment (parent is boundary-less with the child)		Abandonment (parent walls out the child)
HEROIC ROLES	*SCAPEGOAT*	*LOST CHILD*
FALSELY EMPOWERED	FALSELY EMPOWERED/ DISEMPOWERED	DISEMPOWERED
WOULD CARRY EMOTIONS FOR PARENT OTHER THAN SHAME	CARRIES SHAME AND ANY OF THE OTHER EMOTIONS (fear, anger, pain, passion, guilt)	CARRIES SHAME
GETS "VALUE" FROM TAKING CARE OF OTHER PEOPLE	GETS "VALUE" AND "POWER" FROM BEHAVING BADLY IN RELATIONSHIPS	GETS "VALUE" FROM BEING GOOD & PERFECT
IS: LOVE AVOIDANT A GOOD CAREGIVER SEEKS INTENSITY	IS: LOVE AVOIDANT A BAD CAREGIVER SEEKS INTENSITY	IS: LOVE ADDICTED SUBJECT TO EXPERIENCING ANXIETY & DEPRESSION

Adapted from Mellody, P., 2016, used with permission

disappear, creates the Hero or Scapegoat. Abandonment, in which the child/parent boundary is a wall, creates the Lost Child. These roles fill the parents' needs.

The First Enmeshment Role: The Hero

In the Hero Role, the parent falsely empowers the child in order to make him or her counselor or mediator to the parents or parent to a sibling: Daddy's Little Girl or Mommy's Little Boy. In each of these roles, the child is expected to support the parents. Energy flows from the child to the parent instead of the healthy reverse. But it is traumatizing to force a child to take responsibility for others, and doing so creates a counterfeit identity that is falsely empowering and gives the child a distorted sense of his or her value ("The Good God"). These enmeshed children learn that self-esteem and value come from caretaking, a role that follows the child into adulthood. Hero children are driven to succeed by praise and the need for perfection, but develop profound senses of isolation and boredom. Consequently they seek intensity outside their marriages or relationships to feel alive, becoming risk takers, unfaithful spouses, gamblers, motorcycle racers, cocaine addicts, firemen, helicopter pilots, Special Forces operatives, or surgeons.

The Second Enmeshment Role: The Scapegoat

The second enmeshment role is the Scapegoat ("The Bad God")—simultaneously empowered and disempowered. The child becomes a vessel that holds the parents' own shameless thoughts and feelings (which itself is disempowering)—praised as the "Best of the Bad" (itself strangely empowering). The message is what I heard, "We are so disappointed in you." It is easy to understand how any child raised in this environment could take everything personally. When you are blamed as a child, you take the blame as an adult. The autocratic, totalitarian family cannot tolerate a freethinking child: its will must be broken. The simultaneous roles of Hero and Scapegoat are confusing.

The Abandonment Role

Neglect and abandonment are disempowering and covertly shaming. Parents who never wanted children or who ignore them reinforce the message that they are worthless. These children assume the third role, the Lost Child. Forty-six percent of my patients have been emotionally neglected and 54% have been emotionally abused. This prevalence is much higher than that in general medical patients with similar demographics (Chapter 9).[58–60]

Lost children live lonely lives, amusing themselves with fantasy, reading, and video games in constant attempts to shut down and disappear. Because they have been shamed by feelings of inherent defectiveness, they compensate by trying to be perfect in every way to please their parents, but are filled with senses of worthlessness and fear that their insignificance will be discovered. As adults they feel like frauds and live in constant dread of exposure. Fear recognizes fear.[61] When distressed, they have never learned to comfort themselves. Recurrent fears resurface as if they have never been addressed. Emotional abuse provides obvious links to perfectionism, body shame, and plastic surgery. There is never "enough"; there is no time for rest; all comparisons are unfavorable; the search for perfection is ceaseless. Perfectionism becomes just another addiction.

The Outcomes of the Role You Played

The common result of these parental roles is a child who never learns that self-esteem is inherent and not dependent upon actions, caretaking, or perfect behavior.[62] As these roles slide forward into adulthood, they interfere with relationships, intimacy, and happiness. Shame becomes multigenerational. Secrets cannot be worked out, only acted out. The family cannot put words to its pain—alexithymia—and what it cannot feel, it cannot face and treat.[63] It re-creates its

TABLE 3.4 The Innate Characteristics of Children and How Trauma Distorts Them[3]

Children's Attributes	How Abuse or Neglect May Affect Them	How Patients May Manifest the Trauma
Boundlessly Energetic	Children are not taught to contain their energy appropriately Shamed into silence Encouraged to be perfect	Childlike Fearful of confiding to surgeon or staff Expect surgical perfection Pace, fidget, poor control of their actions
Vulnerable	Parents do not provide adequate protection Parents may rage or injure Children develop protective walls and learn that the world is dangerous	Untrusting Unnecessarily fearful May feel victimized May become irrationally fearful during minor treatments
Dependent	Parents do not teach self-care, or how to be helpful to others Parents do not teach when to ask for help Parents may expect children to care for them Children turn parental neglect into self-indictment	Do not talk or listen attentively Keep inappropriate distance from surgeon or staff Are overly dependent on the staff and neglect self-care postoperatively Adult patients may still require parental decisions May neglect routine postoperative care
Undeveloped Thinking Skills	Parents do not validate children's correct observations and encourage mature reasoning Parents do not distinguish truth from error Parents allow children's misapprehensions to go uncorrected Parents do not teach children that not knowing everything is not shameful Children doubt their own thinking skills	Cannot make up their minds "No, tell me what you think I should do" May be unable to hear other opinions May be distrusting or have irrational beliefs (e.g., that everyone notices their noses)
Immature	Parents do not allow children to act their age, and expect inappropriate maturity Parents may encourage immaturity and teach children to be overly dependent on them Parents may expect children to care for them or become surrogate parents	Behave younger than their years Overly dependent on surgeon and staff May rely on parent to make surgical decisions Fail to keep appointments May attempt to be inappropriately controlling

own history. Violent spouses produce violent children. Intolerable feelings convert into acceptable ones: people laugh at things that aren't funny, cry or feel guilt when they should feel anger. Some emotions are family-sanctioned; others are not. It is easy to imagine how such conversions can associate with psychogenic and organic illness, as the Adverse Childhood Events Study and our own research have identified (Chapter 9).

The Innate Characteristics of Children and How They Become Stifled

1. Children are *authentic*, which is why they are so delightful to observe in play. They are characterized by exuberant energy, vulnerability, dependency, nascent reason, and appropriate immaturity. Each of these characteristics can be distorted, creating joyless, shut-down children (Table 3.4).
   Parents intolerant of a child's energy will shame the child into silence; the child will often cope by trying to become "perfect": not childlike but masked, falsely adult.
2. Children are *physically and emotionally vulnerable*. Abuse that inappropriately invades the child's boundaries forces him or her to compensate with walls, which protects against rage and cover fears, but which also isolates the child from his or her own authenticity and from others.
3. Children are *born dependent* and must learn to become appropriately independent. When the child is helpless, attentive parental care nurtures the child's independent self-worth. The parent must gradually support the child into relational independence.

Immature parents who do not care for their children's needs message that the children are worthless. Crying infants who are cooed, rocked, ignored, or beaten each concoct completely different conceptions of their worth and whether the world is safe. Children whose neglectful mothers do not teach them to calm themselves become unable to do so alone. As adults, they cannot be comforted: when their questions are answered and their fears are addressed, the reassurance does not last. The same fears soon re-emerge. Physicians see the effects of this neglect in patients who become childlike following surgery, or in Internet conversations where patients give medical advice to each other or pose questions that should be directed toward their surgeons—or not even asked: ("I am two days following surgery; what is this bump on my nostril?" "What kind of nose would fit my face?" "I am four days following surgery—Am I still swollen?" " I had surgery; can I go to a theme park?" "Should my nose look like this at one month?" "My surgery was two weeks ago. What's wrong?" "It's been a week and I think the surgeon ruined my life; what can I do?"). In one patient-assistance website, at least 75 percent of the questions had been written within the first postoperative week while bandages were in place. Before they have seen the results, these patients are already frightened. Another 15 percent of the questions were unanswerable: "Should I have a rhinoplasty?" Or even sadder: "I feel ugly. What should I do?"

4. Children have *incompletely developed reasoning skills* and must learn to match what they observe with what they think: in other words, make sense of their worlds without distorting the input. Children who don't trust their own perceptions live according to others' assessments and others' judgments. Immature reasoning unguided by non-nurturing parents creates untrusting adults who are intolerant of diverse opinions, fearful of not knowing everything, and unwilling to discover the truth.
5. Children are *appropriately immature* and must be allowed to develop wisdom and judgment commensurate with their ages. Six-year-olds are not equipped to care for their parents, nor should they need seek love by pretending to be helpless and undisciplined. Children must not remain children forever. Children expected to act like adults begin to suffocate their own natural energies and doubt their own judgments; and as adults they will be excessively controlling of themselves and others, unwilling to allow their partners to retain their own individualities. The child allowed to have temper tantrums becomes an uncontained adult with uncontrolled emotions, unable to enjoy functional relationships.

Trauma does not affect all children at all ages in all roles similarly. Key to understanding the trauma ego state is the age at which the role was imposed.

★★★★★

"This is my picture before I had surgery," she said. The pretty teenager in the photograph had a flawless, straight nose. Now she was a tall woman with bright, quick eyes and a helmet of auburn hair. She sat on my examination table sideways, swinging her crossed ankles. She smoothed her skirt as I came in.

"Your nose looked nice," I said.

She paused, her voice small. "It was."

I looked at her. "So why did you have surgery?"

Sigh. The way she hesitated I expected that there was something to learn, if she'd only tell me.

"It was my aunt's idea. She was very pretty. She had my ears fixed, too. She didn't like them." Her eyes clouded. I wondered what other memories were stored there. She opened her mouth again, but nothing came out.

"What don't you like now?" I asked.

A small furrow appeared between her brows. "I don't know. It's the tip, I think. It just doesn't look right. I see myself every day on camera and something is wrong. My agent says I need to have surgery."

She was right: it was the tip. It was also the length, the sunken bridge, and the collapsed sidewalls. I didn't know how she could breathe. I laid her photographs in front of her. Perhaps seeing them would help.

"What do you see in the photographs?" I asked.

For a moment, her eyes rested on me. The small furrow reappeared. "I don't know." She made several noncommittal gestures with her hands.

"It's the tip, I think." She sighed quietly and gave a tiny shake of her head. "I guess I don't know. I just don't know."

Not being able to explain your surgical goals is not only about depression, or education, or the ability to be analytical. It's not really even about body dysmorphic disorder.

Not being able to see your face is the ultimate loss of self.

The Age-Dependent Response to Developmental Trauma

The Wounded Child, the Adapted Wounded Child, and the Adult Adapted Wounded Child

Developmental trauma survivors or, for the purposes of this book, patients, behave in certain inauthentic roles; and when stressed, they regress. Where this regression starts and how far back it goes depends in part upon the age that the trauma occurred.

Trauma Before Age 5: The Wounded Child

When trauma is inflicted on infants or children under five, coping mechanisms and language skills are not sufficiently mature to create adequate defenses. These children cannot reason logically, and so judge instead through perceptions and feelings, not knowing which thoughts belong to themselves and which to their parents. Their home environment remains unmodulated and diffused by outside contact with peers, teachers, or coaches. When these early wounds are reactivated, their unexpressed pain manifests as worthlessness; vulnerability; or rebellious, dependent, overwhelmed, dissociated, chaotic emotions. This is the *Wounded Child*. These raw, intense emotions receive minimal input from the cerebral cortex. Wounded children can only assign limited meanings and adapt in limited ways. When strong feelings occur, it is useful to ask, "How old do I feel right now?"

The emerged Wounded Child manifests symptoms of posttraumatic stress disorder with childish immaturity and vulnerability. It is important to recognize that this is not an act: the patient is actually *becoming* the wounded child, losing his or her identity. Language and behavior become childlike, illustrated in many of our vignettes. This transition is seamless and can easily be missed by the physician not expecting it. Occasionally the wounded child emerges in unexpected circumstances: the clue is incongruous behavior. Sudden, seemingly unjustifiable fear or distrust can be clues to some triggered, unnamed childhood trauma. And just as quickly as it emerges, the wounded child slips back into the chrysalis.

★★★★★

The physician cannot interact with the wounded child in the same way that he or she would act with a patient in an adult adapted state. It is not possible to be "reasonable" or "rational" with a patient thinking with an immature, distraught, trauma-activated brain. One of my patients is a retired Navy Seal who has PTSD from an incident in Vietnam. The terrifying, imprinting experience occurred 40 years ago. He is no longer in Vietnam. Intellectually he knows that he is safe. But the wound remains and cannot be treated by trying to reason with the part of his brain that was hardwired for abstract thinking, not survival. His brain's response to this adult trauma simulates the damage done to a child subjected to repeated emotional or physical abuse or neglect. We are all interrupted by the past.

> *"[My earliest memory] is a fogged-out landscape," writes Stephen King. "[I was] raised by a single parent who moved around a lot . . . and who . . . may have farmed my brother and me out to one of her sisters for a while because she was economically or emotionally unable to cope with us. . . . 'What I do not understand, Stevie,' [my mother] said, 'is why you'd write junk like this in the first place.' . . . She had rolled up a copy of [my first manuscript] and was brandishing it at me. . . . I was ashamed. I have spent a good many years since . . . being ashamed about what I write. . . . Almost every writer . . . who has ever published a line has been accused by someone of wasting his or her God-given talent."*[64]

Trauma From Ages 6 to 9: The Adapted Wounded Child

When trauma is inflicted at approximately ages 6 to 9, the child's coping mechanisms are better, more able to adapt and cope with the abusive environment. The *Adapted Wounded Child* learns how to behave and stay out of trouble by pretending to be an adult—or how an adult looks to a child. The encrustations of adapted behavior may thicken the shell, but the Wounded Child is still underneath. In my patients, that same adaptation manifests as either petulance or constant worry about certain postoperative imperfections or obscure complications. Through unknown mechanisms patients can unintentionally compromise their own outcomes with irrational worry. Virtually all physicians have seen it.

Trauma From Ages 11–16: The Adult Adapted Wounded Child

When the self is wounded from approximately ages 11 to 16, the so-called *Adult Adapted Wounded Child* becomes a parent to the wounded or adapted wounded child, paralleling the child-parent roles that each had earlier adopted. The Adult Adapted Wounded Child feels more in control of his or her environment and behavior and can better identify what the parents desire. Thinking, however, can become rigid, harsh, all or nothing, black or white, perfectionistic, and categorical.

As adults, Adult Adapted Wounded Children who have sustained falsely empowering abuse (Hero or Scapegoat) may become arrogant, grandiose, judgmental, invulnerable, anti-dependent good and perfect, controlling, and walled. Conversely, the child who has sustained disempowering abuse will either act boundaryless or walled, good and perfect, needless and wantless, but also manipulative and passive-aggressive. Our Adapted Wounded Children model themselves in the ways we were raised. If we were treated rigidly and harshly, our Adapted Adult Wounded Children will be rigid and harsh. Real uses the metaphor of a battery that stores energy that we absorb as children and then discharge as adults.[57]

Anyone married to an Adult Adapted Wounded Child faces challenges; it is easy to imagine the tumult in a marriage between two Adapted Adult Wounded Children. Under the grown-up veneer, the Wounded Child cowers. Only functional adults see nuances and can be completely relational, forgiving, and gentle.

TABLE 3.5 Relational Trauma Reactions

Wounded Child *Birth to about 4*	*Adapted Adult-Child* *About age 5 through age 17. Parents the self with criticism, neglect, &* *indulgence*		
	Hero *Falsely Empowered Child*	*Lost Child* *Disempowered Child*	*Scapegoat* *Falsely Empowered / Disempowered Child*
SELF-ESTEEM Less Than	SELF-ESTEEM Better Than Others	SELF-ESTEEM Less Than Others	SELF-ESTEEM Less Than
BOUNDARIES Too Vulnerable	BOUNDARIES Walled in invulnerable	BOUNDARIES Alternates Between No Boundaries & Walls	BOUNDARIES Walled in & invulnerable
REALITY Bad	REALITY Good & Perfect	REALITY Good & Perfect	REALITY Bad/Rebellious
DEPENDENCY Too Dependent	DEPENDENCY Anti-Dependent	DEPENDENCY Needless/Wantless	DEPENDENCY Too Dependent

(Continued)

TABLE 3.5 (Continued)

Wounded Child *Birth to about 4*	*Adapted Adult-Child* *About age 5 through age 17. Parents the self with criticism, neglect, &* *indulgence*		
	Hero *Falsely Empowered* *Child*	*Lost Child* *Disempowered Child*	*Scapegoat* *Falsely Empowered/* *Disempowered Child*
MODERATION Out of Control	MODERATION Out of Control With Being in Control of Others	MODERATION Out of Control With Being Manipulative of Others	MODERATION Out of Control
Overwhelmed, Passive Dissociative	Unavailable Passive/Aggressive All Powerful	Yielding, Enabling Passive/Aggressive Appears Powerless	Unavailable Aggressive

Adapted From Mellody, 2016

Stored Emotions From Relational Trauma and How to Recognize Them (Table 3.5)

Two types of emotions are stored during this childhood abuse and emerge during regression to earlier childhood states. The first is gentler, and occurs when the child understands the source of the abuse but retains his or her boundaries and yet feels empathy for the parent. The parent's energy becomes "carried" by the child, producing an uncomfortable but not disequilibriating emotion.

When, however, the parents' energy is so intense that it collapses the child's boundaries, emotion and shame penetrate so deeply that the child feels like the abuser, not the abused, and collapses into a state of defective worthlessness. This is the destructive "carried shame" transmitted by a caregiver who has behaved shamelessly and unapologetically. The child absorbs that shame and *carries it as if it were the child's own*, defining himself or herself by the parents' same abusive language. This phenomenon reappears in the victim language of an adult patient who says, "You deserted me," "You betrayed me," or "You abandoned me." Genuine emotion is moderate; carried emotion is immoderate. Sadness is real; depression is carried. Fear is real; anxiety is carried. Healthy shame is real; toxic shame is carried.[65]

Patients who have not yet become functional adults have incorporated shell upon shell of beliefs and behaviors that do not represent their authentic selves. Operating as a functional adult feels much better. Instead of looking to others for survival, guidance, and approval, the functional adult looks to self. With proper trauma work, those punishing voices that torment the Adult Adapted Wounded Child do quiet.

★★★★★

These stages of compensatory behavior are possible to recognize. Listen for childish thinking and childish words. The Wounded Child, injured before age 5, thinks illogically and magically, behaves vulnerably, and feels dissociated, overwhelmed, and worthless. He or she cannot self-soothe when distressed. The Adapted Wounded Child, traumatized between ages and 9, understands his or her family better and has learned how to cope with the unique insanities of its system. He or she has learned how to behave, how to transform, and how to function safely and "perfectly." Evolving further, the Adult Adapted Wounded Child feels powerful, grandiose, but walled-in. Many of the most controlling, seemingly gifted people are severely depressed, particularly if the genesis was abandonment. Self-esteem only self-generates when it does not depend on illusion or achievement.

Most patients who come from difficult childhoods behave like Adult Adapted Wounded Children. They feel mature but are instead judgmental, controlling, and perfectionistic, either attacking and neglecting or indulging and boundaryless. Recovery requires uncovering the Wounded Child or the Adapted Wounded Child, identifying the source of the carried shame, returning it to the offender, and allowing the new Functional Adult to re-parent the Inner Child through experiential trauma therapy.[66–68] The fact that this wounding and destructive programming occurs at the survival brain level, not the cortex, and becomes the default pathway for the brain stem and limbic system explains why "talk therapy" or even cognitive behavior therapy may never penetrate the real damage. Trauma is not stored in the cortex. It is the limbic system that scans for potential danger; and when a threat is identified, the memory of that threat *and whatever is associated with it* get stored together. When the traumatic memory, *or the same feeling associated with that memory*, is activated by any of a number of triggers, the patient does not remember the wound, *he or she becomes the wound*, "feeling" these memories frozen in time but not understanding them. Functional MRIs of patients reliving trauma parallel the appearance of those scans taken just after the trauma. Triggered patients feel the distress but do not cognitively understand it, so their cortices fabricate reasons for these awful feelings, and incorporate their surroundings. Their wounds are not in the past. In a medical setting they hover in the surgeon's examination and operating rooms, and the physician becomes the default perpetrator.

The Way in Which You Relate to Others

The final piece of the model connects us to our worlds. Though dysfunctional relational behavior appears along a spectrum, the extremes are easiest to identify as the *Love Addict* and the *Love Avoidant*.[6] (Those who find "Love" in these contexts confusing or ambiguous can substitute *relationship, social engagement,* or *intimacy*.) In the attachment literature, these traits are referred to as Avoidant and Insecure or Anxious styles, respectively.[41, 42, 69, 70] Love Addicts, in particular, have special capacities to create fantasies that significantly complicate the surgeon-patient relationship and may contribute to the unhappiness and emotional intensity felt by patients driven to plastic surgery because of body shame or BDD.

Love Addiction and Love Avoidance

It is not difficult to imagine how living at the extremes of the five core issues can create difficulties in intimate relationships, but imagine what problems they create when the love addict is a patient.

According to Mellody's model, love addicts are parented by distant, walled, abandoning caregivers, causing the child to be shamed by the neglect and parental distance that they experienced, which in turn destroys the child's confidence in his or her ability to self-care. In relationships love addicts search for strong, protective rescuers that they need to survive, or so they think.

The *Love Addict* therefore selects a partner who has the walled, controlled, powerful persona reminiscent of his or her abandoning parents, maintaining the obsessive childhood fantasy that survival depends upon someone else. If the partner leaves, the addict becomes depressed and medicates the pain with depressant substances or behaviors—alcohol, shopping, food—and may attempt revenge.

The *Love Avoidant*, conversely, was raised in a house by boundaryless parents who enmeshed the child and taught him or her to be a care-taking hero. This role diminishes the child's sense of himself or herself and creates a life model in which self-esteem is contingent upon caretaking. To fulfill that role without being enmeshed again as an adult, the love avoidant erects protective walls that modulate or block intimacy. Stephen King recalled of his childhood that he could "build walls like the Dutch build dikes."[64] In order to feel "alive," however, the love avoidant seeks intensity by risky behavior outside the relationship—i.e., gambling, affairs, motorcycle racing, or combat service.

Adult behaviors are learned. If you are a grandiose or disempowered adult, ask yourself: (1) Who was grandiose or disempowered toward you? or (2) Who allowed you to be grandiose or disempowered and approved of it?

Love Addicts and Love Avoidants can be either gender, and someone can be a love avoidant in one relationship and a love addict in another. The "target gender" depends upon the gender of the parent who was either walled off or enmeshing. For example, if a man was enmeshed by his mother, he will be love avoidant to women. If a woman was enmeshed by her mother, she will likewise be love avoidant to women. This principle holds regardless of sexual preference. Thus a lesbian who was abandoned by her mother will be love addicted to women. The gender of the partner depends upon the gender of the influential parent; the addiction or avoidance pattern depends on the history of disempowerment or false empowerment.

How the Physician, Surgeon, or Therapist Can Become an Unwitting Player

In the midst of this bewildering morality play, the provider's confident behavior and apparently unflagging strength may mesh perfectly with the patient's boundaryless vulnerability and sense of defectiveness. Many surgeons can appear to be supremely powerful, nine-foot tall, bulletproof protectors to whom the love addict can assign much more power than the surgeon actually possesses. These patients always expect more flawless results than are humanly achievable and may be angry, feel victimized, and want to "get even" when the impossible does not occur. Because love addicts often see their parents in these physicians, they can hate them when they are triggered—when the result isn't flawless, when surgery is not transformative, when self-worth doesn't appear and only toxic shame remains. Patients who scapegoat their surgeons often accuse them of being what the patients themselves are—or what their parents were.

Even beyond the surgical result, love addicts expect their surgeons to rescue them from their own unhappiness, protect them from pain, and nurture them— exactly the attention that they never received from their parents. Thus the surgeon can become the false savior, the object of an addiction that becomes indistinguishable from alcohol, drugs, sex, gambling, or work. Failure is certain, and so the patient may move to another surgeon, create the same cycle again, and suffer subsequent disappointment. The toxicity of the patient's disappointment fuels his or her victim anger, generating medical board complaints or retaliation through the Internet.

A summary of the ramifications of a dysfunctional childhood is displayed in Table 3.6.

★★★★★

In 1956, Norman Cousins, then editor of the Saturday Review, traveled to Lambaréné, Africa, to visit Albert Schweitzer, aiming to encourage Schweitzer to finish his manuscripts and to speak out in favor of nuclear disarmament. Recognizing that Schweitzer never worried about his legacy, Cousins reflected:

The tragedy of life is not in the hurt to a man's name. . . . The tragedy of life is what dies inside a man while he lives—the death of genuine feeling, the death of inspired response, the death of the awareness that makes it possible to feel the pain or the glory of other men in one's self. Schweitzer's aim was not to dazzle an age but to awaken it, to make it comprehend that moral splendor is a part of the gift of life, and that each man has unlimited strength to feel human oneness and to act upon it.[71]

Narcissism in the Classical Sense: A Player in Body Image Disorders

Physicians, therapists, and onlookers, including the media, frequently label body dysmorphic and other difficult patients as simply narcissistic.[72] The DSM-5 defines

TABLE 3.6 The Inner Child Overview

	Functional Childhood	Dysfunctional Childhood Immaturity		Secondary Symptoms Unmanageability	Relational Problems	Functional Adulthood
	Precious Child	**Wounded-Child**	**Adapted Adult-Child**			**Functional Adult**
Ego State: Emotional	1st Ego-State	2nd Ego-State	3rd Ego-State			4th Ego-State
Age: Physical Age:	Current Age; Birth—18 yrs	Approximately 1–6 yrs old; Approximately 1–6 yrs old	Approximately 7–18 yrs old; Approximately 7–18 yrs old	Depression; Anxiety Disorders	Problems with Intimacy; Enmeshment	Current Age; 18–85 yrs old
	Childhood Trauma causes Immaturity ↑		*Childhood Trauma AND Immaturity drive both unmanageability* ↑	Chemical Addictions; Problems with Spirituality; Sex Addiction	Dishonesty; Problems with Interdependence; Love Addiction	
				Intensity; Physical Illness; Money Disorders	Love Avoidance	
				Eating Disorders; Behavioral Addictions; Raging	*Childhood Trauma Immaturity, AND unmanage ability create Relational Problems* ↑	*Treatment, Recovery, Intimacy and Reparenting can create the Functional Adult*
Core Issues		**Core Issues**				**Core Issues**
Self-Esteem	Vulnerable	Less Than	Better Than			Self-Esteem
Boundaries	Vulnerable	Too Vulnerable	Invulnerable			Healthy Boundaries
Reality	Imperfect ↑	Rebellious	Perfectionist ↑		↑	Accepting Imperfections
Dependency	Dependent	Too Dependent	Needless / Wantless			Healthy Expression of Needs and Wants
Moderation	Spontaneous	Out of Control	Controlling			Spontaneous Moderate

Adapted from Mellody, P. 2016, used with permission

Narcissistic Personality Disorder as indicated by the presence of at least 5 of the following nine criteria:

- A grandiose sense of self-importance
- A preoccupation with fantasies of unlimited success, power, brilliance, beauty, or ideal love
- A belief that he or she is special and unique and can only be understood by, or should associate with, other special or high-status people or institutions
- A need for excessive admiration
- A sense of entitlement
- Interpersonally exploitive behavior
- A lack of empathy
- Envy of others or a belief that others are envious of him or her
- A demonstration of arrogant and haughty behaviors or attitudes

These criteria perfectly describe grandiosity and adapted adult wounded child behavior. But who was Narcissus? Ovid's *Metamorphoses* notes that Narcissus was the son of the nymph Liriope. Anxious to know if her son would live to see a ripe old age, she consulted the seer Tiresias. The prophet answered, "If he never knows himself." Seeing his reflection in a pool of water, Narcissus was engulfed by the beauty of his own image. "He fell in love with an image without reality, and he mistook for reality what was only an image. Narcissus was held spellbound by himself and lay there motionless . . . gazing into his own eyes . . . the beauty of his face, the rosy glow on his snow-white skin, and he admired all that he saw. . . . Foolishly he longed for himself. . . . So Narcissus, pining with love, wasted away and was gradually consumed by the fire of love buried within him. . . . Narcissus laid his weary head upon the green grass as death closed the eyes that wondered at the beauty of the sight that held them."[73]

Narcissus, filled with "such chill pride," was unable to establish an authentic relationship, and instead became captivated and eventually destroyed by the illusory beauty of his own reflection. In *I Don't Want to Talk About It*,[73] therapist Terrence Real agrees with the Renaissance philosopher, Marsilio Ficinio, that Narcissus suffered not from an overabundance of self-love but rather from a deficiency of it. The myth of Narcissus is therefore a parable about the absence of self-esteem. Rather than an internal sense of self-worth instilled by his parents, Narcissus created his sense of himself entirely from the external: his beautiful appearance—one form of "other esteem." Like anyone addicted to reflected glory, Narcissus cannot break free, even at the cost of his own life. Narcissus is not self-obsessed; rather he is image-obsessed and so becomes a metaphor for many of the patients whom we are discussing and for others who never become patients. "Unconditional love and acceptance of self seems to be the hardest task for all humankind. . . . We try [instead] to create more powerful false selves, or we give up and become less than human. This results in a lifetime of cover-up and secrecy . . . the basic cause of human suffering."[18]

The Implications of Parenting on Body Image

The inescapable conclusion is that a significant part of the self, certainly the part that interacts with the family and the world at large, is the product of what happens in childhood: the role that your family of origin assigned, what type of parenting generated it, how you adapted and the developmental age at which you still play that role, and the manner in which you relate to others. The final common pathway for familial abuse or neglect is toxic shame. *Abuse and neglect are the tinder; shame is the fuel.* When people develop shame binds attached to their bodies, both their souls and flesh have been affected; it is not possible to go much farther.

> *In complex brains, the map-making cerebral cortices describe the body and its doings in . . . detail . . ."*[74] *Patients with body image disorders know them in hyperexquisite detail. Bodily feelings are more pressing than sights, smells, or sounds, which are external stimuli that can be revised. "The body-minded brain is indeed a captive of the body and of its signaling.*[75]

Are body image disorders the cause of the shame that these patients feel, or are they the result of that shame? Are the associations of family prevalence, self-esteem issues, associated addictions, obsessive behavior, and depression with body image the result of body dysmorphic disorder or are they all precursors generated by the family of origin? How might the manifestations of body dysmorphic disorder and the human adaptions to childhood trauma figure in body image? Can we make a connection? We will look for further clues.

What This Information Means

The childhood role that you played in your family of origin, where it originated, the developmental age at which you still play it, and the way in which you relate to others influence or impair—for better or worse—the five core components that make up a functional adult: appropriate self-esteem, healthy boundaries, accurate processing of your environment, and competence in caring for yourself and living in moderation. When rearing is suboptimal or traumatizing, these core attributes do not develop normally so that individuals live at the extremes— becoming disempowered and unable to manage themselves, or falsely empowered and grandiose so that rules don't apply to them. Children raised in abusive or neglectful environments feel shamed and defective. Events around them can trigger early wounds and manifest as behavioral coping mechanisms that were protective in childhood but are wholly inappropriate in adult situations. Relationships and happiness are impaired and any feeling of abundance becomes impossible.

Because all trauma is somatic—felt and expressed in the body—can shame shape body image or explain body image disorders?

References

1. Kafka F. *Letter to My Father*. North Carolina: Lulu; 2008.
2. Mellody P. How the Symptoms Sabotage. In: *Facing Codependence*. New York: Harper Collins; 2003:51–60.
3. Mellody P, Freundlich LS. *The Intimacy Factor the Ground Rules for Overcoming the Obstacles to Truth, Respect, and Lasting Love*. San Francisco: Harper Collins; 2003:7–24.
4. Mellody P, Freundlich LS. *The Intimacy Factor the Ground Rules for Overcoming the Obstacles to Truth, Respect, and Lasting Love*. San Francisco: Harper Collins; 2003:11–49.
5. Mellody P, Miller AW, Miller JK. *Facing Codependence: What It Is, Where It Comes From, How It Sabotages Our Lives*. New York: Harper Collins; 1989.
6. Mellody P, Miller AW, Miller JK. *Facing Love Addiction: Giving Yourself the Power to Change the Way You Love*. New York: Harper Collins; 1992.
7. van der Kolk BA, Perry LC, Herman JL. Childhood Origins of Self-Destructive Behavior. *Am J Psychiatry* 1991; 148:12:1665–1671.
8. van der Kolk BA, Pelcovitz D, Roth S, et al. Dissociation, Somatization, and Affect Dysregulation: The Complexity of Adaptation to Trauma. *Am J Psychiatry* 1996; 153:7:83–93.
9. van der Kolk B. Trauma and Memory. In: van der Kolk B, McFarlane AC, Weisaeth L, eds. *Traumatic Stress*. New York: The Guilford Press; 2007:3289–3296.
10. van der Kolk BA. *The Body Keeps the Score: Brain, Mind, and Body in the Healing of Trauma*. New York: Viking (Penguin Group); 2014.
11. van der Kolk B, van der Hart O. The Intrusive Past: The Flexibility of Memory and the Engraving of Trauma. *Am Imago* 1991; 48:425–454.
12. van der Kolk B. The Complexity of Adaptation to Trauma Self-Regulation, Stimulus, Discrimination, and Characterological Development. In: van der Kolk B, McFarlane AC, Weisaeth L, eds. *Traumatic Stress*. New York: The Guilford Press; 2007:182–213.
13. van der Kolk BA, van der Hart O. Pierre Janet and the Breakdown of Adaptation in Psychological Trauma. *Am J Psychiatry* 1989; 146:12:1530–1540.
14. van Zelst C, van Nierop M, van Dam DS, et al. Associations between Stereotype Awareness, Childhood Trauma and Psychopathology: A Study in People with Psychosis, Their Siblings and Controls. *PLoS One* 2015; 10:2:e0117386.
15. Black C. Family Violence. In: *It Will Never Happen to Me: Growing Up with Addiction as Youngsters, Adolescents, Adults*. 2nd edition. Center City [MN]: Hazelden; 2005:102.
16. Black C. *It Will Never Happen to Me: Growing Up With Addiction as Youngsters, Adolescents, Adults*. Center City [MN]: Hazelden; 1981.
17. Black C. Shame Circle. In: *It Will Never Happen to Me: Growing Up With Addiction as Youngsters, Adolescents, Adults*. 2nd edition. Center City [MN]: Hazelden; 2002:65–84.
18. Bradshaw J. *Healing the Shame That Binds You*. Deerfield Beach [FL]: Health Communications; 2005:159–165.
19. Bradshaw JE. *Healing the Shame That Binds You*. Deerfield Beach [FL]: Health Communications; 1988.
20. Bradshaw JE. *Post-Romantic Stress Disorder: What to Do When the Honeymoon Is Over*. Deerfield Beach [FL]: Health Communications; 2014.
21. Herman JL. *Trauma and Recovery: The Aftermath of Violence: From Domestic Abuse to Political Terror*. New York: Basic Books (Perseus Books Group); 1992.
22. Van de Kemp H. Biography of Alexandra Adler. *Psychology of Women* Spring 2003; 30:2.

23. van der Kolk B, McFarlane AC, van der Hart O. A General Approach to Treatment of Posttraumatic Stress Disorder. In: van der Kolk B, McFarlane AC, Weisaeth L, eds. *Traumatic Stress*. New York: The Guilford Press; 2007:428–429.

24. van der Kolk B, van der Hart O, Marmar CR. Dissociation and Information Processing in Posttraumatic Stress Disorder. In: van der Kolk B, McFarlane AC, Weisaeth L, eds. *Traumatic Stress*. New York: The Guilford Press; 2007:282–296.

25. van der Kolk B. The Black Hole of Trauma. In: van der Kolk B, McFarlane AC, Weisaeth L, eds. *Traumatic Stress*. New York: The Guilford Press; 2007:3–23.

26. van der Kolk B. The Body Keeps the Score. In: van der Kolk B, McFarlane AC, Weisaeth L, eds. *Traumatic Stress*. New York: The Guilford Press; 2007:214–242.

27. van der Kolk B. The Body Keeps the Score. In: van der Kolk B, McFarlane AC, Weisaeth L, eds. *Traumatic Stress*. New York: The Guilford Press; 2007:233–234.

28. van der Kolk BA, McFarlane AC, Weisaeth L, eds. *Traumatic Stress: The Effects of Overwhelming Experience on Mind, Body, and Society*. New York: The Guilford Press; 1996.

29. van der Kolk BA. Developmental Trauma Disorder toward a Rational Diagnosis for Children with Complex Trauma Histories. *Psychiatric Ann* 2005; 35:5:401–408.

30. van der Kolk BA. The Compulsion to Repeat the Trauma. *Psychiatr Clin N Am* 1989; 12:2:389–411.

31. van der Kolk BA. Foreword. In: Ogden P, Minton K, Pain C, eds. *Trauma and the Body*. New York: W W Norton & Company; 2006:41–64.

32. Ioannidis JPA. Is It Possible to Recognize a Major Scientific Discovery? *JAMA* 2015; 314:11:1135–1137.

33. Real, T. *Full Respect Living Tool Kit*, www.terryreal.com, 2016.

34. Phillips KA. *The Broken Mirror: Understanding and Treating Body Dysmorphic Disorder*. Revised and expanded edition. New York: Oxford University Press; 2005.

35. Wilhelm S. *Feeling Good About the Way You Look: A Program for Overcoming Body Image Problems*. New York: The Guilford Press; 2006.

36. Neziroglu F, Barile N. Environmental Factors in Body Dysmorphic Disorder. In: Phillips KA, ed. *Body Dysmorphic Disorder: Advances in Research and Clinical Practice*. New York: Oxford University Press; 2017:277–284.

37. Lee KA, Guy A, Dale J, et al. Adolescent Desire for Cosmetic Surgery: Association with Bullying and Psychological Functioning. *Plast Reconstr Surg* 2017; 139:1109–1118.

38. Cyrus KD. Medical Education and the Minority Tax. *JAMA* 2017; 317:1833–1834.

39. Jackson AC, Dowling NA, Honigman RJ, et al. The Experience of Teasing in Elective Cosmetic Surgery Patients. *Behav Med* 2012; 38:129–137.

40. Herringa RJ, Birn RM, Ruttle PL, et al. Childhood Maltreatment Is Associated with Altered Fear Circuitry and Increased Internalizing Symptoms by Late Adolescence. *Proc Natl Acad Sci* 2013; 110:47:19119–19124.

41. Schore AN. Early Superego Development: The Emergence of Shame and Narcissistic Affect Regulation in the Practicing Period. *Psychoanal Contemp Thought* 1991; 14:187.

42. Schore AN. *The Science of the Art of Psychotherapy*. New York: W Norton & Company; 2012.

43. Devinsky O. Right Cerebral Hemisphere Dominance for a Sense of Corporeal and Emotional Self. *Epilepsy Behav* 2000; 1:1:60–73.

44. Buhlmann U, Wilhelm S, McNally RJ, et al. Interpretive Biases for Ambiguous Information in Body Dysmorphic Disorder. *CNS Spectrums* 2002; 7:6:435–443.

45. Kaufman G. *The Psychology of Shame*. New York: Springer; 1989, quoted by Bradshaw in Bradshaw JE. *Healing the Shame That Binds You*. Deerfield Beach [FL]: Health Communications; 1988:xviii.

46. Miller A. *Pictures of a Childhood*. New York: Farrar Straus, Giroux, 1986.

47. Kline CB. *Orphan Train*. New York: Harper Collins; 2013:177.

48. Harder DH, Zalma A. Two Promising Shame and Guilt Scales: A Construct Validity Comparison. *J Pers* 1990; 55:3&4:729–745.

49. Porges SW. *The Polyvagal Theory: Neurophysiological Foundations of Emotions Attachment Communication Self-Regulation.* New York: W W Norton & Company; 2011.

50. Porges SW. *The Polyvagal Theory: Neurophysiological Foundations Of Emotions Attachment Communication Self-Regulation.* New York: W W Norton & Company; 2011.

51. Brown B. *Daring Greatly.* New York: Random House; 2015.

52. Bliss, M. *Harvey Cushing, a Life in Surgery.* New York: Oxford University Press; 2005:317.

53. Vance JD. *Hillbilly Elegy: A Memoir of a Family and Culture in Crisis.* New York: Harper Collins Publishers; 2016:254.

54. Cash TF, Phillips KA, Santos MT, et al. Measuring "Negative Body Image": Validation of the Body Image Disturbance Questionnaire in a Non-Clinical Population. *Body Image* 2004; 1:363–372.

55. Palacio RJ. *Wonder.* New York: Knopf (Borzoi Books); 2012.

56. Real T. *Grandiose Women—Shut-Down Men: An Internet Training Course,* 2016, www.terryreal.com.

57. Felitti VJ, Anda RF. The Lifelong Effects of Adverse Childhood Experiences, Chapter 10. In *Chadwick's Child Maltreatment: Sexual Abuse and Psychological Maltreatment,* 4th edition. Florissant [MO]: STM Learning; 2014.

58. Felitti VJ, Anda RF, Nordenberg D, et al. Relationship of Childhood Abuse and Household Dysfunction to Many of the Leading Causes of Death in Adults. *Am J Prev Med* 1998; 14:4:245–258.

59. Felitti VJ, Anda RF. The Lifelong Effects of Adverse Childhood Experiences. *Chadwick's Child Maltreat: Sex Abuse Psychol Maltreat* 2014; 2:203–215.

60. Kerig PK, Bennett DC, Thompson M, et al. Nothing Really Matters: Emotional Numbing as a Link Between Trauma Exposure and Callousness in Delinquent Youth. *J Traumatic Stress* 2012; 25:3:272–279.

61. Ogden P, Fisher J. *Sensorimotor Psychotherapy: Interventions for Trauma and Attachment.* New York: W W Norton & Company; 2015.

62. Kench S, Irwin HJ. Alexithymia and Childhood Family Environment. *J Clin Psychol* 2000; 56:6:737–745.

63. King S. *On Writing: A Memoir of the Craft.* New York: Scribner; 2000:49–50.

64. Recordati G. A Thermodynamic Model of the Sympathetic and Parasympathetic Nervous Systems. *Autonom Neurosci: Basic Clin* 2003; 103:1.

65. Basham K. Transforming the Legacies of Childhood Trauma in Couple and Family Therapy. *Soc Work Health Care* 2004; 39:3–4:263–285.

66. Collins JK. *The Drama—Free Way.* Minneapolis: Wise Ink; 2016.

67. Frank JD, Frank JB. *Persuasion & Healing: A Comparative Study of Psychotherapy.* Baltimore: Johns Hopkins University Press; 1961.

68. Ogden P, Minton K, Pain C. Attachment: The Role of the Body in Dyadic Regulation. In: *Trauma and the Body.* New York: W.W. Norton & Company; 2006:41–64.

69. Schore AN. *Affect Regulation and the Repair of the Self.* New York: W W Norton & Company; 2003.

70. Cousins, N. *Dr Schweitzer of Lambaréné.* New York: Harper Collins, 1960.

71. Marcus P. Some Preliminary Psychological Observations on Narcissism, the Cosmetic Rhinoplasty Patient and the Plastic Surgeon. *Aust NZ J Surg* 1984; 54:543–547.

72. Real, T. *I Don't Want to Talk About It.* New York: Scribner; 1997.

73. Damasio A. *Self Comes to Mind: Constructing the Conscious Brain.* New York: Vintage Books; 2010:96.

74. Damasio A. *Self Comes to Mind: Constructing the Conscious Brain.* New York: Vintage Books; 2010:128.

4

BODY IMAGE AND BODY IMAGE DISORDERS

"Man is summoned to make his own decisions," writes theologian Harvey Cox, former Hollis Professor of Divinity at Harvard Divinity School, *"so to shove them off on someone else, even God or the church, is a betrayal of his manhood."*

This entire book is about choices and whether we make them for ourselves. Dr. Cox' admonition thus applies perfectly: *"Man is that creature who is created to shame and enacts his own destiny. Whenever he relinquishes that privilege to someone else, he ceases to be a man. . . . To be a man . . . means accepting the terrifying duty of deciding who I will be . . . rather than introjecting the stereotypes that others assigned to me."*[1]

★★★★★

She sat on the edge of my examination table with stocking feet swinging off the edge. Her shoes, which had one of those fancy inlaid golden logos I didn't recognize, were tidily arranged on the floor in front of her.

"I have read your papers in my country. Perhaps you are smart enough to treat me. My first surgery was 20 years ago."

I looked at photographs taken before surgery. Her nose was flawless. Yet she had surgery.

"What were you trying to accomplish?"

She looked past me out the window and shook her head slowly. "I don't know. I was crazy."

DOI: 10.4324/9781315657721-6

Her face was grim.

"But afterward, I was devastated. So I went to a famous surgeon. I always go to famous surgeons. He put cadaver cartilage in my nose, then another surgeon put my own cartilage in, then another surgeon put in artificial material. But that got red and painful, and he took it out."

She leaned over and cupped her forehead with her hands. I noticed that she used a lot of body English. Though she wasn't English, she had it down very well.

She straightened and waved her index finger at her face. "Now my nose is too short, I see too much nostril, my tip is pinched, and my upper lip is very bad."

She held the hand mirror to her face.

"Maybe I need jaw surgery." Her voice drifted off.

"I want you to have a lifetime solution," I said. "An implant won't give that. You will need rib grafts, but in a young woman rib can distort. You might need a second surgery if you want the best result I can provide."

"I don't care about that. Where will you put the scar for the rib?"

I pointed to the place on her lower chest.

"I don't want it there. I want it up here, under my breast."

I shook my head.

"That rib is too big. A smaller rib does not have to be changed so much to fit, so it's not as likely to distort."

Her voice got louder.

"No. The scar has to be hidden. I am not some old woman. I have to wear bikinis. I won't let you scar me."

Suddenly her voice quieted and she gave me her best smile, the one that was supposed to make her look cuter than the Tooth Fairy.

"I'm not here for trouble." She gave me the smile again. I think she was disappointed that I didn't get dizzy.

I nodded appreciatively.

"That's comforting," I said. "I give Maintenance enough to do already."

She stared into the mirror, ignoring my little pleasantry.

"I don't know; my feeling is, you know, maybe I shouldn't be asking for surgery."

One month later she returned with her mother. She leafed through photocopied pages from my publications, critiquing each result while her mother stroked her hair. She turned the pages slowly. She sighed. I had been sitting so long that I began to feel like Robinson Crusoe. Now, 17 years later, I would recognize what was happening. But I operated *anyway. Surgery went smoothly. "It is beautiful. It is my old nose again," she said, embraced me, and flew home.*

Four weeks later she was back. She looked tired. Her eyes were wide and frightened. Her mother accompanied her to make sure I was outnumbered. She carried a little notebook. I could see several pages filled with writing. Both were dressed for serious discussions. The room felt hot and overpopulated.

"Take all the grafts out. My nose is worse. Before you operated, my nose was gracious; now it is ugly. You have ruined my face. I don't look like myself anymore. Men won't look at me. And I am still swollen."

"More surgery isn't safe yet. It's been only one month since surgery."

She doubled over, covering her face with her hands. At first she controlled her crying but soon it got away from her. Her shoulders shook, her chest heaved and then stopped while she held her breath, mascara trickling down her cheeks.

Her mother stood and rubbed her back. "No one should have to suffer like this," she said. Mother stared at me, then wrote something in her notebook. Probably a note to call her attorney. She frowned at me.

"We are chastising you," Mother said. "Aren't you sorry?"

I smiled. "Not yet." But maybe soon.

Suddenly the crying ended. The patient blinked until I came back into focus.

"How could you be so stupid." She stopped to wipe her eyes with her sleeve, assured herself that I was still there, took a deep breath, and sobbed again, stopping to speak when she needed to take a breath. It began to seem scripted.

"I was in love before the surgery. Do you know how love feels? Now he left me. How can you know how awful that is? You have made me age. You have stopped my life. I am hideous."

She sat back and gave me a stare. It was supposed to be piercing, but all she had mastered was petulant.

"I want you to operate today."

I tried to look steadfast. She liked talking about herself.

"I think you will be fine. But it's too soon for revisions." I gave my most reassuring smile.

"At my first operation they gave me a hematoma," she said. "Do you remember that?"

"I do."

"It was not a hematoma," Mother said. "It was a blood clot." She sat back down again.

The patient scowled. "Mother, it was a hematoma."

"Don't listen to her, Doctor," Mother said. She sighed quietly and patted her daughter's back again.

"Sometimes her memory isn't good anymore. It was a blood clot."

The patient pushed out her lower lip like a teenager who'd just been grounded.

"What's the difference in your mind?" I asked Mother.

She made a dismissive gesture. "It's too complicated to explain," she said.

"Because most people consider them the same," I said. Her daughter sat up straighter and passed her eyes between us.

"You are avoiding the subject," her mother said, and leaned forward. "We have questions."

The silence got livelier. She nodded to prompt her daughter.

"My profile is beautiful. It's just what I wanted."

I began to relax.

*****

"But everything else is wrong. You have to make my tip smaller, and flatten the right side, just 2 millimeters."

She turned her head in front of the hand mirror.

"And see, the profiles aren't the same, and my nose is too large for my face, and the top has to be made smaller."

She lowered her head and studied me beneath her brows.

"I understand these things. I am an engineer."

She won't fire me yet, I thought. No one else has been able to tolerate her. Somehow that wasn't comforting.

"If we operate again, I need more details. Study your pictures and write me about what you'd like," I said.

Her six-page letter read like the Unabomber Manifesto. Accompanying photos indicated that another surgeon had made recent changes.

"I must see you. I promise to behave myself this time. I will take tranquilizers."

"The rib scar is very ugly. The left half of the tip is higher. The asymmetry is very marked. I see veins on the tip. My nose is giving me great anxiety. I have had to increase my antidepressants. Before you operated on me, I was very happy [emphasis original]. I have read your operative report. It says 'the mucoperichondrial flaps were re-approximated.' This is not clear to me. How did you shape your spreader grafts? Like the doctor on the Internet?"

"I have labeled the photos. The vertical distance between point A and the base of the columella is approximately 0.7 cm in photograph two but approximately 0.8 cm in photo one. Now, we have a trapezoid ABEF on top of a rectangle EFCD. The most protruding point seems to lie along EF rather than along CD and is closer to an ideal vertical tangent. The distance between points O and N is now 11 mm instead of 10 mm. In some lights the nose appears divided into two parts above and below line EF. I like the new columella, but it is not compatible with the tip."

"But I am confident that you are the only surgeon to help me with my nose."

Body Image Development and Standards

Body image and the extent of one's desire to be attractive are intensely subjective and affected by how each of us interprets our worlds. Rarely is self-esteem better displayed than in anyone's opinion about his or her body.

The body image literature is extensive and thoughtful. What is perhaps most curious is its sizable overlap with the body shame literature. Much "body image" literature deals with body dissatisfaction.[2] It is harder to find data on people who are happy about the way they look than on those who don't, perhaps a commentary on our world—just as it is easier to find more research on depression than on happiness.

We learn early. Even as children, we learn from legends, classical mythology, and nursery rhymes. Witches are never beautiful. Princesses and fairies always are. Deformity symbolizes or accentuates evil. Captain Hook wasn't Captain Hook by accident. The scarred face signifies a gangster. One-armed movie characters are rarely heroes. Hunchbacks, wooden legs, withered hands (Matthew 12:1–9), and bizarre facial distortions become metaphors that have powerful psychological ramifications for the patients who have them. Every hand surgeon recognizes the embarrassment and shame (and, for men, the sense of impotence) that can attach to upper extremity injuries. In fact, early body image research attempted to explain "phantom limbs," sensate extremities still experienced by patients even after amputation. In one experiment, plastic surgery patients were instructed to draw self-portraits before and after surgical correction. Unexpectedly, patients who had the most marked surgical improvements drew images that still resembled their presurgical images, but patients who had more subtle improvements drew self-portraits that were strikingly more attractive.[3] Harvey Cushing intimately understood what appearance epithets can do to the soul: "In May 1927 he wrote a rare letter to *Time* magazine, criticizing its frivolous and cruel derision of an acromeglic who was being exhibited as the 'World's Ugliest Woman' in the Ringling Brothers' circus."[3]

Early researchers Schilder (1935) and then Fisher and Cleveland[4] related body image to "boundaries" that could be respected or penetrated and thereby created body image for which accurate or distorted perceptions could be assigned. Body image became a projection of mental experience. Shontz[5] offered the opposing view: that body image began in the body and was processed in the brain.

These constructs are now considered insufficiently comprehensive: each theory is both right and incomplete. Theoretical body image construction is both "top-down" (rational and cortical) and "bottom-up" (based on sensory perception and brain stem/midbrain function). This distinction is provocative. If body image is shaped by childhood experiences and modified by abuse or neglect—felt somatically—much of our body perception is a midbrain phenomenon. Patients react before they think or feel. The extent to which any trauma wound has influenced a patient's sense of self-worth will add an unconscious element to body awareness and body image and thus affect self-worth, thought processing, and the patient's desire to care for his or her body. The difficulty for all clinicians is recognizing these trauma-based modulators and their triggers.

Common Themes in the Body Image Literature

Key body image principles can be summarized by bullet points.

- Body image and self-esteem are closely linked.
- Western culture places great emphasis on appearance, which especially targets girls and women.
- Body shame is common, especially among women.
- The motivation for improvement often implicates perfectionism, idolatry, or delusional thinking. Societal standards of beauty are transmitted by family, peers, and media, absorbed by individuals, and create body satisfaction or dissatisfaction.
- Family members, particularly parents, profoundly affect body image and can generate body shame.
- The degree to which an individual is susceptible to external beauty standards depends on self-esteem and therefore indirectly upon the child's caregivers.
- Evidence of impaired family functioning is common. Parents influence their children's body images directly and indirectly, by criticism or feeding habits or by examples of their own grooming and dietary behavior.
- Prejudice against obesity begins in very young children, and can influence later employment and even medical examinations.
- Obesity is attributed to genetic factors, stress, sleep, not counting calories, circadian rhythms, and medications. Body shame, neglect, and abuse are almost never cited.
- The printed and electronic media are oppressive and create overpowering thoughts of physical inferiority in susceptible women, who are thus driven to plastic surgery.

- For unknown reasons the degree of deformity does not often correspond to the distress that it generates.
- Some individuals are more susceptible to teasing and more conscious of body image than others. The reasons are unknown.
- Body shame affects happiness, mental health, and social anxiety, and can be associated with deliberate self-injury.[6,7,8,9]
- Physical attractiveness confers status and rank.
- Cultural "attractiveness" is partly evolutionary, and therefore susceptible to both environmental and genetic factors. It takes only 150 milliseconds to decide whether a face is attractive. Correlated with electroencephalographic activity, several studies have indicated that facial aesthetics, emotion, and speech factor equally in determining personal appeal and are processed separately by the brain. Three components of facial attractiveness are critical: averageness, symmetry, and neoteny (juvenile features in an adult).[10]

Body Image in Context and Application

This latter point deserves elaboration. *Averageness* indicates similarity to a typical phenotype for a group and therefore signals genetic diversity (and presumably greater health and disease resistance). *Symmetry* seems obvious; in fact, studies across a number of species have shown that less "fluctuating asymmetry" (i.e., greater symmetry) is associated with both fitness and fertility. It is not simple youthfulness but *neoteny* that is particularly associated with facial attractiveness. A baby's features (large eyes, small nose, round cheeks, smooth skin, glossy hair, and lighter skin tones) correlate with greater perceived attractiveness, more paternal attention, and even a lower incidence of child abuse. A preference for childlike facial features appears consistently across ethnic populations, regardless of sexual orientation.

Attractiveness is also associated with sexual dimorphism—that is, the degree to which a particular face resembles the prototype of his or her sex. In men, this means larger jaws and supraorbital ridges; more prominent cheekbones; smaller eyes; thinner lips; and wider, larger noses. In women, dimorphism indicates prominent cheekbones; smooth, hairless skin; wider eyes; higher, thinner eyebrows; smaller jaws; fuller lips; and shorter, smaller noses.[11]

Therefore although facial attractiveness may not conform to mathematical or Renaissance proportions, it derives nevertheless from species-specific psychological adaptations.[12,13] Artists including Dürer, Alberti, Cousin, Audran, Francesca, Pacioli, Cennini, Savonarola, and da Vinci formulated a series of canons that are still used in art and subsequently in medicine through the influence of the artist-anatomists of the seventeenth through nineteenth centuries. Here are a few that surgeons use:

The head can be divided into halves at a horizontal line through the eyes.
The face can be divided into thirds, with the nose occupying the middle third.

The head can be divided into quarters, with the middle quarters being the forehead and nose, respectively.

The length of the ear is equal to the length of the nose.

The distance between the eyes is equal to the width of the nose.

The distance between the eyes is equal to the width of each eye.

The width of the mouth is 1½ times the width of the nose.

Bashour[10] tabulated the prevalence of each of these aesthetic ideals in groups of Caucasians, blacks, and Han Chinese. Not a single criterion applied to all ethnic groups, and the only one that exceeded 50% prevalence was nasal width equaling one quarter facial width (51.5% in Han Chinese). Even among Caucasians, for whom all rules should apply best because they were created by European artists, only one ("inter-canthal distance equals inter-alar distance") applied to 41% of the population; all others were significantly less prevalent; four did not apply at all.

These guidelines may be useful to portrait artists, but they almost never apply in humans. Yet individuals focused on body image still try to achieve them, surgeons still teach and use them, and both doctors and patients get discouraged and confused when they do not work or when following them creates unnatural deformities.[12]

It is hard to conceive that body dysmorphic disorder might be a favorable evolutionary change, as Stein has noted.[14] Most BDD patients are not driven to be attractive, but rather not to be ugly.

Body Image Beyond the Face

Beyond the face, there are other markers of physical attractiveness. Researchers who use the Waist-to-Hip Ratio (WHR) contend that low-ratio women (i.e., more voluptuous) are universally more attractive. However, it turns out that body mass index (BMI) far outweighs the importance of the WHR. Thinner bodies are perceived to be more attractive than heavier ones, relevant to obesity, considered below. One study has documented that 70% of adolescent girls want to be thinner than they are.[15, 16] Eating disorder researchers have contended that pathological eating is a millennia-old attempt by which women compete for sexual partners. The same logic has been applied to slenderness and muscularity for men. Perhaps the most interesting finding is how commonly eating disorders are comorbid with perfectionism. Rather than search through the millennia, it is not hard to conjecture that the young child, influenced by parental example, abuse, neglect, criticism, or abandonment, can become perfectionistic in order to survive and avoid punishment in a dysfunctional household; and that perfectionism and obsessive body surveillance surface later in carried shame, body dissatisfaction, and pathologic eating.

Twin studies have been contrasted with adoption studies; both provide provocative results. Much literature concludes that genetic influence is "moderate to large," based on the observation that 50% or more of tested individuals within families have body image problems.[17] However, of the 27 studies tabulated, only 14 have body dissatisfaction or weight preoccupation prevalence scores of 50% or greater, and only 6 exceed 60%. At the same time, adoption studies have shown body dissatisfaction prevalences that approximate 60%. A prevalence of 47% body image disturbance in preadolescent and adolescent females has been cited as "moderate genetic influences"; other studies indicate minimal genetic influences. The findings are not reassuringly uniform. A skeptic could argue instead that the axiom "body weight problems are heritable" may be heavily influenced by another observation: childhood abuse and neglect and their coping mechanisms also run in families. Epigenetic factors (genetically transmissible) can also apply. Research in this area is understandably difficult, but when the body image literature and the mental health literature are unable to document high genetic prevalences in twins, adoption studies, or body dysmorphic disorder patients, it is reasonable to speculate that there may be other even more powerful—and common—factors at work.

★★★★★

Neuroimaging findings support this hypothesis. Studies that compare girls and women with and without anorexia nervosa demonstrate increased activity in the fusiform gyrus (active in face and body recognition), left cerebral hemisphere, pre-frontal cortex, and temporal lobe; and even more striking activity in the amygdala and anterior cingulate cortex, coincidentally also active in traumatized and PTSD patients and those with body dysmorphic disorder (Chapters 2, 7). When anorexic women are tested for body distortion imaging, they perceive as accurately as patients without eating disorders.[18] Paradoxically, however, they see their own bodies as too wide.[7, 19] Patients who have undergone bariatric surgery with massive weight loss still see fat bodies in the mirror. Neuroimaging findings document patients' anxiety in seeing their own faces and bodies, but is it not also possible that some underlying cause could account for both the anxiety and the body dissatisfaction?

The Effect of Body on Self-Image

Personality and physical characteristics each influence body image. Adults react more favorably to cute children; obese children are more often rejected and teased. However, researchers note that healthy self-worth provides "resilience" to such teasing, just as those without self-esteem or social support become more vulnerable. Yamamia's research indicates that exposure to thin model images for only five minutes can increase body dissatisfaction.[20] However, not all women are the same, and those with self-esteem are resistant to becoming body dissatisfied. Those observations make sense: self-worth and resilience are always antidotes. Nurturing parents teach their children boundaries, which enables them to judge incoming criticism and disregard it when indicated. Perfectionistic patients are especially at risk and manifest their body images through grandiosity or unhappy disempowerment. "Self-worth" is often tagged as a principal factor in individual body image.[7, 21]

McKinley repeatedly links "self-worth" to body dissatisfaction.[22] More frequent body surveillance is associated with lower body satisfaction and more eating problems. Similarly, higher body shame correlates with more frequent body surveillance, lower satisfaction, lower psychological well-being, and more eating disorders. Men diagnosed with "body dysmorphia" have elevated prevalences of mood and anxiety disorders, obsessive compulsive behavior, substance abuse, and impairment in social and occupational functioning. The subgroup that also uses anabolic steroids also displays other high-risk behavior: recreational drug use, unsafe injection practices, or unprotected sexual behavior.[23]

Cultural and Gender Differences

There are differences within cultures and sexual orientations. As a rule, American and European women are more dissatisfied than African American and Latino women. Lesbian women have higher body surveillance than heterosexual women. African American women suffer more skin tone shame than Caucasians.[24–26] Gay men manifest more body dissatisfaction than heterosexual men, especially with regard to muscularity. Gay men and heterosexual women appear to be those most unhappy with their bodies.[27] Finally, younger women have higher levels of body shame than middle-aged women;[28, 29] and body image dissatisfaction in young women predicts depression and self-esteem as they age. Writers who allege that women who seek cosmetic surgery are only dupes of unscrupulous surgeons may not remember the centuries-old desire in both men and women to be attractive, whether by perfumes, makeup, dress, or body modification by scarification, tattooing, foot binding, earlobe or lip stretching, or body piercing. Although much of the information about body attitudes comes from self-administered questionnaires without clinician input, the results are believable and should not be lightly dismissed.[7]

Body dissatisfaction does not disappear once it is established, except perhaps in women over age 60, who appear to become more satisfied with their bodies as they age.[30] Perhaps most interesting is the observation that body surveillance and body shame correlate with other health indicators, like smoking and high-risk sexual behavior. This is not unexpected based on the Adverse Childhood Events study and our own research on the childhoods of plastic surgery patients (Chapter 9).

The Effect of Body Shame

Shame is distinct from dissatisfaction, and carries with it the added sense of humiliation and inferiority—of being "less than" others—that encompasses how a person perceives others' reactions. In turn, shame drives social exclusion and anxiety, each of which can be modulated by the family environment.[8]

There is, however, good news: patients with positive body images are also optimistic, have adequate social support, good coping mechanisms, stable body weights, and assured senses of self-worth.[21, 31–33] Relate these characteristics to the developmental model in Chapter 3: Functional adults have self-esteem, good boundaries, and appropriate reality; live in moderation; and care for themselves. Thus one's attitude toward oneself encompasses both body and environment. A sense of abundance only manifests in a balanced life and makes the qualities that we call "resilience" possible.

Tylka examines the subject from the opposite perspective: What are the characteristics of positive body image?[34] It turns out that they mirror the traits of functional adults: appreciation for their bodies' unique appearance and functioning; unconditional acceptance from family and peers; recognition that personality and inner qualities trump external appearances; optimism; healthy social networking; awareness of the fantasy of idealized media images; good self-care; and belief that a higher power has conferred specialness on each of them.[35] It is easy to match these characteristics to the five core traits discussed in Chapter 3 and to the characteristics that define resilience (Chapter 10).

Also optimistic is Wood-Barcalow's study, which indicates that negative body image can be overcome by "protective filtering" (i.e., intact boundaries), interpersonal support, associating with others who have good body images, and conceptualizing beauty very broadly (i.e., realistically).[36]

> *"So we beat on, boats against the current, borne back ceaselessly into the past." With this sentence Fitzgerald concludes* The Great Gatsby,[37] *the story of several friends whose intertwined lives do just that. Our histories only define us if we let them.*

Body Image Development and Obesity

Body image develops early. Even infants respond to videos of other infants and at age 2 begin to recognize themselves in mirrors and photographs. At ages 4 to 6, when children start to demonstrate pride and feel embarrassment or healthy shame, they also start to compare themselves to other children. This is also the age at which childhood abuse or neglect can wound and influence the child's sense of self-worth, abilities to perceive reality, trust others, and protect themselves.[38–41] Even preschoolers recognize obesity among their peers and adults, and girls become more attuned to body image than boys. By age three, children already have negative attitudes about obesity and rate thin or average sized figures as nicer, smarter, more popular, cuter, and quieter than chubby figures.[42] Despite this awareness and stigmatization, US childhood obesity is currently 17%, and extreme obesity 5.8%.[43–47] Preschoolers already understand that body weight is controllable, and therefore ascribe negative attributes to their overweight peers.

What these children do not yet recognize is that obesity is only controllable when it is a problem, not a solution.

Adults studying this problem are not much ahead. Experts still hope to identify abnormal causative genes or brain abnormalities, or rely on new food and nutrition studies, limited restaurant portions, sugar taxes, and development of more low-calorie items as solutions to obesity:[44, 47, 48]

> NBC Nightly News reported on Friday that FDA . . . announced a major revamp for nutritional labels. . . . The rules better correspond with updated dietary guidelines and health research. . . "calories from fat" will be eliminated.
>
> (*AMA Wire*, May 20, 2016)

> The *Los Angeles Times* reports that US adults who are obese now outnumber those who are merely overweight. . . . 67.6 million Americans over the age of 25 were obese as of 2012, and an additional 65.2 million were overweight.
>
> (*AMA Wire*, June 23, 2015)

Etiologic explanations and treatments for obesity parallel almost entirely those for body dysmorphic disorder, alcoholism, and smoking; and researchers have indeed observed that obese people's brains show addiction-like responses to some foods.[45] Genetic sequence variations, mutations in the hypothalamic leptin-signaling pathway, and other metabolic factors continue to be investigated, though the incidences of documented abnormalities are in the low percentages.[47] Unfortunately, the family is rarely considered, even though its prevalence among obese individuals is 100 percent.

Despite better education about each of these health risks, their incidences continue to rise, suggesting that simply ignoring adverse effects is not the reason that people do not change behaviors. They eat excessively, drink, and smoke even though they know better, suggesting that each of these behaviors is only a problem to their observers. "Fat acceptance"—increasing toleration and justification of excessive weight—fuels the problem.[47]

Media influences, glorifying excessive thinness and Barbie doll figures are commonly cited in the literature as major factors, but how much impact the media has also depends upon the child's sense of self-worth, boundaries, and reality processing. If the media is truly that powerful, why doesn't every girl develop an eating disorder? Why are 35% of men and 40.4% of women in the US population obese (BMI over 30) or morbidly obese (BMI over 40 in 5.5% of men and 9.9% of women)?[48] There have to be other factors. In fact, longitudinal media exposure and adolescent body image studies have not found significant correlations.[49] My speculation is that if the test subjects were divided according to their self-esteem, lower senses of self-worth would correspond to greater media influences and poorer body images.

Literary, Familial, Peer, and Societal Influences

Children's stories and cartoons are also influences. The Lost Boys in Disney's *Peter Pan* each had comical appearances (obesity, prominent ears, overbite), but Peter was slender and athletic, and Wendy, John, and Michael were each attractive or cute, reinforcing the subliminal association between goodness and beauty.[7] However, stimulus is only one side; susceptibility (self-esteem, boundaries, and reality) is the other—a truism that applies to all addictions and unregulated behaviors. Exposure to media or literary ideals does not automatically create body or self-dissatisfaction. In the body image literature, boundaries are termed "autonomy"—the ability to accept or resist external pressures and ideals. Even the power of peer pressure has been questioned. A study in 12-year-old girls[50] documented that body dissatisfaction preceded peer influence by one-to-two years. Not surprisingly, adolescents who see themselves unfavorably join peers who feel the same way.

Surgeons who treat children and adolescents with congenital anomalies recognize that adaptation to deformity is a family project. The observation that different children with equivalent facial deformities can attribute a higher or lower importance to them is a real life example that any deformity does not automatically correspond to the amount of distress that the patient or family feels.[51] I have seen this phenomenon in the broad behavior spectrum of teenagers referred for deformities associated with cleft lip and palate. Some are young people who avert their gazes and cannot speak for themselves, accompanied by controlling, aggressive, guilt-ridden parents; and others are patients with open, smiling, relational faces who can articulate their surgical goals who have already established themselves as leaders among their peers. The parents who support them are relaxed and connected but defer surgical decisions to the patients. The difference depends entirely upon the importance and significance placed on the deformity by the parents and the degree to which carried shame spills over onto their children.

★★★★★

During adolescence parents become increasingly influential as they model good or bad eating habits or the importance of physical perfection. I have had patients whose mothers forced them to diet even as young children, or gave them laxatives and enemas if they gained weight. As I have taken more childhood histories, I have been impressed by the number of cosmetic surgery patients who described previous or current, treated or untreated, eating disorders that began in adolescence. Even research on adolescent girls notes the critical accompanying factors of self-esteem, depression, and perfectionism.[52] The more body-focused girls are, the more likely they are to be depressed. Children learn to mirror their parents' body dissatisfaction and absorb it—carry it—as their own. Parental criticism of a child's weight or body shape impacts body dissatisfaction and may create body shame binds that can persist into adulthood.[53] What these young people fear most is peer rejection based on their physical appearances, a destructive logic generated in abusive homes; [54] those raised by non-nurturing caregivers already know how rejection feels.

Anderson, Gooze, Lemeshow et al. demonstrated in a survey of 977 subjects that adolescent obesity was 2.45 times higher among subjects with poor-quality maternal relationships.[55] Andrews documented another fascinating finding in a study of 70 burned adults, in which there was no relationship between burn severity and depression.[56] I have noted the same in my own patients. *Opportunity is not the same as susceptibility.* The same findings appear in groups with psoriasis, vitiligo, or craniofacial anomalies.[21] Other researchers have found that the quality of life that burn patients recover depends largely on the quality of life before the burn. Associated with those patients are good self-esteem, attentive and loving families, and the ability to remain optimistic—mirroring the factors that protect against PTSD in battle.[57] We have found a different relationship in our patients, in which the severity of childhood abuse or neglect did not correlate with patient resilience (Chapter 9). Our more resilient patients did not necessarily have easier childhoods.

★★★★★

Patients vary widely in how they interpret the reactions of others. Recall from Chapter 3 that any patient's reality depends upon what individuals "make up" from sensory input and how they react to it. The patient who believes that "strangers stare at me because of my nose and think I am ugly" has chosen to interpret undefined observations in a punishing way. How we string together our observations, beliefs, and responsive feelings depends on what we were taught, experienced, and observed at very young ages. The patient who values appearance highly often assumes that everyone else feels and judges the same way. This is where it can get confusing. If we assume that all information processing is "top-down," beginning with rational thoughts, it becomes impossible to understand those patient ideas and behaviors that are, in fact, "bottom-up"—when patients react before they think. There are a lot of them.

Adolescent boys seem to have it easier, probably because of peer influence, but how much peers matter depends heavily on parental attitude and feedback. Muscularity and athleticism appear to be more important than physical beauty for boys; sports and team collegiality may therefore be protective.[58]

★★★★★

"What is it that keeps this world as decent and hopeful as it is? It is the men and women who in a time when you might expect them to be cynical, disillusioned, discouraged and out of faith, are not. . . . Faith is man's inner self-committal to convictions and causes and persons that seem to him supremely true and worthwhile."

Here Harry Emerson Fosdick, the minister who stimulated the "modernist" (i.e., non-fundamentalist) movement in the American Protestant church, quotes George Bernard Shaw.[59] *"The real opposites of faith are cynicism, disillusionment; the sense of futility . . . that life . . . means nothing. . . . What a man believes may be ascertained not from his Creed, but from the assumptions on which he habitually acts."*
We can indeed escape our pasts.

★★★★★

No one knows how often parental teasing, criticism, or ridicule create or intensify body image disorders because most studies were not designed to answer that question. Parental criticism is often noted but not tabulated, which suggests that it was considered an incidental finding. Verbal abuse is only destructive when boundaries function poorly. Porous boundaries leave self-esteem, reality processing, self-care, and living in moderation each at risk. It follows that adolescents who like their own appearances also like those of their peers and family.[7, 60]

Most overweight children or adolescents were not overweight at birth or early in their lives. My own clinical experience supports Felitti's observation that weight increase, obesity, or anorexia occurred suddenly at some eventful time, which most patients can date precisely: following sexual abuse, abandonment, divorce, increased alcohol or drug abuse by the parents, a difficult relocation, sudden poverty, or the cumulative effect of chronic parental depression.[61] Obesity and eating disorders become compensatory behaviors for underlying intrafamilial abuse or neglect. This schema is not compatible with the concept that overweight patients are simply lazy, with poor willpower and "prone to overeating."[62] Childhood abuse prevalences are high in morbidly obese adults.[63–65] Do obesity and eating disorders also occur with the same incidence among people raised in nurturing, loving households? Apparently no one knows, but I suspect that they do not.

Body Image in Adults

Less research has been performed on adults over 30, but some does exist, usually cross-sectional and not longitudinal studies (which would have provided useful information about individuals' body images over time), but some conclusions can still be drawn.

Even for adults, media pressures remain, and aging men and women are less likely to be portrayed as attractive and sexual, with a few exceptions. Bodies of adult actors are less exposed than those of younger actors. Aging adults may be portrayed as asexual, lonely, or depressed.

But that is Hollywood's output; how it is absorbed by each adult depends upon the adult. There is some evidence that many women do not become more body dissatisfied as they age.[30] Opposing this optimistic finding are reports that more than 50% of men and women over the age of 40 felt *ashamed* (italics mine) of their appearances.[66] This body shame does not diminish with age.[32] When dissatisfaction does occur, weight seems to be its primary focus. Even in adulthood, teasing is associated with increased body dissatisfaction; spousal criticism correlates with worse body esteem, and spousal praise correlates with better body esteem, regardless of body size or BMI.[67] As in youth, men are generally more body image satisfied than women, and when dissatisfaction does appear, it is usually linked to a desire to look younger. These are, however, associations, not predictors, because so much depends on the boundaries of the receiving party and his or her resilience.

★★★★★

The degree to which body image links to self-esteem is extremely variable, a phenomenon that plastic surgeons notice daily in their practices. The literature indicates that body dissatisfaction is associated with low self-esteem for both men and women.[68] Body dissatisfaction can be predicted by individual self-esteem, weight teasing, and comparison to media body ideals.[69] Especially sensitive individuals develop "self-schema," salient concepts of their appearances. Self-discrepancy theory proposes that any difference between an individual's own body image and their media influences can create chronic vulnerability, body dissatisfaction, and depression.[70, 71]

The key is how much "other esteem" patients receive from their physical appearances. Those who have the sense of individual preciousness from a very early age are less troubled than those whose self-esteem is not internal but based on externals.

Where is the boundary at which healthy interest in appearance and self-care becomes excessive or self-hating? When does body dissatisfaction turn to body shame ("I am ugly." "I am a freak.")?[72] The question is not rhetorical. In the DSM-5, the difference appears to be whether the imperfection is visible to others and how much distress it causes; but each depends upon the eye of the observer and the sensitivity of the individual, both broad variables. "The major conceptual inadequacy is the lack of any underlying unifying framework."[66] I agree. In the context, however, of nurturing or traumatic childhood development and its effect upon anyone's ability to become a functional adult, the relationships seem much clearer.

★★★★★

"My son is going to be an opera singer." She let each word ring in its own space. "He takes lessons."

Her son looked about 45. He'd have to hurry. He might be able to sing, but he was long-legged and lithe and looked more like one of the dancers for Cirque du Soleil. Right now he was sitting on the examination table, chewing gum and staring at his cell phone.

"Stand up when the doctor comes into the room." He nodded absently. He didn't move.

"Clarence." She paced each syllable. He ignored her.

"He's pathetic," she said. *"It must be his generation. I did everything for him."*

She folded her arms.

"Sit up straight when you speak to the doctor." Without looking he gave me a languid handshake and continued to study his phone. He chewed his gum.

"We are here to see about a rhinoplasty." She tipped her head back and stared through her glasses the way a lizard looks at a grasshopper. I resisted the stare.

"Where did you go to medical school?" She knew the answer from the diplomas in the waiting room. This was just my audition. I smiled encouragingly. I was pretty sure that she had spent most of her life considering herself and little else.

"That's a wonderful career, opera singing," I said. *"Who is your voice coach?"*

He sat silently. I had no way of knowing if he'd heard me.

"We have traveled a very long way to see you because you are a subspecialist. My son requires a subspecialist. I believe that he needs a cephalic trim. Will you do a cephalic trim?" She struck her imperious pose.

I turned to him. *"So, what do you dislike about your nose?"*

He spoke without looking up.

"I'm not sure." His voice was tight and strident, like a child talking to someone else's parent.

"Tell him, Clarence." There was no response, yet there was an exceptional intimacy between them. His eyes had clouded over. Maybe his blood was congealing, like mine. I thought of Tennessee Williams' line in Cat on a Hot Tin Roof: *"It's no use; we talk in circles and have nothing to say to each other."*

She continued. *"His nose needs to be shorter, like this."* She turned and lifted his tip with her index finger.

A tiny grimace flickered across his face and then disappeared. He had been through this exercise before. She stroked his hair and spoke to him in the voice you use with a puppy.

"He'll always be my little baby."

She continued.

"And I want it understood: if he has to undress before surgery, I will remove his underwear, not the nurses."

I was beginning to understand the real problem—at least part of it.

"Is that right—what your mother is telling me about your nose?" I said.

I heard her voice again. So far, this was like some odd ventriloquist act. I asked him and she answered. He didn't even move his lips.

"Doctor, pay attention. His tip is too wide and ugly. It needs to be much narrower and should look like this—see how I'm pinching it? It needs to be thin. He can't look like his father."

She showed me. He didn't move.

"Tell him the rest, Clarence." Her back stiffened. He stared at his phone.

"All right, dear, be an idiot." She pivoted toward me. "Doctor, we don't want a bump on our nose."

The Familial Environment and Body Image

A young child's parents are gods. The child depends on them for food, clothing, shelter, love, acceptance, and protection. By observing them, children form their own understandings of male, female, and parental behavior. The drive for parental approval, therefore, is profoundly strong. When parents are excessively critical or demand perfection and do not allow their children to be spontaneous, vulnerable, and imperfect, body image suffers, as does the child's self-esteem and his or her ability to become a functional, independent adult.

The literature reinforces these findings. When parents criticize the child's appearance, it affects the child's body image. When parents prize thinness or muscularity, it affects their children's' attitudes toward eating and exercise. The degree to which parents help their children develop appropriate boundaries will determine how sensitive their children are to appearance or parental criticism through their childhoods and into the adolescent years.

Teasing about weight is common and destructive. However, there are other types of trauma not always emphasized the body image literature. Explicitly unfavorable messages about appearance or other verbal abuse or emotional neglect do not occur in an otherwise perfect household. Parents who do not help their children develop their own senses of self-worth usually lack it themselves. The misconception that goodness and approval depend on perfect appearance flags non-nurturing parenting. Emotional abuse, emotional neglect, and living with an alcoholic or drug-addicted parent are the most common types of childhood trauma among the patients in my practice compared to a general medical population (Chapter 9).[73–75] Each trauma type creates feelings of shame and defectiveness that can drift into adulthood and create what we later observe as absent self-esteem, perfectionism, obesity, failure to trust, excessive sensitivity to teasing, or eating disorders.[76] These are not random or independent outcomes, but rather products of poorly functioning home environments. "Beyond a person's perceived satisfaction or dissatisfaction with his or her body, affect also plays an important role . . . feelings of anxiety, distress . . . and shame, often expressed as the result of failing to meet perceived cultural ideals of appearance"[77]—or failing to meet parental expectations and achieve parental approval, I would add. Sadly, those women driven to achieve media-defined appearance ideals hold the subliminal belief that achieving them will improve their lives.

Sexual Abuse and Body Image

As the successful professional woman emerged from anesthesia after a routine and successful operation, she began to struggle violently in the operating table, wrestling away from the nurses and anesthesiologist who were trying to keep her from falling. Straining against them, she began to scream. "Let go of me. Let go. No taking shirts off. No taking shirts off." With her cortical function impaired by the anesthesia and the sensation of being overpowered and on her back, she propelled back to her sexually abused wounded child, and spoke with the immature language that she used at the time. When I asked her later how the abuse had affected her life, she realized that she had become untrusting, unwilling to marry, driven to excellence and perfectionism in her career, and remote from social contacts. These are the lightning flashes of childhood trauma.

Sexual abuse is a profoundly intimate physical boundary violation and the strongest type of body-connected abuse, often worsened by caregivers who will not believe or protect the child. Added to the sexual abuse are therefore emotional abuse and neglect, a dreadfully powerful combination. We have found that many types of abuse and neglect do not occur discretely but in predicable groups (Chapter 9).

The connection between childhood sexual abuse, body image, and body shame is a broad topic and will be discussed further in Chapter 6. The relevant points in the body image literature can be summarized.

- Sexual abuse may occur by itself, may be accompanied by eating disorders or self-harming behavior, and is often associated with borderline personality disorder.
- The link between childhood sexual abuse and borderline personality disorder appears to be mediated by guilt and shame.
- Borderline personality disorder also correlates with body image disturbances. Childhood sexual abuse generates negative adult body images. Patients recount histories of sexual abuse and explicitly seek multiple types of aesthetic surgery to transform themselves into people who were never abused.
- Patients who have been sexually abused and also have body dysmorphic disorder seek more types and more extensive aesthetic surgery than those who have not been abused. In fact, they find the surgical experience paradoxically pleasurable.

- Childhood sexual abuse is particularly associated with bulimia nervosa and binge-eating disorder, as well as adulthood obesity.
- In some studies, physical and emotional abuse are even more strongly tied to eating disorders than childhood sexual abuse.
- Patients with histories of sexual abuse have more negative body perceptions than those with nonsexual traumatization or without trauma histories.[76, 77, 78]
- Sexually abused children and adolescents can dissociate from their bodies or turn on their bodies in anger and confusion. Their sense of what is "me" and what is "outside me" becomes poorly defined. Both self-harm and anorexia provide ways of turning on their bodies. "My body betrayed me. . . . Therefore I hate my body."[79]
- Childhood sexual abuse and borderline personality disorder are associated with a variety of self-harm behaviors, including cutting and burning. This association has been found largely in abused females, not males. In effect, these patients treat their bodies with the same cruelty and indifference as did their aggressors.[80, 81]
- The strongest mediator between childhood sexual abuse and eating disorders is body shame. Girls who have been sexually abused may become disgusted with their bodies and try to change them through surgery or deliberate self-injury.
- The overwhelming emotional pain of childhood sexual abuse can be temporarily relieved by self-harm; because alexithymia is so common in childhood sexual abuse victims, self-injury may be a form of reconnecting their emotions to physical sensations.[80]
- Many childhood abuse survivors have altered pain sensations and may report a sense of disembodiment from themselves.
- When sexually abused girls dissociate from their bodies, their bodies no longer belong to them, which decreases their self-perceived disgust, inadequacy, or shame.

There will be more to say about childhood sexual abuse and its ramifications subsequently, but these observations become part of a cohesive whole if they are placed in the context of all types of childhood abuse and neglect. Emotional abuse is broadly considered to be even more destructive than physical or sexual abuse, explained in part by how comparatively often emotional abuse can occur. Children can be criticized, insulted, berated, and shamed more frequently than they can be sexually abused. Of all the patients whose childhoods I have surveyed for childhood abuse or neglect, very few patients report only one type of abuse: the median number of positive answers was 2.9. Traumatized children do not grow up in households where everything is perfect except for sexual abuse.

★★★★★

It is not difficult to imagine how Winston Churchill's neglectful mother and verbally abusive father might have powered his drive and personality. Churchill quotes a letter that his father wrote him upon admission to Sandhurst: *"Do not think I am going to take the trouble of writing you long letters after every folly and failure you commit. . . . I am certain that if you cannot prevent yourself from leaving the idle, useless, unprofitable life you have had during your school days and later months you will become a mere social wastrel, one of the hundreds of the public-school failures, and you will degenerate into a shabby, unhappy, and futile existence."*

How Children Cope With the Family Environment

If childhood abuse and neglect are starting points and the common final pathway is defectiveness or shame, and if children learn to cope in this environment and eventually medicate their pain with addictions, everything falls into line. Obesity is self-medication. Eating disorders and alexithymia become medications, as do cutting or self-harming, factitious injuries, promiscuity, risky sexual behavior, perfectionism, alcohol or drug abuse, and even elective aesthetic surgery. These addictions may look like problems to the outsider, but they are solutions to the patient, which is why they are so refractory.

The compulsive desire for surgery can be so strong that the very act of surgery becomes meaningful, even if there is no patient benefit. One grateful long-term reconstructive patient sent Christmas cards every year and copies of new recordings that she released until I refused to revise a scar that I could not see. "I don't care if you can't see it; I want the surgery anyway," she told me. She left in anger and sent a letter explaining how I had abandoned and degraded her. She has never returned. The surgical act itself carried such symbolism that whether it achieved anything was irrelevant. I had deprived her of symbolic caring and a way of erasing shame.

Regrettably, traditional methods of treating the traumas of childhood sexual abuse have not been remarkably effective. In one study, failure to improve in four months of treatment was twice as high among childhood sexual abuse victims than among those with eating disorders, and the treatment dropout rate was three times higher.[82] Trauma work is specialized and differs from traditional talk therapy. The trauma damage is not embedded in the cortex but in the midbrain, which must be a primary focus of treatment.

Female Genital Surgery and Body Image

Of particular relevance at the time of this writing is a significant increase in requests for elective labiaplasty, in which surgeons most commonly reduce the size of the labia minora. The ostensible indication is discomfort and chafing with clothing and embarrassment when nude, particularly now that women's clothing has been made thinner and more revealing.[83] Yet some studies add different dimensions. In most of the illustrated cases in the plastic surgery literature, the labia are normal size.[84, 85] Surveys of women seeking labiaplasty indicate that they have had "more media exposure" to labia "in advertisements and the Internet" than those who are not seeking labiaplasty.[85] Well, of course, but how exactly does this happen? A woman cannot be searching for Christmas recipes and accidentally find photos of labia; she has to be looking for them, which indicates a particular body interest that not every woman has. Why? Compared to controls in this particular study, fewer women seeking labiaplasty were involved in romantic relationships and many were dissatisfied with their lives. Other studies indicate that the majority of older women seeking labiaplasty are in unhappy relationships or between relationships. This must be significant.

Another recent paper gathered qualitative data through semi-structured interviews.[85] Their most provocative findings were that (1) Eighty-six percent of patients were already aware that their labia were normal size, but wanted surgery anyway; (2): Fifty-seven percent reported that their post-surgical labial appearance was still not "perfect," by which they meant absolutely symmetrical without visible labia (i.e., childlike); (3): Even women who received positive postoperative comments about their new labial appearance did not accept them and continued their preoperative avoidance behaviors. That finding suggests that there are other factors at play.

Today the surgery has been expanded to include teenagers and women under 25, the majority of whom have avoided sexual intimacy because of shame about their labial appearances or because of parental concern. This is an important observation because it recognizes the non-functional, (cosmetic) indications for labiaplasty, much less often used to justify it.[86] As a result of "media exposure," the majority of teen patients request labiaplasty to treat asymmetry, although in the series referenced, only 17% were unilateral procedures, and although asymmetry is common and self-correcting during adolescence. While I understand that some young women, for example competitive swimmers, might feel self-conscious, that cannot be the majority of teenagers requesting the surgery. By what standard must labia be symmetrical? What do the parents who sign their daughters' consents believe?

Newer still is labia majora or minora augmentation with injectable fillers or fat grafts to reduce signs and symptoms of aging and menopause. Postoperatively the majority of patients were satisfied, but the authors' scoring technique measured both appearance and symptoms; most patients did not report symptom relief, suggesting that their satisfaction was largely appearance-based.[87] In a literature review of labia majora augmentation, the authors cite a decrease in "sexual self-esteem" as the motivation for surgery; in those studies surveyed that documented patient satisfaction, all patients were satisfied.[88]

The American College of Obstetrics and Gynecologists has recommended preoperative patient education about normal labial anatomy, mental and emotional maturity assessment, body dysmorphic disorder screening, and discussion of non-surgical options; some gynecologists have advised against the procedure.[89] Some gynecologists report that young women now seek consultation to be reassured that they are anatomically normal (Nikola Curtis, M.D., personal communication, 2018). Relevant to this advice is work by Veale and co-authors, who determined that 18% of their study group met BDD criteria.[90, 91]

★★★★★

I fully recognize that the subject is not simple, and I am sympathetic to women of any age who desire labiaplasty for discomfort, embarrassment, or "sexual self-esteem." Veale has established in separate patient groups that the prevalence of childhood abuse or neglect was not high in the labiaplasty patients studied (which surprises me),[91] and that eight of nine patients who qualified for body dysmorphic disorder preoperatively did not qualify postoperatively—in other words, were improved by the surgery.[92, 93] A 92% patient satisfaction rate was documented in one multicenter study,[94] and improvement in sexual functioning in another.[95] This is very positive information (though only based on short-term data) but counterintuitive to the majority of data that we have on postoperative satisfaction in body-image-shamed patients, which is usually low. It is not clear why labiaplasty patients, based on what we know today, might be different. Perhaps correcting an anatomical source of shame may be therapeutic, or perhaps symptomatic relief really is the only driving issue. We need more information.

Though plastic surgeons have their individual operative criteria, preoperative assessment of labiaplasty patients will always be incomplete without a history that includes childhood, particularly sexual, trauma. Women who have been fondled as children frequently consider their genitalia as "dirty" (Pia Mellody, personal communication, 2016). Sexual abuse in plastic surgery patients is not an obscure finding. In my own practice, the prevalence in 175 patients was 22% (Chapter 9). When the question has been asked as a preoperative labiaplasty screen, prevalences are less than 0.5%. This data is likely to be inaccurate because it was obtained preoperatively in patients motivated to have surgery and naturally hesitant to be candid.

The connection does not need to be this obvious. Parents who use their children to meet the parents' emotional needs can romanticize and sexualize the parent/child relationship. When a parent with unresolved sexual issues has a bond with one of his or her children that becomes more important or intimate than the spousal relationship, the child can be emotionally sexually abused. It is not hard to conjecture that some patients seeking labiaplasty have been sexually abused and that their motivation for labiaplasty may be to reduce or minimize one sign of adult sexual appearance. Some labiaplasty patients have sexual abuse histories (Janice Lalikos, M.D., personal communication, 2016). While some women's indications for labiaplasty may be only what they tell their surgeons, we don't know that yet. It is important for surgeons and for the patients themselves to understand all their motivations, and in particular to recognize that labiaplasty is potentially more than a technical exercise designed to produce symmetry or meet arbitrary beauty standards. We have larger responsibilities as surgeons.

Feeding Disorders, Obesity, and Body Image

Recent figures from the Centers for Disease Control indicate that 14% of 2–5-year-olds were obese, compared with 18.4% of 6–11-year-olds and 20.6% of 12–19-year-olds. Among adults, obesity prevalence is approximately 39.8% in the United States (2015–2016 data). There are associated observations that elaborate this phenomenon:

- Overweight children, even at preschool ages, are at higher risk for teasing
- Overweight children are less frequently liked by their peers
- Overweight children have lower self-esteem
- Overweight young people are more likely to be dissatisfied with their body images
- Most obese girls express low levels of body satisfaction
- Overweight adults are ashamed of their body sizes and overvalue their bodies[96]
- Overweight adults have higher levels of mood disturbances and illness
- Overweight adults often overestimate or underestimate their body sizes
- Cognitive behavior therapy in obese individuals does not produce weight loss

The question not so often asked is, why are these individuals obese? The common bias is a simple lack of willpower, lower access to healthy foods, especially among lower income groups, or eating the wrong types of foods. Periodically the Food and Drug Administration releases its guidelines, the most recent of which advise reduced salt and fat intake. Is overeating simply the response to a deregulated food industry or plentiful advertising?[62] If that is so, why aren't more people obese? Is overeating just weakness? Or are these patients medicating pain with food? If so, why?

★★★★★

Overweight people die one year earlier than expected and . . . moderately obese people die up to three years prematurely, research suggests. . . . The meta-analysis also found obesity is nearly three times more deadly for men than it is for women.

(*AMA Wire*, July 14, 2016)

Presumably this is news to someone, though that is hard to imagine. Until now, obese patients only had to worry about ridicule from childhood, staring, teasing, criticism for lack of willpower, heart disease, hypertension, diabetes, venous ulcers, gout, and hyperlipidemia. They can't buy clothes or shoes easily, they don't fit into airplane seats, and maintaining a morbidly obese weight is almost a full-time job. Now the overweight also have to worry about dying early.

If it is the media's fault, then the media might as well be culpable for both obesity and anorexia. What is not well understood is that eating disorders are solutions. A recent autobiographical bestseller makes the same points.[97]

Anorexia nervosa shares overlapping global characteristics with obesity, childhood sexual abuse, and body dysmorphic disorder: obsession, perfectionism, mirror checking, body image disturbance, denial, feelings of disgust, shame, and self-consciousness, depression, and poor self-esteem. Like its teammates, anorexia is notoriously difficult to treat without eventual relapse. Less often described about any of these entities is their cause. In a study of 84 women with posttraumatic stress disorder (PTSD) after childhood sexual abuse and co-incident eating disorders, Dyer, Borgmann, Kleindienst, Feldman, et al.[98] document coincident negative body image that affects both the cognitive-affective and behavioral components of body image.[99] Self-acceptance was poor. The PTSD component alone accounted for all of the body image disturbances. This conclusion supports the thesis that trauma is the starting point for many body image and addictive disorders, which in turn do not appear *de novo* but are rather outcomes or compensatory behaviors that stem from childhood experiences. Poor self-esteem, intrafamilial discord, and associated mental health conditions are not, therefore, coincidental.

Treatment of Body Image Disorders

Treatment of body image disorders can be either "top-down" (Cognitive Behavior Therapy [CBT]) or "bottom up" (Experiential). Both have been successful although, as with much clinical research, long-term outcomes are hard to find. CBT does not routinely explore the developmental origins of excessive body image investment, but rather the patient's attitude and behavior toward it.

CBT typically follows a careful pattern:

- Identify the patient's overvalued ideas about shape and weight and their damaging effect on self-esteem
- Enhance underdeveloped self-worth
- Examine compensatory shape checking and avoidance behaviors
- Examine distortions in body image thoughts and emotions
- Provide the patient with insight into the causes for these distortions
- Teach the patient to identify triggers provoking unhealthy behavior
- Address mood, perfectionism, self-esteem, and interpersonal problems

This schema has proved to be effective at 60-week follow-up. Jarry and Cash have documented improvements maintained at 4.5 months.[100] Others have noted similar successes.[7, 101–103] If one accepts the concept that body image disorders develop, at least in part, from childhood abuse and neglect, and therefore encompass thoughts, feelings, images, and auditory, visual, and other somatic components produced by the neglect, it follows that working directly with sensory and somatic memories would be most effective. Treatment variations have components: insight and identification of current feelings; attention to bodily sensations associated with them; and accessing and releasing unconscious memories and emotions that are not readily accessible by the traditional talk therapy aimed at cortical function.[104]

What This Information Means

The ubiquitous common final pathway for childhood abuse and neglect is toxic shame. Body dissatisfaction therefore differs from body shame, which has unique manifestations and becomes the driver for depression and unhealthy or even addictive behavior.[105] Traumatized individuals who continually self-monitor their appearances frequently develop body shame, dissatisfaction, depression, and somatic symptoms.[106] But are all these individuals the same? Can we learn anything about body dysmorphic disorder from their experiences? Do functioning adults with self-esteem, boundaries, reality, and self-caring, moderated lives still develop body shame, or just those who survive trauma?

That's where the thread leads next.

Note

* Meacham, J. *Franklin and Winston: An Intimate Portrait of an Epic Friendship*. New York: Random House, 2003, pp. 12–13.

References

1. Cox HG. *On Not Leaving It to the Snake*. London: SCM Press Ltd.; 1964:ix–xvii.
2. Godart NT, Flament MF, Perdereau F, et al. Comorbidity Between Eating Disorders and Anxiety Disorders: A Review. *Eat Disord and Anxiety Disord* 2002; 32:3:253–270.
3. Bliss, M. *Harvey Cushing, a Life in Surgery*. New York, New York: Oxford University Press; 2005:317.
4. Fisher S, Cleveland SE. *Body Image and Personality*. 2nd edition. New York: Dover Publications; 1968.
5. Shontz F, *Perceptual and Cognitive Aspects of Body Experience*. New York: The Guilford Press; 1969.
6. Cash TF, Smolak L, eds. *Body Image: A Handbook of Science, Practice, and Prevention*. New York: The Guilford Press; 2011.
7. Grogan S. *Body Image: Understanding Body Dissatisfaction, in Men, Women, and Children*. London: Routledge; 2008.
8. Gilbert P, Miles J, eds. *Body Shame: Conceptualization, Research and Treatment*. East Sussex [UK]: Routledge; 2002.
9. Russek LG, Schwartz GE. Feeling of Parental Caring Predict Health Status in Midlife: A 35-Year Follow-Up of the Harvard Mastery of Stress Study. *J Behav Med* 1997; 20:1:1–13.

10. Bashour M. History and Current Concepts in the Analysis of Facial Attractiveness. *Plast Reconstr Surg* 2006 Sep 1; 118:3:741–756.

11. Gilbert P, Price JS, Alan S. Social Comparison, Social Attractiveness, and Evolution: How Might They Be Related? *New Ideas Psychol* 1995; 13:2:149–165.

12. Constantian MB. Planning Rhinoplasty: Abstract Concepts and Aesthetics. In: Constantian MB, ed. *Rhinoplasty: Craft and Magic*. St. Louis: Quality Medical Publishing; 2009:279–316.

13. Scott I, Swami V, Josephson SC, et al. Context—Dependent Preferences for Facial Sexual Dimorphism in a Rural Malaysian Population. *Evol Hum Behav* 2008; 29:4:289–296.

14. Stein DJ. Evolutionary Psychiatry and Body Dysmorphic Disorder. In: Phillips KA, ed. *Body Dysmorphic Disorder: Advances in Research and Clinical Practice*. New York: Oxford University Press; 2017:243–252.

15. Tischner I, Malson H. Understanding the "Too Fat" Body and the "Too Thin" Body: A Critical Psychological Perspective. In: Rumsey N, Harcourt D, eds. *The Psychology of Appearance*. Oxford [UK]: Oxford University Press; 2012:306–319.

16. Smolak L. Body Image Development in Childhood. In: Cash TF, Smolak L, eds. *Body Image*. 2nd edition. New York: The Guilford Press; 2011:73.

17. Suisman JL, Klump KL. Genetic and Neuroscientific Perspectives on Body Image. In: Cash TF, Smolak L, eds. *Body Image: A Handbook of Science, Practice, and Prevention*. New York: The Guilford Press; 2011:29–38.

18. Cash TF, Deagle EA. The Nature and Extent of Body-Image Disturbances in Anorexia Nervosa and Bulimia Nervosa: A Meta-Analysis. *Int J Eat Disord* 1997; 22:2:107–125.

19. Gardner RM. Perceptual Measures of Body Image for Adolescents and Adults. In: Cash TF, Smolak L, eds. *Body Image: A Handbook of Science, Practice, and Prevention*. New York: The Guilford Press; 2011:146–153.

20. Yamamia Y, Cash TF, Melnyk SE, et al. Women's Exposure to Thin and Beautiful Media Images: Body Image Effects of Media-Ideal Internalization and Impact-Reduction Interventions. *Body Image* 2005; 2:1:74–80.

21. Moss TP, Rosser B. Adult Psychosocial Adjustment to Visible Differences: Physical and Psychological Predictors of Variation. In: Rumsey N, Harcourt D, eds. *The Psychology of Appearance*. Oxford [UK]: Oxford University Press; 2012:273–292.

22. McKinley NM. Feminist Perspectives on Body Image. In: Cash TF, Smolak L, eds. *Body Image: A Handbook of Science, Practice, and Prevention*. New York: The Guilford Press; 2011:48–55.

23. Pope HG. Body Image Disorders and Abuse of Anabolic-Androgenic Steroids Among Men. *JAMA* 2017; 317:1:23–24.

24. Balsam KF, Molina Y, Blayney JA, et al. Racial/Ethnic Differences in Identity and Mental Health Outcomes among Young Sexual Minority Women. *Cultur Divers Ethnic Minor Psychol* 2015; 21:3:380–390.

25. Franco DL, Roehrig JP. African American Body Images. In: van der Kolk B, McFarlane AC, Weisaeth L, eds. *Traumatic Stress*. New York: The Guilford Press; 2007:225.

26. Robert A, Cash TF, Feingold A, et al. Are Black-White Differences in Females' Body Dissatisfaction Decreasing? A Meta-Analytic Review. *J Consult Clin Psychol* 2006; 74:6:1121–1131.

27. Siever MD. Sexual Orientation and Gender as Factors in Socioculturally Acquired Vulnerability to Body Dissatisfaction and Eating Disorders. *J Consult Clin Psych* 1994; 62:2:252.

28. McLean SA, Paxton SJ, Wertheim EH. Factors Associated with Body Dissatisfaction and Disordered Eating in Women in Midlife. *Int J Eat Disord* 2010; 43:6:527–536.

29. Lewis DM, Cachelin FM. Body Image, Body Dissatisfaction, and Eating Attitudes in Midlife and Elderly Women. *Eat Disord* 2001; 9:29–39.

30. Grogan S. Body Image Development in Adulthood. In: Cash TF, Smolak L, eds. *Body Image: A Handbook of Science, Practice, and Prevention.* New York: The Guilford Press; 2011:93–100.

31. Markey CN, Markey PM, Birch LL. Understanding Women's Body Satisfaction: The Role of Husbands. *Sex Roles* 2004; 51:3–4:209–216.

32. Tiggemann M, Lynch JE. Body Image across the Life Span in Adult Women: The Role of Self-Objectification. *Development Psychol* 2001; 37:2:243–253.

33. Weiderman MW. Body Image and Sexual Functioning. In: Cash TF, Smolak L, eds. *Body Image.* 2nd edition. New York: The Guilford Press; 2011:271–278.

34. Tylka TL. Positive Psychology Perspectives on Body Image. In: Cash TF, Smolak L, eds. *Body Image: A Handbook of Science, Practice, and Prevention.* New York: The Guilford Press; 2011:56–66.

35. Bellew R. The Role of the Family. In: Rumsey N, Harcourt D, eds. *The Psychology of Appearance.* Oxford [UK]: Oxford University Press; 2012:239–254.

36. Wood-Barcalow NL, Tylka TL, Augustus-Horvath CL. "But I Like My Body": Positive Body Image Characteristics and a Holistic Model for Young Adult Women. *Body Image* 2010; Mar 7; 2:106–116.

37. Fitzgerald, FS. *The Great Gatsby.* New York: Harper Collier; 1982.

38. Gilbert R, Widom CS, Browne K, et al. Child Maltreatment 1: Burden and Consequences of Child Maltreatment in High-Income Countries. *The Lancet* 2009; 373:68–81.

39. Gilsdorf JR. The Good-Enough Parent. *JAMA* 2016; 316:20:2089.

40. Ginzburg K, Arnow B, Hart S, et al. The Abuse-Related Beliefs Questionnaire for Survivors of Childhood Sexual Abuse. *Child Abuse Negl* 2006; 30:8:929–943.

41. Giovannelli TS, Cash TF, Henson JM, et al. The Measurement of Body-Image Dissatisfaction-Satisfaction: Is Rating Importance Important? *Body Image* 2008; 5:2:216–223.

42. Musher-Eizenman DR, Holub SC, Barnhart-Miller A, et al. Body Size Stigmatization in Preschool Children: The Role of Control Attributions. *J Pediatric Psychol* 2004; 29:8:613–620.

43. Flegal KM, Kruszon-Moran D, Carroll MD, et al. Trends in Obesity among Adults in the United States 2005 to 2014. *JAMA* 2016; 315:21:2284–2291.

44. Burke MA, Heiland FW. Evolving Societal Norms of Obesity: What Is the Appropriate Response? *JAMA* 2018; 319:3:221–222.

45. Guth E. Counting Calories as an Approach to Achieve Weight Control. *JAMA* 2018; 319:3:225–226.

46. Livingston EH. Reimagining Obesity in 2018: A JAMA Theme Issue on Obesity. *JAMA* 2018; 319:3:238–240.

47. Yanovski SZ, Yanovski JA. Toward Precision Approaches for the Prevention and Treatment of Obesity. *JAMA* 2018; 319:3:223–224.

48. Zylke JW, Bauchner H. The Unrelenting Challenge of Obesity. *JAMA* 2016; 315:21:2277–2278.

49. Levine MP, Chapman K. Media Influences on Body Image. In: Cash TF, Smolak L, eds. *Body Image: A Handbook of Science, Practice, and Prevention.* New York: The Guilford Press; 2011:101–109.

50. Ricciardelli LA, Mellor D. Influence of Peers. In: Rumsey N, Harcourt D, eds. *The Psychology of Appearance.* Oxford [UK]: Oxford University Press; 2012:255.

51. Feragen KB. Congenital Conditions. In: Rumsey N, Harcourt D, eds. *The Psychology of Appearance*. Oxford [UK]: Oxford University Press; 2012:353–371.

52. Wertheim EH, Paxton SJ. Body Image Development in Adolescent Girls. In Cash TF, Smolak L, eds. *Body Image: A Handbook of Science, Practice, and Prevention*. New York: The Guilford Press; 2011:76–84.

53. Smolak L. Appearance in Childhood and Adolescence. In: Rumsey N, Harcourt D, eds. *The Psychology of Appearance*. Oxford [UK]: Oxford University Press; 2012:123–141.

54. Massie H, Szajnberg N. My Life Is a Longing: Child Abuse and Its Adult Sequelae: Result of the Brody Longitudinal Study from Birth to Age 30. *Int J Psychoanal* 2006; 87:471–496.

55. Anderson SE, Gooze RA, Lemeshow S, et al. Quality of Early Maternal-Child Relationship and Risk of Adolescent Obesity. *Pediatrics* 2012; 129:132–140.

56. Andrews RM, Browne AL, Drummond P, et al. The Impact of Personality and Coping on the Development of Depressive Symptoms in Adult Burn Survivors. *Burns* 2010; 36:1:29–37.

57. Wisely J, Gaskell S. Trauma—with Special Reference to Burn Injury. In: Rumsey N, Harcourt D, eds. *The Psychology of Appearance*. Oxford [UK]: Oxford University Press; 2012:372–397.

58. Wertheim EH, Paxton SJ. Body Image Development in Adolescent Girls. In: Cash TF, Smolak L, eds. *Body Image*. 2nd edition. New York: The Guilford Press; 2011:76–84.

59. Fosdick HE. *What Is Vital in Religion: Sermons on Contemporary Christian Problems*. New York: Harper & Brothers; 1955:50, 113.

60. Ricciardelli LA, Mellor D, Influence of Peers. In: Rumsey N, Harcourt D, eds. *The Psychology of Appearance*. Oxford [UK]: Oxford University Press; 2012:253–272.

61. Felitti VJ, Jakstis K, Pepper V, et al. Obesity: Problem, Solution, or Both? *Perm J* 2010; 14:1:24–31.

62. Lawson V. Appearance Concerns, Dietary Restriction and Disordered Eating. In: Rumsey N, Harcourt D, eds. *The Psychology of Appearance*. Oxford [UK]: Oxford University Press; 2012:320–349.

63. Grilo CM, Masheb, RM, Brody M, et al. Childhood Maltreatment in Extremely Obese Male and Female Bariatric Surgery Candidates. *Obes Res* 2005; 13:1:123–130.

64. Rodhe P, Ichikawa L, Simon GE, et al. Associations of Child Sexual Abuse and Physical Abuse With Obesity and Depression in Middle-Aged Women. *Child Abuse Neglect* 2008; 32:9:878–887.

65. Zeller MH, Noll JG, Sarwer DB, et al. Child Maltreatment and the Adolescent Patient with Severe Obesity: Implications for Clinical Care. *J Pediatr Psychol* 2015; 40:7:640–648.

66. Tiggemann M, Slevec J. Appearance in Adulthood. In: Rumsey N, Harcourt D, eds. *The Psychology of Appearance*. Oxford [UK]: Oxford University Press; 2012:153.

67. McLaren L, Kuh D, Hardy R, et al. Positive and Negative Body–Related Comments and Their Relationship with Body Dissatisfaction in Middle–Aged Women. *Psychol Health* 2004; 19:2:261–272.

68. Davis C, Katzman MA. Chinese Men and Women in the United States and Hong Kong: Body and Self-Esteem Ratings as a Prelude to Dieting and Exercise. *Int J Eat Disord* 1998; 23:1:99–102.

69. van den Berg P, Paxton SJ, Keery H et al. Body Dissatisfaction and Body Comparison with Media Images in Males and Females. *Body Image* 2007; 4:257.

70. Dittmar H, Halliwell E, Stirling E. Understanding the Impact of Thin Media Models on Women's Body—Focused Affect: The Roles of Thin—Ideal Internalization and

Weight—Related Self—Discrepancy Activation in Experimental Exposure Affects. *J Soc Clin Psychol* 2009; 28:1:43–72.

71. Markus H. Self—Schema and Processing Information about the Self. *J Pers Soc Psychol* 1977; 35:2:63.

72. Rumsey N, Harcourt D, eds. *The Psychology of Appearance.* Oxford [UK]: Oxford University Press; 2012:117–178.

73. Felitti VJ, Anda RF. The Lifelong Effects of Adverse Childhood Experiences, Chapter 10. In: *Chadwick's Child Maltreatment: Sexual Abuse and Psychological Maltreatment,* 4th edition. Florissant [MO]: STM Learning; 2014.

74. Felitti VJ, Anda RF, Nordenberg D, et al. Relationship of Childhood Abuse and Household Dysfunction to Many of the Leading Causes of Death in Adults. *Am J Prev Med* 1998; 14:4:245–258.

75. Felitti VJ, Anda RF. The Lifelong Effects of Adverse Childhood Experiences. *Chadwick's Child Maltreat: Sex Abuse Psychol Maltreat* 2014; 2: 203–215.

76. Salwen JK, Hymowitz GF, Bannon SM, et al. Weight-Related Abuse: Perceived Emotional Impact and the Effect on Disordered Eating. *Child Abuse Neglect* 2015; 45:163–171.

77. Menzel JE, Krawczyk R, Thompson JK. Attitudinal Assessment of Body Image for Adolescents. In: Cash TF, Smolak L, eds. *Body Image: A Handbook of Science, Practice, and Prevention.* New York: The Guilford Press; 2011:154–172.

78. Sack M, Boroske-Leiner K, Lahmann C. Association of Nonsexual and Sexual Traumatizations with Body Image and Psychosomatic Symptoms in Psychosomatic Outpatients. *Gen Hosp Psychiatry* 2010; 32:315–320.

79. Delinsky SS. Body Image and Anorexia Nervosa. In: Cash TF, Smolak L, eds. *Body Image.* 2nd edition. New York: The Guilford Press; 2011:279–288.

80. van der Kolk BA. The Compulsion to Repeat the Trauma. *Psychiatric Clin N Am* 1989; 12:2:389–411.

81. Young L. Sexual Abuse and the Problem of Embodiment. *Child Abuse Neglect* 1992; 16:89–100.

82. Rodriguez M, Perez V, Garcia Y. Impact of Traumatic Experiences and Violent Acts upon Response to Treatment of the Sample of Colombian Women with Eating Disorders. *Int J Eat Disord* 2005; 37:4:299–306.

83. Hunter JG. Commentary on: Factors That Influence the Decision to Seek Labiaplasty: Media, Relationships, and Psychological Well-Being. *Aesth Surg J* 2016; 36:4:479–481.

84. Sharp G, Mattiske J, Vale KI. Motivations, Expectations, and Experiences of Labiaplasty: A Qualitative Study. *Aesth Surg J* 2016; 36:8:920–928.

85. Sharp G, Tiggemann M, Mattiske J. Factors That Influence the Decision to Undergo Labiaplasty: Media, Relationships, and Psychological Well-Being. *Aesth Surg J* 2016; 36:4:469–478.

86. Hamori C. Teen Labiaplasty: A Response to the May 2016 American College of Obstetricians and Gynecologists (ACOG) Recommendations on Labiaplasty in Adolescents. *Aesth Surg J* 2016; 36:807 [sjw099].

87. Fasola E, Gazzola R. Labia Majora Augmentation with Hyaluronic Acid Filler: Technique and Results. *Aesth Surg J* 2016; 36:10:1155–1163.

88. Jabbour S, Kechichian E, Hersant B, et al. Labia Majora Augmentation: A Systematic Review of the Literature. *Aesth Surg J* 2017; 37:1:1157–1164.

89. Rogers RG. Most Women Who Undergo Labiaplasty Have Normal Anatomy: We Should Not Perform Labiaplasty. *Am J Obstet Gynecol* 2014; 211–281.

90. Veale D, Eshkevaria E, Ellison N, et al. A Comparison of Risk Factors for Women Seeking Labiaplasty Compared to Those Not Seeking Labiaplasty. *Body Image* 2014; 11:1:57–62.

91. Veale D, Eshkevart E, Ellison N, et al. Psychological Characteristics and Motivations of Women Seeking Labiaplasty. *Psychol Med* 2014; 44:3:555–566.

92. Goodman MP, Placcik OJ, Benson RH III. A Large Multi-Center Outcome Study of Female Genital Plastic Surgery. *J Sex Med* 2010; 7:4:1565–1577.

93. Goodman MP, Placik OJ, Matlock DL. Evaluation of Body Image and Sexual Satisfaction in Women Undergoing Female Genital Plastic/Cosmetic Surgery. *Aesth Surg J* 2016; 36:9:1048–1057.

94. Turini T, Roxo ACW, Serra-Guimarães F, et al. The Impact of Labiaplasty on Sexuality. *Plast Reconstr Surg* 2018; 141:1:87–92.

95. Veale D, Naismith I, Eshkavari E, et al. Psychosexual Outcome after Labiaplasty: A Prospective Case-Comparison Study. *Int Urogynecol J* 2014; 25:6:831–839.

96. Matz PE, Foster GD, Faith MS, et al. Correlates of Body Image Dissatisfaction among Overweight Women Seeking Weight Loss. *J Consul Clin Psychol* 2002; 70:4:1040–1044.

97. Mitchell A. *It Was Me All Along: A Memoir.* New York: Clarkson Potter [Penguin Random House Company]; 2015.

98. Dyer A, Borgmann E, Kleindienst N, et al. Body Image in Patients with Posttraumatic Stress Disorder after Childhood Sexual Abuse and Co-Occurring Eating Disorder. *Psychopathol* 2013; 46:186–191.

99. Foa EB, Ehlers A, Clark DM, et al. The Posttraumatic Cognitions Inventory (PTCI): Development and Validation. *Psychol Assess* 1999; 11:2:303–314.

100. Jarry JL, Cash TF. Cognitive-Behavioral Approaches to Body Image Change. In: Cash TF, Smolak L, eds. *Body Image: A Handbook of Science, Practice, and Prevention.* New York: The Guilford Press; 2011:415–423.

101. Cash TF, Strachan MT. Cognitive-Behavioral Approaches to Changing Body Image. In: Cash TF, Pruzinsky T eds. *Body Image: A Handbook of Theory, Research, and Clinical Practice.* New York: The Guilford Press; 2002.

102. Rosen JC, Orosan P, Reiter J. Cognitive Behavior Therapy for Body Image in Obese Women. *Behav Ther* 1995; 26:25–42.

103. Jenkinson E. Therapeutic Interventions: Evidence of Effectiveness. In: Rumsey N, Harcourt D, eds. *The Psychology of Appearance.* Oxford [UK]: Oxford University Press; 2012:551–567.

104. Levine PA. *Trauma and Memory: Brain and Body in a Search for the Living Past: A Practical Guide for Understanding and Working with Traumatic Memory.* Berkeley [CA]: North Atlantic Books; 2015.

105. Andrews B, Hunter E. Shame, Early Abuse, and Course of Depression in a Clinical Sample: A Preliminary Study. *Cogn Emot* 1997; 11:4:373–381.

106. Scaer RC. *The Body Bears the Burden: Trauma, Dissociation, and Disease.* 2nd edition. New York: Routledge; 2007:63, 72, 75–104.

The Fruits

How We Suffer and Medicate

5

THE WAYS WE SUFFER

Body Shame and the Astounding Spectrum of Its Ravages

"All children, except one, grow up. . . . Wendy knew that she must grow up. You always know after you are two. Two is the beginning of the end."

The author of *Peter Pan* was ironically a melancholy man, the son of a distant father and a mother tortured by the deaths of three of her children. Barrie took it upon himself to keep his mother's spirits bright by telling her stories—(Recall the caretaking role of the child who has no childhood in Chapter 3). Barry's own marriage was unhappy, and he later took prescribed heroin for chronic insomnia. *Peter Pan* is as much a story of Barrie's own abandonment and lost childhood as it is of childhood forever:

Long ago, [Peter said, speaking to Wendy] I thought like you that my mother would always keep the window open for me; so I stayed away for moons and moons and moons, and then flew back; but the window was barred, for my mother had forgotten all about me and there was another little boy sleeping in my bed.[1]

A Critical Key: Body Shame Versus Body Dissatisfaction

Sagas have their pivot points. For two months during the summer of 1862, Abraham Lincoln had been holding a draft of the Emancipation Proclamation, waiting for the right time to issue it. After the Northern defeats at Harper's Ferry, Seven Days, Cedar Mountain, and twice at Manassas, it seemed as if that opportunity would

DOI: 10.4324/9781315657721-8

never come. But the battle of Antietam changed everything. Five days later Lincoln issued his Proclamation, which changed the very nature of the Civil War from an effort to pull the Union together into one that would redefine it completely.[2]

I am hardly Abraham Lincoln, but the pivot point in my struggle to understand the deep and seemingly irrational dissatisfaction of some surgical patients came from Bernice Andrews' research distinguishing *body shame* from *body dissatisfaction* and locating body shame squarely between childhood abuse and depression, where it is often complicated by eating disorders.[3] This was a critical missing piece linking childhoods and body image.

That publication and her follow-up work established that even patients without histories of early childhood abuse or neglect connect body shame directly to recurrent depressive episodes.[3–6] The fact that her research was done by face-to-face interviews and not self-administered questionnaires only strengthens her findings. In Andrews' 1997 study, 51% of patients reported physical or sexual abuse in childhood, and half had suffered both types. Thirty-five patients with primary diagnoses of depression were inventoried both for adverse childhood experiences and then asked, "Have you ever felt ashamed of your body or any part of it?" Patients who answered affirmatively were asked to elaborate. They described self-consciousness about appearance, shame in exposing body parts, efforts to conceal themselves, and "mortification" when others commented on their appearances. The correlation between childhood abuse and body shame was .46 (moderately positive correlation); both men and women with childhood trauma histories had significantly higher body shame scores than those without trauma histories. Gender differences were not found. Those patients with more extreme and chronic depression had higher shame scores than those with only episodic depression.

Patients were asked to localize their body shame. Seventy-five percent were concerned with overall shape: some thought that they were too fat, some too thin. Specific body areas included legs, thighs, breasts, and chest, but 17% involved facial features, skin, and nails. How strikingly this area data resembles body dysmorphic disorder.

Body Shame in the Literature

The mental health literature distinguishes three types of shame: Body Shame, Characterological Shame (What kind of person I am: e.g., social competence, assertiveness, communication ability, hygiene, and life success or failure), and Behavioral Shame (How I behave: poor social conduct, unwarranted aggressiveness, unreliability, poor relationships with the opposite sex, alcohol abuse, inadequate self-care, or suicide attempts).[7] Two-thirds of the entire study group had either behavioral shame or characterological shame in addition to body shame. However, *body shame had the strongest relationship to early abuse*; neither behavioral nor characterological shame were significantly correlated. Marital violence histories were also common, and the women who had suffered childhood trauma blamed either their character or their own behavior—i.e., they deserved the abuse.[8, 9]

Franzoni, Gualandi, Caretti, et al. established correlations between body shame, alexithymia (difficulty in identifying and describing feelings), childhood trauma, dissociation (a hallmark of PTSD), and eating disorders.[10] In 143 eating disorder patients, the authors found strong correlations among alexithymia, dissociation, body shame, and trauma histories. These authors and others[11] have pieced their findings into a logical causative order: Childhood physical and sexual abuse lead to body shame, dissociation, emotional dysregulation, alexithymia, and eating disorders. In fact, it would be hard to reassemble these observations into any other sequence that makes better etiologic sense—for example, to argue that eating disorders lead to body shame and sexual abuse; yet the parallel schema is commonly used to explain body dysmorphic disorder. While depression itself could generate shame and body dissatisfaction, regression analysis always placed shame at the core.

Noll and Frederickson examined the feminist view that cultural objectification of women as sexual objects creates body shame, which in turn may generate eating disorders.[12] They found what they were looking for: self-objectification and increased body shame in women correlates with dieting, even among women who are not overweight. But women varied in the degree to which they are susceptible to outsiders' opinions. In other words, some women had better boundaries than others and better senses of their own self-worth. If that weren't true, of course, every woman would have an eating disorder.

★★★★★

Fitzgerald describes the dual damaging melancholy of boundaries and walls in this section of *The Great Gatsby*: "Cordelia and Grace and Carol are sitting, jammed in together, whispering and giggling. I have to sit . . . by myself because they aren't speaking to me. It's something I said wrong, but I don't know what it is because they won't tell me. Cordelia says it will be better for me to think back over everything I've said today and try to pick out the wrong thing. That way I will learn not to say such a thing again. When I've guessed the right answer, they will speak to me again. It's for my own good."[13]

★★★★★

These associations spread in other directions. Didie, Kuniega-Pietrzak, and Phillips[14] examined a group of 99 patients with body dysmorphic disorder, and found that the severity of body dysmorphic disorder correlated with their degree of unhappiness and delusionality. In fact, body dysmorphic men were actually more invested in their appearances than controls, but body dysmorphic women were not, which fits the context of the importance that many—perhaps most—women pay to their appearances, self-objectified by a male-dominated culture or not. Also relevant is the finding that all BDD patients felt less physically healthy. Women were less interested in their own fitness and health; and women in particular were less aware of being ill—i.e., more dissociated from their bodies and less able to self-care. This data begs the question of whether appearance is really the target issue or whether there is some unifying underlying force that creates appearance obsession, dissociation from self-care, and poor body image all together.

Wenninger and Heiman explored the profoundly destructive effects of childhood sexual abuse, and noted after a broad range of tests that abuse survivors (more than half of whom had been abused more than five years, 47% by different abusers) were more depressed, had poorer sexual functioning, were more averse to sexual arousal, had more pain during intercourse, more sexual partners, more self-destructive behavior, more use of recreational or illicit drugs, and a 62% prevalence of self-mutilation.[15] Not surprisingly, these unfortunate patients also had more negative body images, particularly with regard to sexual attractiveness.[16] A correlation between childhood trauma and high-risk behavior was also found in the Adverse Childhood Events study (Chapter 9). Other researchers have also noted correlations among dissociation, alexithymia, self-hatred, and PTSD symptoms in victims of sexual abuse.[17]

In a group of 240 outpatients with psychosomatic complaints, Sack, Boroske-Leiner, and Lehmann[18] found a childhood trauma prevalence of 67.5%, which would be a stunning number except for the Adverse Childhood Events Study,[19] documenting a prevalence of 64% in over 17,000 educated, employed, middle-class patients, and the 80% prevalence in my own plastic surgery practice (Chapter 9). In both men and women the authors found large differences among traumatized patients with regard to body dissatisfaction, other psychological symptoms, somatoform complaints, and dissociative symptoms. Sexual abuse survivors, especially those with coexistent borderline personality disorder (BPD), even reacted negatively to body-related words in the Emotional Stroop Test.[20, 21]

★★★★★

Sir William Osler himself, the archetypal diagnostician, was fascinated by illnesses for which there was no apparent explanation—in this case PTSD in a World War I soldier: "His work on the functionally impaired centered on . . . a man who had been disabled in 1916. . . by 'typhoid spine.'[22] They could find nothing organically wrong with the soldier—Osler had several sets of x-rays done, but the slightest touch caused him excruciating pain. . . . [He] was taken off an ambulance at six in the morning. At ten that night Meakins had a call from Osler. . . . 'The SOB is walking.' "[23]

★★★★★

"Oh, you're great. You're wonderful. You're wonderful. Thank you so much for treating me."

I had barely entered the examination room when she rocketed off the table and embraced me. I tried my enigmatic smile because I didn't know what else to do. It seemed to help. She settled back on the table and we looked at each other. She had the wide eyes of a child on Christmas morning. Her hair was suspiciously blonde and disarrayed, and she was dressed perfectly for going on safari. Her skin was pale. I couldn't detect any makeup, but that's not so necessary on safari.

She was a therapist who had broken her nose in sports. Previous surgeries had not corrected its asymmetry nor opened her airway. I explained her deformities. She loved each observation. I explained the surgery. She agreed ecstatically. I discussed potential complications. She thought complications would be exciting. Unless I confessed to being an axe murderer, she was going to schedule surgery.

Postoperatively it was a different story. The patient lived in a constant state of hyperarousal, torturing herself with fantastically unlikely possibilities, unable to reassure herself, and unable even to retain our reassurances for more than a few minutes before the same worries resurfaced. In three to four phone calls a day, these were her questions, even though she was 50 years old and had already undergone several nasal surgeries:

"I might have scratched my nose while I was sleeping and moved my septum. Do you think so?"

"I accidentally hit my nose with my hand and now I think I might have a sinus infection."

"I know it has been a month since surgery but I think my nose is ripping. Maybe I am sleeping in the wrong position."

"I don't know if I mentioned it, but there is a place on the right that still protrudes more than the other side."

"I bumped my nose with a Styrofoam cup. Maybe I broke it again."

At her next visit, she completed the Adverse Childhood Events questionnaire. Her abuse had been both physical and sexual. I asked about her family and why she had chosen her career. She started to tell me, beginning with the same phrase that so many patients use.

"Well, it wasn't my parents. My parents were wonderful."

She smiled brightly again. I waited. Then she looked down at her folded hands as if they were something new and unusual. Her voice began to constrict till it was barely audible.

"But my father." I waited. Her voice became a whisper. "He had a bad temper."

She paused to button her sweater carefully. The pace of her words slowed.

"He took it out on my mother." She went back to studying her fingers.

I dropped my voice to be almost as soft as hers. "Did he take it out on you?"

She began nodding slowly, and then spoke, as if she suddenly remembered that she should say something.

"Oh, yes." Her voice drifted off again.

"And then I had this uncle." Suddenly both hands clenched and one fist rose to her throat. She closed her eyes. Her chin tipped upward. Her voice was quiet and deliberate.

"He grabbed me from behind and said he'd slit my throat." She slid her fist across her neck miming the blade's movement.

The silence was deep enough to be audible. Suddenly she looked at me, took in a long breath, and smiled. I felt the wall go up.

"But, you know, every family . . . Right?" Her voice trailed as she shrugged off the memories.

Like Jay Gatsby and so many other patients, this productive woman reinvented her parents with the maturity that she had as a child, describing them as so many patients do: "Just wonderful." The loving family was only a Potemkin Village.

Where Body Shame Fits

How can we place body shame into the mental health, plastic surgical, and developmental perspectives that we have already investigated? First, it is important to recognize that *body shame is not body dissatisfaction*. Body shame is always about self-worth. Perhaps the best way to explain the difference is to define *body dissatisfaction* as unhappiness with some aspect of body shape or facial feature that may in turn reflect societal or cultural value, but that does not diminish the individual.[24] The toxicity of *body shame*, on the other hand, can connote deficiency, humiliation, inferiority, vulnerability, wickedness, helplessness, powerlessness, or betrayal. With body shame there is always the element of inadequacy. Body shame cannot co-exist with healthy self-esteem.

Recall from Chapter 3 that shame can either be healthy or toxic. Healthy shame is what most of us call "embarrassment" or "guilt," the occasional necessary reminder of our humanity. Carried shame is not intrinsic but rather generated by a caregiver who has acted shamelessly without acknowledging his or her behavior. The child picks up the shame as if it were his or her own and experiences the sensation of intense worthlessness. That is why it is so easy to connect body shame to childhood abuse and neglect. Adult patients may sustain deforming trauma, burns, or disease, but *shame does not automatically follow disfigurement*. Body dissatisfaction may follow the patient who seeks reconstructive surgery, but diminished self-worth does not automatically accompany visible deformities. Like soldiers who enter battle with healthy senses of their own intrinsic value, solid boundaries, and undistorted reality and survive without developing PTSD, patients who sustain disfiguring injuries or disease can still retain their self-worth. They instinctively recognize that how they look does not define who they are. Perhaps because body image can be so fragile, people who retain their self-esteem despite significant physical injuries become unusually memorable to their caregivers. Physicians and nurses consider them to be their most remarkable patients. I have been privileged to know many.

Body shame, therefore, is rooted in abusive experiences and imparts a sense of vulnerability, fear, and helplessness. It is the degree of self-esteem that a patient carries that accounts for the common observation that the size of the deformity does not always correlate with the amount of distress that it creates. The premorbid sense of self-worth makes all the difference. Shame-motivated patients cannot attain self-worth from surgery.

Abuse, Neglect and Body Shame

Childhood physical and sexual abuse are profound physical boundary violations that impact the way the child experiences his or her body.[25] The carried shame that the child experiences often generates a lifestyle devoid of self-care and moderate living, and may also involve depression, self-hatred, self-mutilation, addictions, disfigurement, and eating disorders. Dose-response relationships apply: the highest rates of violent marital relationships and depression occur in those patients who have suffered the worst developmental trauma.[26, 27] Those who were repeatedly assaulted are most likely to blame their own characters: something is wrong with them that makes them bad and unlovable, justifying the abuse.

This dense self-blame can manifest as helplessness and inherent unworthiness that accounts for the self-injurious and suicidal behavior in some trauma victims. Andrews inventoried a series of mothers and their daughters for body shame.[3–6, 28, 29] High body shame levels were always associated with childhood sexual and physical abuse in the mothers and daughters. The body shame relationship remained even when the data were corrected for self-esteem and body dissatisfaction: carried shame became the critical determinant.

In these women's daughters, body shame expanded into anorexia and bulimia. We shall consider those problems presently. Although body shame quite often related directly to sexually relevant breasts, buttocks, stomach, and legs, shame about other body areas was not so directly implicated. In severe sexual trauma—such as violence or rape in adulthood—body shame did not occur unless there had also been childhood abuse. The childhood component was critical.

This connection between childhood abuse and adult depression is easy to understand because toxic shame always has a somatic connection. Every type of abuse or neglect links to the body in some way, either by inflicting fear or pain, denying needs, or negating the importance of the individual.[30]

*****

"I have been tired of this face for a long time. I look at it as little as possible—even when I shave. . . . I feel that this is a face, not like Helen of Troy's that launched a thousand ships, but only has launched millions of tickets. . . . I would like to have a façade behind a façade, and therefore I especially dislike my face. I never did like it, even when it was 'pretty.' I liked only what I hoped was behind that face. . . . What I thought I was inside, not what I appeared to be from skin side."

So writes Errol Flynn in his autobiography.[31] The son of a famous father and disapproving mother, Flynn grew up wildly unsupervised in the South Pacific. Though himself famous and accomplished, he recounts a life of excesses and poor self-care and is candid about his own profound unhappiness and undefined self-image:

"I essentially disliked women. . . . My principal emotion was that I was hoaxed by life, that I had become something other than what I set out to be. Now my name was simply associated with sex. I was a male Mae West, as it were. . ., My big house, my yard, my bank accounts, seemed hollow. None of these could take the place of self-respect, which I had lost. . . . I sat on the edge of the bed with the muzzle of the gun directly in my mouth, pointed at the roof. . . . I sat that way for quite a while. . . . Disconsolation went through me in waves. . . . But there must have been a stronger life force in me than I could emotionally or intellectually resist. . . . Instead of killing myself I bought a new boat."

Natural History of Body Shame

Body shame is not evanescent but chronic. Patients' lives became permeated with body appearance obsession, especially as it relates to the opinions of outsiders. Patients conceal, avoid, and ruminate. "The older you get," one woman said, "the more you discover what other people think you have . . . wrong with you, so when you get to 18 or 19, you cannot walk out the door."[32] Body shame always implies outside valuation and therefore can only occur in patients with poor boundaries and absent self-worth who generate their self-esteem through external sources. Accordingly, these patients become perfectionistic and obsessed or compulsively attack their bodies through self-mutilation. If I am body *dissatisfied*, I am imperfectly human but valuable. If I am body *shamed*, I am exposed, inferior, threatened, betrayed, and deficient. Body shame implies vulnerability that converts self-worth to self-hatred. That is the essential difference.

Andrews cautions that her observations were limited to working-class mothers and daughters living in deprived inner-city areas. However, Felitti's research in a general, middle-class medical population at Kaiser Permanente, and my own in an elective, largely aesthetic plastic surgery practice only confirm Andrews' findings.[33, 34] The sad truth is that childhood trauma, body shame, and depression are classless.

Anorexics, so numerous in the mothers examined in these studies, commonly arise in families dominated by perfectionism, self-image, and respectability. Even before I immersed myself in the mental health literature, I was surprised by how many of my patients revealed histories of eating disorders, in particular anorexia. Patients were typically perfectionistic, controlling, dissociated, and poorly communicative, and when their parents accompanied them, often tyrannical, rigid fathers and obsessive mothers whose sole interests were their children's (usually daughters') appearances. The family members were powerfully enmeshed and boundaryless. In turn, my anorexic patients controlled their families by starving and weight loss, but their visible focus was endless cosmetic surgery.

The body image literature repeatedly links the family to the body-shamed individual, and the body-shamed individual to compensatory behaviors (eating disorders or self-harm when the trauma was physical or sexual abuse).[32] This makes sense. Of all the common addictive compensatory behaviors that people use to medicate their pain (eating, gambling, sex, work, alcohol or drugs), the two that relate directly and most intensely to the body are eating disorders (which can control, punish, deprive, or flood the body) and deliberate self-injury. It is easy to imagine how vulnerable, perfectionistic trauma survivors driven by toxic shame could attach their self-worth to their bodies and manifest what we observe as body dysmorphic disorder or addictive plastic surgery.[35] Perfectionism, obsessive compulsive behavior, eating disorders, depression, suicidality and deliberate self-injury often coexist with body dysmorphic disorder, as does a history of childhood abuse or neglect.[36–38] Each associated disorder interprets the way body shame manifests and medicates in a different toxic way.

★★★★★

Evidence bubbles through the body shame literature to support this thesis. Body shame is defined as a cognitive sense of self-blame, uselessness, worthless, or ugliness with behavioral components (gaze aversion, defensiveness, social anxiety, seeking cover, concealing, depression, disengagement) and a parasympathetic stress response. The statements that patients make ("I am fat and ugly"; "I am a failure"; "I had surgery to be more perfect"; "I had surgery so people would love me") are all highly personal, deeply internal, visceral emotions. Toxic shame is not voluntary, but rather an inner-directed sense of unworthiness that can date from two years of age within the family unit and long before media pressures have exerted their influences.[39, 40]

Without necessarily meaning to do so, many authors describe the shame milieu in terms of self-esteem and the presence or absence of qualities that nurturing, functional family units impart. "Having qualities that one thinks others will value is especially related to self-esteem . . . more so than having quality that one values oneself."[41] "The more safe people feel . . . and cared for, the easier it may be to process . . . potentially shameful events: making mistakes, failing or disfigurements."[42] "Symptoms of anxiety are believed to create a negative image in the eyes . . . of perceived bodily appearances and functioning . . . The fear of creating negative impressions activates . . . anxiety. Rumination could play a major role in linking shame to other problems such as depression."[43] "It is being shamed by those we most depend on to mirror and affirm the sense of attractiveness that carries the most risk of being internalized. . . . People who have very high external shame [are] deeply distressed by rejection . . . fear negative evaluation and criticism and have a variety of anxiety disorders . . . social awkwardness . . . concealment, and avoidance behaviors." "Shame and humiliation have been bracketed together."[44] "Some people . . . seek medical intervention to change their bodies . . . and looks."[45] "People with visible differences show lower levels of self-esteem and higher levels of depression, anxiety, and social disability."[46] "Some children and families show remarkable resilience. . . . Variations in distress associated with disfigurement may be related to early parent-child interactions."[47] "Narcissism . . . perfectionism, low self-esteem, self-directed hostility, and low levels of perceived control . . . often moderate . . . the severity and outcome of eating disorders."[48]

The Betrayal of Imposed Surgery

I believe that a case can be made that repetitive, compulsive plastic surgery that continues, even after multiple complications, represents another type of deliberate self-injury, no different than wrist-cutting except that the agent is a surgeon—self-injury by proxy. We surgeons have to recognize the phenomenon earlier: we have to know better.

Virginia Blum explores the cosmetic surgery culture in *Flesh Wounds*.[49] All the same themes are there: body shame, self-esteem, equivalence of value and appearance, aesthetic surgery on normal noses, surgery imposed by boundaryless parents, associated eating disorders, perfectionism, verbally abusive parents who feel the need to perfect their children through surgery, poor maternal attachment, adoption or abandonment creating an obsession with imagined physical flaws, the link between abandonment and imaginary facial flaws, surgery to erase signs of childhood abuse, the irresponsible surgeon-abuser, and the never-ending compulsion for more operations. Her book's meta-message is not very flattering to patients, and especially not to surgeons. Women are gullible and made to feel ugly by the media and sometimes by their families, then exploited by surgeons even when the patient's features are normal. But patients buy into the myth: "To be attractive means . . . to get what you want."[49] Blum is scornful of the prevailing mental health view that body dysmorphic disorder may be biological, and that brain scans may reveal its origins. She also very astutely makes the connection between self-cutting, deep-seated, intolerable, inexpressible shame, eating disorders, and plastic surgery. She is right. As one patient confided to me, "I am never so happy as when I am recovering from plastic surgery."

The author's own experience was a regrettably common one. Without her knowledge, Blum's mother made an appointment for her daughter to have a rhinoplasty, reinforcing the author's sense of imperfection, worthlessness, and failure at not having developed normally. "Your body came out wrong." The patient herself did not dislike her nose but was overpowered. This is parental betrayal, now called "body dysmorphic disorder by proxy."[50]

★★★★★

Even decades later, Blum recalls the surgeon as a repulsive and manipulative monster. "He was an ugly man with a large, sagging face; his eyes seemed almost attached above an enormous nose. Thatches of gray and dark hair erupted unevenly from his head. This is how I remember him at least . . . the slayer of my nose." The surgeon preyed on her mother's fantasy that surgery would transform her daughter into a beauty. "My mother considered it parentally irresponsible not to . . . make me *marketable* [italics mine]. . . . If you are the child of critical parents, you are especially at risk."[49] Some years later, Blum underwent a revision operation from a surgeon who also criticized her chin.

Though I have a brighter view of plastic and reconstructive surgery than the author, she is quite right that everything is wrong with this story. Her body did not belong to her mother. Any parent soliciting or forcing surgery on a child is violating a boundary; betrayal is hard to forget. Recent research has indicated that betrayal alone, even in the absence of a perceived life threat, can produce PTSD.[51] Some adult patients who had rhinoplasties as teenagers cannot remember the name of the doctor, the city, or the hospital, but still remember that a parent forced the surgery. The patient's rightful anger can last for decades. Sometimes the surgeon can determine motivation by seeing the patient alone first.

★★★★★

The psychiatrist's daughter sat alone in the examination room with her arms folded tightly across her chest. She studied me with gimlet eyes. Her mouth was set defiantly. Her parents paced in the waiting room. That usually means it is a good idea to leave them there. I had been told that she wanted a rhinoplasty.

"What do you dislike about your nose?" I said.

She hesitated. "You tell me. My parents said you can make me pretty."

She paused and arched her back. Maybe she wanted to arm wrestle.

"You're the expert," she said.

I smiled for something to do.

She crossed her arms the other way and set her shoulders. She was doing her best to look tougher than Genghis Khan.

"I'm bored," she said. "Plus you've got nothing to say. What do plastic surgeons know?" I hoped she was being ironic.

"I know you don't want surgery," I said.

Something dark and unidentifiable passed behind her eyes. She looked directly at me.

"Bingo. I'm just along for the ride." Her voice quieted. "Maybe you're not so stupid."

"Well that's easy, then," I said. "I'll tell your parents we're not doing anything."

Her eyes changed again, but the rest of her stayed tight. I felt compassion for her. She wanted to run for the fence but knew she'd be caught.

The parents returned. Father took my hand; the other grasped my shoulder. The grip was strong, his gaze impenetrable. I'd probably admit to anything if I were sitting on his couch. He was comfortable in the kind of serene way people have when they are getting what they are due. His voice was loud in the small room.

"So, what are you going to do for my little girl?"

He was dressed as if he'd been sitting all day in a wrinkled navy suit with wide lapels, no tie, shirt open at the collar, and sandals. No socks. It was January. I was impressed. His wife shuffled behind in a gray smock and low heels.

"Talk," he said. "What's the plan?"

"There isn't any plan. We're not doing surgery," I said. "Right now, your daughter isn't ready. If she changes her mind, I'll see her again."

Something stirred behind his face. Evidently that was the wrong answer. He straightened and tipped his head so he could see me through the bottoms of his glasses. He let go of my hand.

"You must be kidding." He spaced his words for emphasis. "We are an old-fashioned family. In our family, the children do what the parents want."

I looked at his daughter. I could feel her starting to close down.

I smiled, even friendlier than a man selling retirement annuities. "I'm sure that's true. But I am not an old-fashioned surgeon. I won't operate until she asks me."

He looked at me like an aardvark looks at a termite.
"You're a nitwit." He spun on his heel and marched out. His wife fol-
lowed. She stuck her tongue out. As his daughter passed, she turned and
spoke so quietly that I had to lean forward to hear.
"This isn't over. But it's over for now."

★★★★★

Any decision to perform aesthetic surgery is an agreement between surgeon and patient, not between surgeon and parent. It is not the parents' job to find flaws or to transform their sons or daughters into something else, no matter how pure the motivation. Surgeons can do the same by pointing out imperfections that the patient has never noticed.

Kathy Davis writes from the feminist viewpoint, but touches all the same themes: a societal standard that connects goodness and beauty but that crushes women's self-esteem and creates a "general female propensity toward feelings of self-worthlessness."[52] Women are never good enough. Her examples of body shame are painful to read: "Hunched forward and with eyes downcast, she begins in a halting and barely audible monotone to explain that she is 'unhappy with what she has.' ... Her breasts are so small that she is ashamed." My patients recount stories of being misfits in a family where all the sisters were more beautiful. This is surgery to gain maternal approval; it is surgery to lose or retain the "family face." It is surgery to combat criticism and loneliness. And yet the abused return again and again seeking approval. "I actually never heard one word from them like, 'Don't you look great.' Not since the operation, never. That is what I really find difficult. ... I guess it means ... that I just did not belong to the family anymore."[52]

Is this perfectionism, is it obsessive compulsive disorder, is it depression, or is it body dysmorphic disorder? I hope that it is becoming clearer that it does not matter where you end up. The starting point is always the same. Its genesis and mediator is developmental trauma, its result is toxic shame, and its manifestations depend on how a particular shame bind becomes attached and is expressed.

The Self-Injury Literature and the Compulsion to Repeat Trauma

About 30 years ago I was called to the Emergency Room to treat a young woman who kept slashing her forearms. I was so ignorant of what I was actually seeing that when I asked why she did it, she dipped her head in silence. None of the wounds ever needed repair; they were only deep scratches. Once she realized that she had to see me anyway she would come directly to my office, tiptoe to the waiting room window, and wordlessly extend her bleeding forearms like a child bringing presents to her teacher. Her alexithymia was profound. Her face never showed emotion: not fear, not relief, not gratitude. Her voice had no prosody. Our conversations were brief, uniform, and dreamlike. I felt as if I were speaking in an empty room. She had a Ph.D. but was homeless. After I had bandaged her three times, she sent me a letter saying that she was going to kill me. At least the letter didn't explode. She never elaborated her reasoning. Some months later, this tortured young woman was found murdered in a lonely alleyway in Chicago.

Surgeons had no sophisticated diagnoses for what they were seeing then. But we all too often diagnose only what we know how to treat. In this case, the diagnosis was superficial, self-inflicted lacerations. What escaped me was its meaning to the patient.

Early Recognition of Self-Injury

Threads emerged in the earliest literature. In 1967, Graff and Mallin,[53] psychiatrists at Hahnemann Medical College, reported a group of 21 patients, all women except one, admitted for cutting their wrists. Until that time, self-injury had been lumped with attempted suicide; these physicians made a critical separation (See Table 5.1).

Excerpts of their data are tabulated below (Table 5.1). The patients were usually in their 20's, mostly unmarried, mostly college graduates, commonly the oldest female child in the family. The authors' opinions of both parents were poor, particularly the mothers, many of whom. Were judged to be perfectionistic, compulsive, and depressed, with poor self-images. Their families had identified some abnormality in 40% of the patients before the age of three. Seventy-five percent had cut themselves before the age of 25. Fifty-five percent had cut themselves more than 20 times. Ninety-five percent had been hospitalized more than twice, 25 percent more than three times. Many were sexually promiscuous; almost as many were sexually inexperienced. Most were not alcohol abusers, though most abused drugs. The majority always expressed anger turned toward themselves, and all had poor interpersonal relationships. Nightmares and uncontrollable tantrums were common; today PTSD would be suspected. Their mothers were viewed as cold, obsessive, verbally abusive, controlling, and perfectionistic. The patients' fathers were distant, abandoning, and hypercritical, but passive toward their wives. Although the authors could not document thought disorders, low self-esteem, feelings of shame and inadequacy were consistently present.

Regrettably, these uniform descriptions of parental abusive and neglectful behavior were dismissed by the authors as manifestations of the patients' character disorders. Instead, the diagnoses were "adjustment reaction of adolescence" (10%), "psychoneurosis" (10%), "emotionally stable personality" (35%) "sociopathic personality" (5%), and "schizophrenia" (40%).

It is easy to lose focus once cutting it is suspected or diagnosed because the image itself is so powerfully disturbing. Try this: Instead of thinking of a "cutter," picture a 23-year-old woman who hates her parents, hates herself, is perfectionistic,

Characteristic	Percent	Characteristic	Percent	Characteristic	Percent
Age Mean—23 years		Position in Sibship		Psychological Diagnosis	
Range—13–42 Years		First Child	30	(More than One May Be Given for Each)	
		Second Child	40	Impulsive	35
Marital Status		After Second Child	30	Perfectionist & Compulsive	25
Single	75			Depressive	25
Married	25	Age at First Cut		Psychosis	10
Marriageable Age	55	11–15	20	Borderline	10
		16–20	30	Fear of Desertion	10
Education		21–25	25	Aggressive	10
High School Student	30	26–38	25	Poor Self-Image	10
High School Graduate	15				
Attended College	40	Total Number of Cuts		Reasons For Cutting	
College Graduate	15	0–5	20	Pleasure and Relief	25
		5–10	25	Anger	20
View of Father		11–20	30	Depression	20
Poor	60	21–24	10	Unstated	35
Indifferent	30	More Than 40	15		
Good	10			Sexual Experience	
		Number of Hospitalizations		Promiscuous	50
View of Mother		One	5	Little	10
Poor	85	Two	55	None	40
Indifferent	5	Three	15		
Good	10	More Than Three	25	Alcohol Yes	30
				No	70
Age at Time of 1st Problem		Clinical Diagnosis			
(if identified)		Adjustment Reaction		Drugs Yes	75
1–3	40	of Adolescence	10	No	25
6–8	15	Psychoneurosis	10		
Adolescent	35	Emotionally Unstable		Expression of Anger	
Unreported	10	Personality	35	Turns Against Self	60
		Sociopathic Personality	5	Outward	40
		Schizophrenia	40	Interpersonal Relations Yes	0
				No	100

Adapted from Graff H, Mallin R. The syndrome of the wrist cutter. *Amer J Psychiat* 1967; 124:1:36–42.

depressed, angry, promiscuous, has poor interpersonal relations, abuses drugs, and has been hospitalized at least twice since her teen years for self-injury—now tell me what you see. The image cries "child abuse." How much progress might we have made if the patients' allegations had been taken at face value and the parental effect had been recognized.

There is more revealing information in this early report. About half of the patients were able to describe the reasons for their cutting. Forty percent of those noted that the experience was pleasurable and painless. Tension would increase and quickly become uncontrollable until the cutting released it. The trigger was almost always a parental visit.

Support From Individual Patient Histories

A single case report was remarkable in some details. The patient was 21 years old and had just cut herself for the first time. The authors described the provocative incident as "an incestuous encounter with the husband of her 40-year-old half-sister." Today we would call that rape by a family member. Even as a child, the patient feared her parents, who were verbally and physically abusive and neglectful. She felt unwanted and "inadequate" and had been a sickly child, always on the outside looking in. She would vomit after being ridiculed by peers—the vagal response to overwhelming threat (Chapter 7). This young woman believed that her sexual promiscuity was a desire for physical contact at any price. Pain from sports or rough physical contact was pleasurable. Recall the cosmetic patients I have described who enjoy the discomfort of the postoperative period—their "happiest times."

The authors make the critical observation that these patients' abnormal behavior began before they could speak. Many were ignored or rejected by their parents. They correctly connected the patients' obsessive thoughts and behavior to their bodies and indicated that "Therapy, to reach them, must be through physical, preverbal messages," a principle that has become the most powerful therapeutic avenue for complex trauma.[54, 55] The authors remarked that most patients were women, a characteristic that continues today. They speculated that the reason that men did not cut themselves derived from how they were treated by their mothers. There are, however, consistent gender differences in trauma response: women are more likely to fly or freeze, men are more likely to fight.[55, 56] Men traumatized in childhood are more likely to abuse others; women are more likely to submit to abuse or turn on themselves.[57] This gender characteristic may in part explain why stories of hostile men dominate the body dysmorphic literature and constitute the most terrifying cases to plastic surgeons. My own data has not indicated that men are necessarily more numerous; but that their aggressive, dangerous behavior does make them more memorable.

★★★★★

Subsequent reports confirmed and expanded Graff and Mallen's observations. They are exceedingly troubling. Physical abuse was present in 60% of patients in one study.[58] Sexual abuse was common. Most patients were depressed. Many had eating disorders. "Disgust" (an overpowering visceral emotion), "emptiness," and self-hatred were almost uniformly present.[59] The authors also note that 60% of the cutting episodes occurred during menstruation (presumably because of its sexual connotation), and that many of these patients had been helpless victims of frightening surgical experiences at very young ages—for example, painful restraint after orthopedic surgery. The cutting ritual, however, unlike the childhood trauma, was completely controlled: the patient determined the time, the extent, and how quickly the bleeding was controlled.

The same themes persist in other reports.[60, 61] Most patients had "disrupted families," low self-esteem, abandonment, isolation, incestuous sexual abuse, poor social support, depression, anger, suicidal ideation, and parental hatred. Perhaps most striking is the age at which self-injury began: 20% in the Graff and Mallen group began as preteens;[53] three of the patients in Pattison and Kahan's study began before the age of six.[60]

Women Who Hurt Themselves

Dusty Miller has thoroughly described the self-injury syndrome in *Women Who Hurt Themselves*,[57] and makes two insightful observations. First, she links obsessive addictions to drugs, alcohol, eating disorders, self-injury, gambling, sex (and, I would add, work) to childhood abuse and neglect. Second, she recognizes the commonly obsessive connection to cosmetic plastic surgery and links all of this behavior to the profound shame that develops in childhood. "Women who hurt themselves, men who hurt themselves, and adolescents who hurt themselves are seeking through their preferred addictions to escape the pain of childhood suffering."[57] This is precisely correct but it is not easy to trace those bonds. Reading the various branches of the addiction, shame, trauma, and body image literature is like watching the members of a large family each describe their hobbies. But Miller is right: they are intimately connected.

In the many patients that Miller describes, abuse is profound and ubiquitous. These tortured individuals develop shame cores that manifest in predictable behavior. Self-esteem is absent; protective boundaries do not exist; life experiences are processed in shaming and self-destructive ways; life is lived without moderation or self-protection. Miller terms the self-abuse cycle "Trauma Reenactment Syndrome," which has four distinguishing characteristics: (1) The sense of being at war with one's own body; (2) compulsive, excessive secrecy; (3) inability to self-correct [inadequate boundaries or self-care]; and (4) a constant struggle for situational and relationship control. The latter characteristic is particularly significant: because the abused child felt powerless, the decision to cut, starve, or medicate would seem self-empowering. Each cycle is a reenactment of childhood trauma that is familiar, painful, paradoxically pleasurable and applicable to additive plastic surgery.

The Compulsion to Reenact

The drive for repeated surgery compels some patients. I recall a man who had undergone nine nasal surgeries over a 30 year by several famous surgeons with good outcomes. Yet he pleaded with me to move a tiny piece of rib from one nostril to the other. Strictly speaking, he was not delusional. The cartilage could be moved. He said that the fragment caused pain and tingling, and while his wife prayed the rosary he begged me to give him "peace of mind," even though he knew his pain would remain. "I won't cause you any problems," he said. "Just please do this for me." Here is where surgeons get caught. The compulsion is not vanity; it is toxic shame from which the surgeon represents rescue.[30, 62] "When the therapist fails to live up to these idealized expectations . . . the patient is often overcome with fury. Because the patient feels as though her life depends upon her rescuer, she cannot afford to be tolerant; there is no room for human error."[63] Under the best circumstances the trauma never goes away, but it can lose its terrible grip.

Reenactment Is Always About Unfinished Business

Miller, herself a survivor of deliberate self-injury, describes each cycle as follows: the woman feels unbearable rage or shame, particularly after a family interaction; she hurts herself and then feels disgusted by what she has done, and so punishes herself through further self-injury. Tension that increases during the shaming period dissipates until the next cycle begins.

Additional supporting data for Miller's clinical scenario is not hard to find and predictably disturbing. Van der Kolk, Perry, and Herman followed 74 patients over a four-year span and correlated suicide attempts and deliberate self- injury with childhood sexual and physical abuse, among which the correlation with sexual abuse was the strongest.[64] The more severe the abuse history, the more likely patients were to continue self-destructive behavior even after treatment. Similarly, the more severe the trauma, the earlier cutting began and the more extensive it was; as the children grew, suicide attempts and anorexia followed milder forms of self-injury.

The age at which the trauma occurred determined how well it was managed. Withdrawal, hyperarousal, depression, self-anger, and dissociation may co-occur. Recall that alexithymia, shame, childhood trauma, and body shame are closely associated.[10, 65]

Those patients who were both sexually abused and neglected and could not remember feeling special or loved by anyone as children were least able to control their behavior. Van der Kolk reports that the patients most refractory to treatment recounted that as children they never felt safe; real and perceived abandonment was the common thread.[66] This latter point is particularly remarkable because emotional neglect is one of seven out of ten data points in our Adverse Childhood Events study in which my plastic surgery patients have prevalences significantly higher than Kaiser Permanente's general medical population (Chapter 9). Again we circle back to self-worth, reality, and self-care. The emptiness of the Lost Child is profoundly destructive.

★★★★★

She straddled my examination table with one leg tucked under her, the other swinging, coughing and wiping her nose. Both parents sat in chairs next to her. Mother had a clipboard in her lap, ready for my answers to her questions. I introduced myself. Mother gave an automatic facial expression, without meaning, to me at least. Father sat while he shook my hand and said hello. He had one of those Hollywood elocution voices.

What had troubled me about his daughter's intake sheet was that, at age 15, she was already on five psychotropic medications: Wellbutrin, Clonidine, Adderall, Vistaril, and Seroquel. I needed to speak to her alone. Mother remained starched and ironed and riveted together. Father sipped his coffee from a paper cup, looking over the rim, his gaze moving slowly over the photographs on the walls.

"I'd like to examine your daughter alone and then we will go over everything," I said. Her father nodded, rose as if he had lost all interest, and left. Mother stared as if she were a condor being asked to abandon her egg. She looked as if she wanted to argue with me but apparently thought better of it and walked out, closing the door sharply behind her.

I sat in front of her daughter.

"You're on a lot of medicines."

"I know." She paused and smiled proudly.

"I have two psychopharmacologists who prescribe them for me."

"Why do you take Clonidine?"

"For my panic attacks."

"How do you know when to take it?"

She coughed and blew her nose. "I guess when I'm going to panic." She coughed again.

I shook my head. "Why didn't you cancel your appointment and stay in bed? You're sick."

She put her thumb in her mouth and began to suck it. I noticed that she bit her nails.

"My parents said I had to come. I need more nose surgery."

I sighed quietly. "Okay. Why do you take Seroquel?"

She spoke around her thumb.

"I'm bipolar."

I paused. This was a game she'd played before: the doctor lobs questions over the wall and she answers, if she wishes. I felt like I were listening to a player piano.

"You take Vistaril 'as needed.' How do you know when to take it?"

She seemed to be musing. "You know. When I need it."

So far, she had been using words like a squid uses ink.

"That's too bad. You're so young. How long have you been on these medicines?"

She stared at me impassively. "Two years."

Questioning her was hard, but not yet as hard as pulling a camel through the eye of a needle.

"What happened then?"

Something was opening. I wasn't sure what, so I kept watching. Then she spoke softly, as if she were thinking aloud.

"I am a cutter."

I could feel her starting to close down but I decided to keep pressing, now that the ice had cracked.

"That's very tough," *I said gently.* "Usually cutters live in very bad circumstances and have had rough lives."

She stared as if I had just started speaking in tongues.

"I want you to understand." *I paused.* "This is not your fault."

She began to study my face so I continued.

"Trauma is somatic. That means it's stored in your body somewhere."

"Can it make me hurt myself?" *she said. She seemed interested.*

"It can, but you can do something about it," *I said.*

She looked toward the room where her parents waited. Her thumb disappeared into her mouth again.

"This is between you and me," *I said.* "I won't discuss it with your parents, but think about it." *She inclined her head to thank me, without commenting on whether she believed what I said.*

"Now tell me about your nose."

Outside it had begun to spit rain. Her parents paraded in silently, composed and defiant.

Her father still looked as hard and polished and expensive as he had earlier. Mother hadn't gotten friendlier. She looked at her clipboard and then stared at me, rougher than barbed wire. She cleared her throat and looked over the tops of her glasses.

"I want to know everything the last doctor did that was a mistake," *she said. She held up her clipboard, ready to write. Father dipped his head in acknowledgment. His daughter trailed her fingers along the exam table paper.*

"Nothing was a mistake," I said. "Everything was current acceptable practice. It just didn't help your daughter. I will give you my ideas, but it is too soon for surgery. The tissues haven't healed, and I need to know more from your daughter about what she would like.

"She is also on a lot of medications for a young adult. This isn't the time to add the stress of surgery. Let's talk in six months when life may be going better for her." I feared it wouldn't, but so far I had gotten farther listening than talking.

Her mother didn't seem to know what else to say, so she focused on being peevish and impenetrable. If I were marooned with her for three days, she could probably turn me into Prufrock.

★★★★★

I thought over what I knew, which didn't take that long, and what I didn't, which seemed nearly endless. What awful memories were stored in that young woman's brain, phantoms so bad that it was better to be numb? She had learned that what she couldn't feel wouldn't torture her. The long-term effect of this self-denial and dissociation is loss of reality, the sense that nothing matters. But we are meant to feel, so even the pain of self-injury can seem better than disconnection from the body. A longitudinal study in 84 girls with confirmed histories of sexual abuse indicated that the girls had more cognitive deficits, were more depressed, more dissociated, more sexually troubled, more obese, more likely to drop out of school, less healthy, and much more likely to self-mutilate.[67] It is this body disconnection that is the target of yoga, theater, eye movement desensitization and reprocessing (EMDR), somatic experiencing,[68, 69] and other therapies.[55, 70]

The detached, dysphoric pain of toxic shame cannot be easily soothed, and children whose abuse began very early in childhood discover that relief only comes from another physical trauma, a competing pain. It is thus important to recognize that childhood abuse victims do not self-injure to manipulate others; the pain is felt in silence and the cutting is done in secrecy, often amplifying the child's fear, helplessness, and shame.[71, 72] "I had not practiced medicine clinically in years. . . . I was desperate to feel anything, or to feel nothing, or somewhere in between. Yes, I wanted to obliterate. . . . But each day I choose to fight, and each day I feel just a little bit better. About myself, my relations to others, and what I can bring to this world. . . . I can start by staring this self-injury secret straight in the face and writing about it."[73] Regrettably, self-injury is so common that a treatment and research center has recently arisen at Cornell University (Cornell Research Program on Self-Injury and Recovery).

Deliberate self-harm is now called Nonsuicidal Self-Injury (NSSI) in the DSM-V, and has been classified as a Condition for Further Study, though it remains one of the criteria for Borderline Personality Disorder.[74]

Borderline Personality Disorder

Miller, who has devoted her career to treating self-injury patients, specifically highlights women with Borderline Personality Disorder because they were her most profoundly symptomatic patients.[57]

As I list the DSM-V criteria for Borderline Personality Disorder, compare them not only to self-injury patients and patients compelled to repeat trauma, but also to those who suffer from various addictions, including compulsive plastic surgery and body dysmorphic disorder. Finally, relate them to the characteristics of immature, or Adapted Wounded Child behavior (Chapter 3).[62,75,76]

These are the abbreviated criteria for Borderline Personality Disorder, DSM-5:[77]

- Impairment in self-functioning: Excessive self-criticism, chronic emptiness, poor self-esteem, unstable life course [recall Self-Esteem, Boundaries, Life Lived In Moderation]
- Impaired empathy, excessive sensitivity to criticism, fear of abandonment if relationships are too close [recall Love Avoidants]
- Emotional lability, intense anxiety, tension, or panic, fear of the future, fear of losing control, fear of rejection [recall Boundaries and Reality processing]
- Frequent depression, pessimism, and shame [recall Self-Esteem and Reality]
- Impulsivity, impaired directed behavior, desire to self-harm [recall Boundaries, Self-care, Living in Moderation]
- Indulgence in risky behavior without regard to consequences [recall Self-care, Love Avoidant]
- Thoughts of self-injury or suicide [recall Self-care]
- Hostility to teasing or insults [recall Self-esteem, Boundaries, Reality]

What can be so disarming about borderline patients is how normal they can appear to those outside the family and casual acquaintances.[78] Yet to their children, they shame, rage, destroy favorite toys, talk to themselves, never apologize for inappropriate behavior, punish independence, fear abandonment but threaten their children with it, discipline inconsistently, expect subservience to their needs, are unjustifiably untrusting of their children and unconfident of their goodness, worry, and expect perfection, but only from others. "The look" in their eyes frightens their children, some of who may cut themselves.[79,80] They depersonalize: even a sister can be described as "that girl," or her own mother as "your grandmother." As a result, their children become hypersensitive to impending attacks.[21,76,78,81,82] Throughout her life, my mother would rage or "ostracize" me for reasons usually understood only by her. The dominant vestige of this behavior is my excessive sensitivity to prosody: to this day, any volume or pitch increase, particularly in a woman's voice, triggers an instant reflex twinge. The content is almost irrelevant.

Even seven-month-old infants respond to the highly distressed or emotional content of voices through activation of their right superior temporal sulci, whereas happy prosody activates the right inferior frontal cortex. The mother's patient cooing, what Darwin and others called "the sweet music of the species," tunes the brain.[83]

★★★★★

Judith Herman and Bessel van der Kolk, who have so effectively posited the critical links among childhood trauma, PTSD, brain and body physiology, and the lifelong wasteland that complex trauma can create, established a connection between Borderline Personality Disorder (BPD) and childhood trauma nearly 30 years ago.[64, 81] In a cohort of 21 BPD patients contrasted with 23 non-Borderline but closely diagnostically related patients, borderline patients had experienced significantly more childhood trauma than those without borderline traits (81% vs. 52%). There was also a dose-response curve: patients with borderline traits but without BPD had intermediate amounts of childhood trauma exposure. Of particular significance to the effect on the Wounded Child is how early the trauma began: 57% of BPD patients had experienced physical or sexual abuse or witnessed domestic trauma by the age of six, compared to only 13% without BPD traits. The BPD patients exceeded other groups in both total trauma prevalence and more types of trauma through the preteen and teenage years: by age 12, 81% of BPD patients had witnessed childhood trauma, nearly three times the prevalence in those without BPD. By age 18, the differences had lessened, though the BPD patients' trauma exposure still exceeded the non-BPD patients by 36% (81% vs. 52%).

★★★★★

Musing about the convoluted intricacies of Gatsby's plan to re-ignite a relationship with Daisy, Nick Carraway says, "[Gatsby] had waited five years and bought a mansion where he dispensed starlight to casual moths—so that he could 'come over' some afternoon to a stranger's garden. . . . Suddenly I wasn't thinking of Daisy and Gatsby anymore. . . . A phrase began to beat in my ears with a sort of heady excitement: 'There are only the pursued, the pursuing, the busy, and the tired.'"[13]

★★★★★

Childhood Trauma and Self-Harming Adult Behavior

Virtually every paper that looks for a connection between childhood trauma and adult adversity finds one. Childhood sexual abuse and incest create significant PTSD, accompanied by hypervigilance, fear, intrusive flashbacks, dissociation, drug and alcohol abuse, self-mutilation, and suicide attempts,[30] behavior problems, sexualized behavior, and absent self-esteem.[84] The same is true for emotional abuse and neglect, which correlate with internalized shame and bipolar disorder.[85–87] In a study of 233 patients followed over an average of 7.5 years, sexual abuse correlated with a two- to four-fold risk of adult psychosis.[88, 89]

And that isn't the end. Imagine almost any self-medicating or self-harming behavior that impairs a functional life, and someone has probably connected it to childhood trauma. Patients seeking couples sexual therapy have a high prevalence of childhood sexual abuse.[90, 91] Ninety-seven percent of 456 adults patients (mean age 40 years) with dissociative disorders (amnesia, depersonalization, identity fragmentation, de-realization, mixed identity, and identity disorder) had at least one episode of childhood sexual or emotional abuse.[92] Sexual abuse and witnessing violence as a child increase the chances of being unemployed or fired as an adult,[93, 94] and increase the risks of being bullied, bullying, panic disorder, agoraphobia, and of suicide.[95–98] Similarly, emotional abuse and witnessing violence directly correlated with compulsive buying.[93] Childhood sexual abuse correlated strongly with sexually violent behavior in a population of psychotic adults,[99] for whom the lifetime risk of PTSD was a stunning 98%.[100]

★★★★★

The bad news continues. Childhood physical abuse is associated with a higher prevalence of suicidality in depressed women[101] and in patients with bipolar disorder.[102, 103] Alexithymia, associated with childhood trauma, shame, and body image disorders,[10, 104] directly connects with depression, substance abuse disorders, anorexia nervosa, bulimia nervosa, panic disorder, somatoform pain disorder,[105] dissociation and Internet addiction,[106] and Complex Regional Pain Syndrome.[107]

From the obstetrics and gynecology literature we have an interesting observation that relates directly to what many physicians see but cannot interpret without understanding its trigger. Amina White, who advises routine inquiry about childhood abuse and rape as part of any patient history, notes that normal altered bodily sensations during pregnancy may trigger disturbing reminders of past sexual abuse and precipitate the hallmarks of PTSD: intrusive, recurrent memories, avoidance of reminders of the traumatic event, autonomic arousal, and mood alteration.[91] The unique triggers of pregnancy include fetal movement, body changes, and the routine breast and pelvic examinations intrinsic in prenatal care. In fact, data suggest that PTSD is higher among pregnant than non-pregnant women in the United States.[108, 109] Childhood abuse survivors who lose bladder or bowel continence during childbirth may be triggered to flashbacks of similar loss of control during childhood abuse.[110] Similarly, abuse survivors have greater levels of mental dissociation during labor, greater postpartum depression, and impaired maternal-infant bonding, which in turn are associated with disturbances in cognitive, behavioral, and emotional infant development, a disquieting transgenerational propagation.[111–113]

How Relational Childhood Trauma May Generate Compulsive Adult Behavior

How can we make a narrative out of these observations? Let us begin by accepting the long-held assumption that adverse childhood experiences can roil under the surface throughout life. This observation is an early one that influenced the treatment methods of Charcot, Janet, and Freud.

Let us also recognize that people who have been traumatized compulsively and perhaps unwittingly re-expose themselves to circumstances reminiscent or repetitive of the initial trauma.[114] Violent criminals reenacting their victimization have often been physically or sexually abused as children.[115–117] Significant percentages of abused children bite, burn, or cut themselves.[118] Childhood neglect impairs the ability to modulate physiological arousal. Physicians commonly see this behavior in patients who cannot reassure themselves or who cannot recall comforting medical advice even moments after it is given. At stressful times or faced with danger, both children and adults seek comforting, increased attachment, even if its only source is an abuser.[119] The drive for attachment prevails over memories of the trauma, so that the abused paint over the behavior and make excuses for it, a common phenomenon in abusive marriages. The more the victim organizes her life around her abuser, the less opportunity she has to build a healthy supportive network. When the abuse recurs, the victims protect themselves by dissociating from the incident so that they can deny that it happened; what follows is a sense of numbness and constriction, depression, self-blame, and learned helplessness. There is no forgiveness; there is no reconciliation. Chronic hyperarousal becomes the physiologic response to repetitive trauma.[120]

★★★★★

Trauma pain is medicated by varying activities, addictions, or deliberate self-injury.[121, 122] In my own field, patients who are the most driven to repetitive surgeries have histories of multiple prior operations, depression, high prevalences of childhood trauma, and low levels of postoperative satisfaction.[123, 124] They do not fear surgery appropriately. Their drive for more operations overwhelms their ability to assess surgical risks. Many have histories of multiple complications, yet they return again and again for more, often to the surgeons who created the initial problem and whom they no longer trust. Not one patient has been able to give me an adequate explanation for this behavior. The unconvincing rationale is, "I guess because the next surgery was free." Is their conduct a marker for compulsive trauma repetition, re-victimization, cutting, self-destructive behavior, or traumatic bonding to the surgeons who injured them? Presently no one knows, but the parallels are provocative.

Individuals whose lives suggest behavior that is not healthily self-protective and prudent may flag persistent childhood abuse or neglect that can corrupt the physician-patient relationship. These patients' responses to adversity are biased toward hyperarousal and re-experiencing. Triggers that are not apparent to the surgeon can provoke unexpectedly strong emotional responses, unjustified fear of abandonment, and seemingly irrational anger that may be impossible to manage.

What This Information Means

Trauma sequelae are not observations that surgeons freely make. Instead, we see disempowered patients who do not know what they want or seek endless surgeries, are unjustifiably untrusting, or driven by shame. When stressed, they believe that they have been victimized and cannot regulate their emotions. They become our most memorable and difficult patients, which is why we must recognize their characteristics earlier, understand their motivations, and guide them appropriately.

When we discuss body image disorders, are we talking about body shame, PTSD, obsessive compulsive disorder, borderline personality disorder, eating disorders, deliberate self-injury, or body dysmorphic disorder? It doesn't seem to matter. Associated childhood trauma seems to be the ultimate driver of each of these unhealthy behaviors. As the trauma digs roots and grows in trauma survivors' lives, one or another of these unattractive blooms may become its manifestation, depending in part upon the location of the toxic shame bind. The dizzying similarity among all these disorders is not an accident. Antecedent developmental trauma is always at the core. Self-esteem is absent; patients are boundaryless, unable to process reality normally; imagine criticism or humiliation where it does not exist; and lead dysregulated, immoderate lives devoid of appropriate self-care. The similarities among these conditions are striking. Sometimes the only difference among them is the particular pathologic outcome being assessed. It doesn't seem possible to understand or effectively treat obesity, borderline personality disorder, deliberate self-injury, eating disorders, BDD, or any of the addictions without recognizing the impact of individual childhood events or the self-harming habits that they foster. That's where the thread leads next.

References

1. Barrie JM. *The Annotated Peter Pan: The Centennial Edition*. New York: W W Norton & Company; 1937.
2. Thomas EM. Robert E. *Lee: A Biography*. New York: W W Norton & Company; 1995.
3. Andrews B. Bodily Shame in Relation to Abuse in Childhood and Bulimia: A Preliminary Investigation. *Br J Clin Psychol* 1997; 36:41–49.
4. Andrews B, Qian M, Valentine JD. Predicting Depressive Symptoms with a New Measure of Shame: The Experience of Shame Scale. *Br J Clin Psychol* 2002; 41:29–42.
5. Andrews B. Bodily Shame as a Mediator Between Abusive Experiences and Depression. *J Abnormal Psychol* 1995; 104:2:277–285.
6. Andrews B. Shame, Early Abuse, and Course of Depression in a Clinical Sample: A Preliminary Study. *Cogn Emot* 1997; 11:373–381.

7. Tantleff-Dunn S, Lindner DM. Body Image and Social Functioning. In: Cash TF, Smolak L, eds. *Body Image*. 2nd edition. New York: The Guilford Press; 2011:263–271.

8. Hundt NE, Holohan DR. The Role of Shame in Distinguishing Perpetrators of Intimate Partner Violence in U.S. Veterans. *J Trauma Stress* 2012; 25:191–197.

9. Snell JE, Rosenwald RJ, Robey A. The Wifebeater's Wife. *Arch Gen Psychiatry* 1964; 11:107–112.

10. Franzoni E, Gualandi S, Caretti V, et al. The Relationship Between Alexithymia, Shame, Trauma, and Body Image Disorders: Investigation Over a Large Clinical Sample. *Neuropsychiatr Dis Treat* 2013; 9:185–193.

11. DeBardaris D, Serroni N, Campanella D. Alexithymia and Its Relationships with Dissociative Experiences, Body Dissatisfaction, and Eating Disturbances in a Non-Clinical Female Sample. *Cogn Ther Res* 2009; 33:5:471–479.

12. Noll SM, Frederickson BL. A Mediational Model Linking Self-Objectification, Body Shame, and Disordered Eating. *Psychol Women Quar* 1998; 22:623–636.

13. Fitzgerald, FS. *The Great Gatsby*. New York: Harper Collier; 1982.

14. Didie ER, Kuniega-Pietrzak T, Phillips KA. Body Image in Patients with Body Dysmorphic Disorder: Evaluations of and Investment in Appearance, Health/Illness, and Fitness. *Body Image* 2010; 7:66–69.

15. Wenninger K, Heiman JR. Relating Body Image to Psychological and Sexual Functioning in Child Sexual Abuse Survivors. *J Traumatic Stress* 1998; 11:3:543–562.

16. Weaver TL, Resnick HS, Kokoska MS, et al. Appearance-Related Residual Injury, Posttraumatic Stress, and Body Image: Associations Within a Sample of Female Victims of Intimate Partner Violence. *J Traumatic Stress* 2007; 20:6:999–1008.

17. Briere J. The Long-Term Clinical Correlates of Childhood Sexual Victimization. *Ann NY Acad Sci* 1988; 528:1:327–334.

18. Sack M, Boroske-Leiner K, Lahmann C. Association of Nonsexual and Sexual Traumatizations with Body Image and Psychosomatic Symptoms in Psychosomatic Outpatients. *Gen Hosp Psychiatry* 2010; 32:315–320.

19. Felitti VJ, Jakstis K, Pepper V, et al. Obesity: Problem, Solution, or Both? *Perm J* 2010; 14:1:24–31.

20. Sanders B, Becker-Lausen E. The Measurement of Psychological Maltreatment: Early Data on the Child Abuse and Trauma Scale. *Child Abuse Neglect* 1995; 19:3:315–323.

21. Witthoft M, Borgmann E, White A, et al. Body-Related Attentional Biases in Patients with Posttraumatic Stress Disorder Resulting from Childhood Sexual Abuse with and without Co-Occurring Borderline Personality Disorder. *J Behav Ther Exp Psychiatr* 2015; 46:72–77.

22. Osler W. *The Principles and Practice of Medicine: Designed for the Use of Practitioners and Students of Medicine*. New York / London: D. Appleton and Company; 1912.

23. Bliss M. *William Osler: A Life in Medicine*. New York / Oxford [UK]: Oxford University Press; 1999, 449.

24. Livingston EH. Reimagining Obesity in 2018: A JAMA Theme Issue on Obesity. *JAMA* 2018; 319:3:238–240.

25. Dorahy MJ, Clearwater K. Shame and Guilt in Men Exposed to Childhood Sexual Abuse: A Qualitative Investigation. *J Child Sex Abuse* 2012; 21:155–175.

26. Felitti VJ, Anda RF. The Lifelong Effects of Adverse Childhood Experiences, Chapter 10. In: *Chadwick's Child Maltreatment: Sexual Abuse and Psychological Maltreatment*. 4th edition. Florissant [MO]: STM Learning; 2014.

27. Epstein RM. Responding to Suffering. *JAMA* 2015; 314:24:2623–2624.

28. Andrews B, Hunter E. Shame, Early Abuse, and Course of Depression in a Clinical Sample: A Preliminary Study. *Cogn Emot* 1997; 11:4:373–381.

29. del Rosario PM, White RM. The Internalized Shame Scale: Temporal Stability, Internal Consistency, and Principal Components Analysis. *Pers Individ Diff* 2006; 41:1:95–103.

30. Herman JL. *Trauma and Recovery: The Aftermath of Violence: From Domestic Abuse to Political Terror.* New York: Basic Books (Perseus Books Group); 1992.

31. Flynn E. *My Wicked, Wicked Ways.* New York: Cooper Square Press; 2003:342, 345.

32. Andrews B. Body Shame and Abuse in Childhood. In: Gilbert P, Miles J, eds. *Body Shame: Conceptualization, Research and Treatment.* East Sussex [UK]: Routledge; 2002:256–266.

33. Andrews B, Brewin CR, Rose S, et al. Predicting PTSD Symptoms in Victims of Violent Crime: The Role of Shame, Anger, and Childhood Abuse. *J Abnormal Psychol* 2000; 109:1:69–73.

34. Felitti VJ. Reverse Alchemy in Childhood: Turning Gold into Lead. *Health Alert* 2001; 8:1:1–11.

35. Wolf N. *The Beauty Myth: How Images of Beauty Are Used Against Women.* New York: Anchor Books (Doubleday); 1991.

36. Troop NA, Redshaw C. General Shame and Bodily Shame in Eating Disorders: A 2.5-Year Longitudinal Study. *Eur Eat Disorders* 2012; 20:373–378.

37. Bienvenu OJ, Samuels JF, Riddle MA, et al. The Relationship of Obsessive-Compulsive Disorder to Possible Spectrum Disorders: Results from a Family Study. *Biol Psychiatry* 2000; 48:287–293.

38. Rodhe P, Ichikawa L, Simon GE, et al. Associations of Child Sexual Abuse and Physical Abuse with Obesity and Depression in Middle-Aged Women. *Child Abuse Neglect* 2008; 32:9:878–887.

39. Gilbert P, Price JS, Alan S. Social Comparison, Social Attractiveness, and Evolution: How Might They Be Related? *New Ideas Psychol* 1995; 13:2:149–165.

40. Sperry S, Thompson JK, Sarwer DB, et al. Cosmetic Surgery Reality TV Viewership: Relations with Cosmetic Surgery Attitudes, Body Image, and Disordered Eating. *Ann Plast Surg* 2009; 62:1:7–11.

41. Gilbert P, Miles J, eds. *Body Shame: Conceptualization, Research and Treatment.* East Sussex [UK]: Routledge; 2002:38.

42. Gilbert P, Miles J, eds. *Body Shame: Conceptualization, Research and Treatment.* East Sussex [UK]: Routledge; 2002:13.

43. Gilbert P, Miles J, eds. *Body Shame: Conceptualization, Research and Treatment.* East Sussex [UK]: Routledge; 2002:16.

44. Gilbert P, Miles J, eds. *Body Shame: Conceptualization, Research and Treatment.* East Sussex [UK]: Routledge; 2002:24.

45. Gilbert P, Miles J, eds. *Body Shame: Conceptualization, Research and Treatment.* East Sussex [UK]: Routledge; 2002:28.

46. Thompson A, Kent G. Adjusting to Disfigurement: Processes Involved in Dealing with Being Visibly Different. *Clin Psychol Rev* 2001; 21:5:663–682.

47. Kent G, Thompson AR. The Development and Maintenance of Shame in Disfigurement: Implications for Treatment. In: Gilbert P, Miles J, eds. *Body Shame: Conceptualization, Research and Treatment.* East Sussex [UK]: Routledge; 2002:103–116.

48. Goss K, Gilbert P. Eating Disorders, Shame and Pride: A Cognitive-Behavioural Functional Analysis. In: Gilbert P, Miles J, eds. *Body Shame: Conceptualization, Research and Treatment.* East Sussex [UK]: Routledge; 2002:219.

49. Blum VL. *Flesh Wounds: The Culture of Cosmetic Surgery.* Los Angeles: University of California Press; 2003.

50. Greenberg JL, Limoncelli KE, Wilhelm S. Body Dysmorphic Disorder by Proxy. In: Phillips KA, ed. *Body Dysmorphic Disorder: Advances in Research and Clinical Practice*. New York: Oxford University Press; 2017:95–102.

51. Kelley LP, Weathers FW, Mason EA, et al. Association of Life Threat and Betrayal with Posttraumatic Stress Disorder Symptom Severity. *J Trauma Stress* 2012; 25:408–415.

52. Davis K. *Reshaping the Female Body: The Dilemma of Cosmetic Surgery*. New York: Routledge; 1995.

53. Graff H, Mallin R. The Syndrome of the Wrist Cutter. *Am J Psychiat* 1967; 124:1:36–42.

54. Mellody P, Miller AW, Miller JK. *Facing Codependence: What It Is, Where It Comes From, How It Sabotages Our Lives*. New York: Harper Collins; 1989.

55. van der Kolk BA. *The Body Keeps the Score: Brain, Mind, and Body in the Healing of Trauma*. New York: Viking (Penguin Group); 2014.

56. Olff M, Langeland W, Draijer N, et al. Gender Differences in Posttraumatic Stress Disorder. *Psychol Bull* 2007; 133:2:183–204.

57. Miller D. *Women Who Hurt Themselves: A Book of Hope and Understanding*. Cambridge [MA]: Basic Books [Perseus Books Group]; 1994.

58. Rosenthal RJ, Rinzler C, Wallsh R, et al. Wrist-Cutting Syndrome: The Meaning of a Gesture. *Am J Psychiatry* 1972; 128:11:1363–1368.

59. Bradshaw JE. *Post-Romantic Stress Disorder: What To Do When The Honeymoon Is Over*. Deerfield Beach [FL]: Health Communications; 2014.

60. Pattison EM, Kahan J. The Deliberate Self-Harm Syndrome. *Am J Psychiatry* 1983; 140:7:867–872.

61. Simpson CA, Porter GL. Self-Mutilation in Children and Adolescents. *Bull Menninger Clin* 1981; 45:5:428–438.

62. Bradshaw J. *Healing the Shame That Binds You*. Deerfield Beach [FL]: Health Communications; 2005:159–165.

63. Herman JL. *Trauma and Recovery: The Aftermath of Violence: From Domestic Abuse to Political Terror*. New York: Basic Books (Perseus Books Group); 1992:137.

64. van der Kolk BA, Perry LC, Herman JL. Childhood Origins of Self-Destructive Behavior. *Am J Psychiatry* 1991; 148:12:1665–1671.

65. Zlotnick C, Mattia JI, Zimmerman M. The Relationship between Posttraumatic Stress Disorder, Childhood Trauma and Alexithymia in an Outpatient Sample. *J Traumatic Stress* 2001; 14:1:177–188.

66. van der Kolk BA. *The Body Keeps the Score: Brain, Mind, and Body in the Healing of Trauma*. New York: Viking (Penguin Group); 2014:141.

67. Trickett PK, Noll JG, Putnam FW. The Impact of Sexual Abuse on Female Development: Lessons from a Multigenerational, Longitudinal Research Study. *Dev Psychopathol* 2011; 23:2:453–476.

68. Levine PA, Frederick A. *Waking the Tiger: Healing Trauma*. Berkeley [CA]: North Atlantic Books; 1997.

69. Levine PA. *In an Unspoken Voice: How the Body Releases Trauma and Restores Goodness*. Berkeley [CA]: North Atlantic Books; 2010.

70. Levis DJ. A Review of Childhood Abuse Questionnaires and Suggested Treatment Approaches. In: Kalfoğlu EA, Faikoğlu R, eds. *Sexual Abuse: Breaking the Silence*. Rijeka, Croatia: InTech.; 2012:1.

71. van der Kolk BA. The Compulsion to Repeat the Trauma. *Psychiatric Clin NAm* 1989; 12:2:389–411.

72. van der Kolk BA. Foreword. In: Ogden P, Minton K, Pain C, eds. *Trauma and the Body*. New York: W W Norton & Company; 2006:41–64.

73. Fortescue EB. Mercy. *JAMA* 2015; 314: 1231–1232.

74. Kerr PL, Muehlenkamp JJ, Turner JM. Nonsuicidal Self-Injury: A Review of Current Research for Family Medicine and Primary Care Physicians. *J Am Board Fam Med* 2010; 23:2:240–259.

75. Mellody P, Freundlich LS. *The Intimacy Factor: The Ground Rules for Overcoming the Obstacles to Truth, Respect, and Lasting Love*. New York: Harper Collins; 2003.

76. Mason PT, Kreger R. *Stop Walking on Eggshells: Taking Your Life Back When Someone You Care about Has Borderline Personality Disorder*. Oakland [CA]: New Harbinger Publications; 1998.

77. American Psychiatric Association. *Desk Reference to the Diagnostic Criteria from DSM-5*. Washington, DC: American Psychiatric Publishing; 2013:131, 325–326.

78. Zanarini MC, Frankenburg FR, Khera GS, et al. Treatment Histories of Borderline Inpatients. *Comp Psychiatry* 2001; 42:2:144–150.

79. Lawson R, Waller G, Sines J, et al. Emotional Awareness among Eating-Disordered Patients: The Role of Narcissistic Traits. *Eur Eat Dis Rev* 2008; 16:44–48.

80. Ledoux JE, Romanski L, Xagoraris A. Indelibility of Subcortical Emotional Memories. *J Cogn Neurosci* 1989; 1:238–243.

81. Herman JL, Perry JC, van der Kolk BA. Childhood Trauma in Borderline Personality Disorder. *Am J Psychiatry* 1989; 146:4:490–495.

82. Melges FT, Swartz MS. Oscillations of Attachment in Borderline Personality Disorder. *Am J Psychiatry* 1989; 146:9:1115–1120.

83. Schore AN. *The Science of The Art of Psychotherapy*. New York: W W Norton & Company; 2012:395.

84. Kendall-Tackett KA, Williams LM, Finkelhor D. Impact of Sexual Abuse on Children: A Review and Synthesis of Recent Empirical Studies. *Psychol Bull* 1993; 113:1:164–180.

85. Felitti VJ, Anda RF. The Lifelong Effects of Adverse Childhood Experiences. *Chadwick's Child Maltreat: Sex Abuse Psychol Maltreat* 2014; 2:203–215.

86. Dong M, Anda RF, Felitti, VJ, et al. The Interrelatedness of Multiple Forms of Childhood Abuse, Neglect, and Household Dysfunction. *Child Abuse Neglect* 2004; 28:7:771–784.

87. Fowke A, Ross S, Ashcroft K. Childhood Maltreatment and Internalized Shame in Adults With a Diagnosis of Bipolar Disorder. *Clin Psychol Psychother* 2012; 19:450–457.

88. Thompson AD, Nelson B, Yuen HP, et al. Sexual Trauma Increases the Risk of Developing Psychosis in an Ultra High-Risk "Prodromal" Population. *Schizophrenia Bullet* 2014; 40:3:697–706.

89. Thompson JK, Wonderlich SA. Child Sexual Abuse and Eating Disorders. In: Thompson JK, ed. *Handbook of Eating Disorders and Obesity*. Hoboken, NJ: Wiley; 2004:679–694.

90. Berthelot N, Godbout N, Hebert M, et al. Prevalence and Correlates of Childhood Sexual Abuse in Adults Consulting for Sexual Problems. *J Sex Marital Ther* 2014; 40:5:434–443.

91. White A. Responding to Prenatal Disclosure of Past Sexual Abuse. *Obstet Gynecol* 2014; 123:6:1344–1347.

92. Gaon A, Kaplan Z, Dwolatzky T, et al. Dissociative Symptoms as a Consequence of Traumatic Experiences: The Long-Term Effects of Childhood Sexual Abuse. *Isr J Psychiatry Relat Sci* 2013; 50:1:17–23.

93. Sansone RA, Chang J, Jewell B, et al. Childhood Trauma and Compulsive Buying. *Intl J Psychiatry Clin Pract* 2013; 17:73–76.

94. Sansone RA, Leung JS, Wiederman MW. Five Forms of Childhood Trauma: Relationships with Employment in Adulthood. *Child Abuse Neglect* 2012; 36:676–679.

95. Copeland WE, Wolke D, Angold A, et al. Adult Psychiatric and Suicide Outcomes of Bullying and Being Bullied by Peers in Childhood and Adolescence. *JAMA Psychiatry* 2013; 70:4:419–426.

96. Panter-Brick C, Goodman A, Tol W, et al. Mental Health and Childhood Adversities: A Longitudinal Study in Kabul, Afghanistan. *J Am Acad Child Adolesc Psychiatry* 2011; 50:4:349–363.

97. Panter-Brick C, Grimon MP, Kalin M, et al. Trauma Memories, Mental Health, and Resilience: A Prospective Study of Afghan Youth. *J Child Psychol Psychiatry* 2015; 56:7:814–825.

98. Warshaw MG, Dolan RT, Keller MB. Suicidal Behavior in Patients with Current or Past Panic Disorder: Five Years of Prospective Data from the Harvard/Brown Anxiety Research Program. *Am J Psychiatry* 2000; 157:11:1876–1877.

99. Bosqui TJ, Shannon C, Tiernan B, et al. Childhood Trauma and the Risk of Violence in Adulthood in a Population with a Psychotic Illness. *J Psychiatric Res* 2014; 54:121–125.

100. Knickman J, Krishnan R, Pincus H. Improving Access to Effective Care for People with Mental Health and Substance Use Disorders. *JAMA* 2016; 316:16:1647–1648.

101. McHolm AE, MacMillan HL, Jamieson E. The Relationship between Childhood Physical Abuse and Suicidality among Depressed Women: Results from a Community Sample. *Am J Psychiatry* 2003; 160:5:933–938.

102. Leverich GS, Altshuler LL, Frye MA, et al. Factors Associated with Suicide Attempts in 648 Patients with Bipolar Disorder in the Stanley Foundation Bipolar Network. *J Clin Psychiatry* 2003; 64:5:506–515.

103. Larsson S, Aas M, Klungsoyr O, et al. Patterns of Childhood Adverse Events Are Associated with Clinical Characteristics of Bipolar Disorder. *BMC Psychiatry* 2013; 13:97:1–9.

104. Lumley MA, Mader C, Gramzow J, et al. Family Factors Related to Alexithymia Characteristics. *Psychosomatic Med* 1996; 58:211–216.

105. Zackheim L. Editorial—Alexithymia: The Expanding Realm of Research. *J Psychosomatic Res* 2007; 63:345–347.

106. De Berardis D, D'Albenzio A, Gambi F, et al. Alexithymia and Its Relationships with Dissociative Experiences and Internet Addiction in a Nonclinical Sample. *CyberPsychol Behav* 2009; 12:1:67–69.

107. Margalit D, Har LB, Brill S, et al. Complex Regional Pain Syndrome, Alexithymia, and Psychological Distress. *J Psychosomatic Res* 2014; 77:273–277.

108. Huth-Bocks AC, Krause K, Ahlfs-Dunn S, et al. Relational Trauma and Posttraumatic Stress Symptoms among Pregnant Women. *Psychodyn Psychiatry* 2013; 41:2:277–302.

109. Seng JS, Low LK, Sperlich M, et al. Prevalence, Trauma History, and Risk for Post-Traumatic Stress Disorder among Nulliparous Women in Maternity Care. *Obstet Gynecol* 2009; 114:4:839.

110. Irwin JL, Beeghly M, Rosenblum KL, et al. Positive Predictors of Quality of Life for Postpartum Mothers with a History of Childhood Maltreatment. *Arch Womens Ment Health* 2016; Aug 12. [Epub ahead of print] PubMed PMID: 27518635.

111. De Venter M, Smets J, Raes F, et al. Impact of Childhood Trauma on Postpartum Depression: A Prospective Study. *Arch Womens Ment Health* 2016; 19:2:337–342.

112. Kerr DCR, Capaldi DM, Pears KC, et al. A Prospective Three Generational Study of Fathers' Constructive Parenting: Influences from Family of Origin, Adolescent Adjustment, and Offspring Temperament. *Dev Psychol* 2009; 45:5:1257–2375.

113. Stein A, Craske MG, Lehtonen A, Harvey A, Savage-McGlynn E, Davies B, Goodwin J, Murray L, Cortina-Borja M, Counsell N. Maternal Cognitions and Mother—Infant Interaction in Postnatal Depression and Generalized Anxiety Disorder. *J Abnorm Psychol* 2012 Nov;121:4:795.

114. Horowitz MJ, Becker SS. The Compulsion to Repeat Trauma. *J Nerv Ment Dis* 1971; 153:1:32–40.

115. Kim EY, Park J, Kim B. Type of Childhood Maltreatment and the Risk of Criminal Recidivism in Adult Probationers: A Cross-Sectional Study. *BMC Psychiatry* 2016; 16:294.

116. Groth AN. Sexual Trauma and the Life Histories of Sex Offenders. *Victimology* 1979; 4:6.

117. Hilberman E. Overview: The "Wife-Beater's Wife" Reconsidered. *Am J Psychiatry* 1980; 137:11:1336–1347.

118. Green AH. Self—Destructive Behavior in Battered Children. *Am J Psychiatry* 1978; 135:579.

119. Cloitre M, Stovall-McClough C, Zorbas P, et al. Attachment Organization, Emotion Regulation, and Expectations of Support in a Clinical Sample of Women with Childhood Abuse Histories. *J Traumatic Stress* 2008; 21:3:282–289.

120. Infurna FJ, Rivers CT, Reich J, et al. Childhood Trauma and Personal Mastery: Their Influence on Emotional Reactivity to Everyday Events in a Community Sample of Middle-Aged Adults. *PLoS One* 2015; 10:4:e0121840.

121. Lang CM, Sharma-Patel K. The Relation between Childhood Maltreatment and Self-Injury: A Review of the Literature on Conceptualization and Intervention. *Trauma Violence Abuse* 2011; 12:1:23–37.

122. Langberg D. *Suffering and the Heart of God: How Trauma Destroys and Christ Restores.* Greensboro [NC]: New Growth Press; 2015.

123. Constantian MB, Lin CP. Why Some Patients Are Unhappy: Part 1: Relationship of Preoperative Nasal Deformity to Number of Operations and a History of Abuse or Neglect. *Plast Reconstr Surg* 2014; 134:4:823–835.

124. Constantian MB, Lin CP. Why Some Patients Are Unhappy: Part 2. Relationship of Nasal Shape and Trauma History to Surgical Success. *Plast Reconstr Surg* 2014; 134:4:836–851.

6

THE WAYS WE MEDICATE

Addictions and Behaviors Most Relevant to Body Image

In 1954, 49-year-old Norman Cousins, for 30 years editor of the *Saturday Review*, became acutely ill with what was diagnosed as a progressive autoimmune disease, compounded by ankylosing spondylitis (a potentially crippling spinal arthritis) and was told that he had one chance in 500 of recovery. Though he followed his doctors' advice in broad strokes, he took charge of his own recovery by taking large doses of vitamin C and laughing uncontrollably by watching comedies: he called the strategy "internal jogging."

In six months Cousins regained the ability to walk and within two years returned to full-time work.

> *"I knew that pain could be affected by attitudes,"* he wrote in Anatomy of an Illness. *"The fact that stress does not come from germs and viruses does not make its effects any the less serious. Apart from severe illness, it can lead to alcoholism, drug addiction, suicide, family breakdown, joblessness. . . . The patient's worry and fears are converted into genuine physical symptoms that can be terribly painful or even crippling. . . . Most people become quickly panicky about almost any pain. . . . Pain is part of the body's magic. . . . It is the way the body transmits a sign to the brain that something is wrong. Leprous patients pray for the sensation of pain."*[1]
> All trauma is indeed somatic.

*****

DOI: 10.4324/9781315657721-9

"You don't have valet parking." she said, looking at her watch.

"This is New Hampshire." I said. "It's probably illegal. We don't even have Pony Express."

A moment of disapproval crossed her face.

"I've never been to a surgeon who doesn't have valet parking."

She sat stiffly on my examination room chair, a slender blonde woman in a blousy, ankle length, faded tie-died dress and rough-out leather sandals with thick heels. I guessed she was 35. Her single pony tail was tied in a ribbon. She wore sunglasses like a headband. Her face was tired. If she told me that she had just crossed the Dust Bowl in a covered wagon I would have believed her.

"Wait," she said. She jumped from her chair, pulled a bottle of water from her purse, which was only slightly smaller than a steamer trunk, and unscrewed the top.

"I drink eight of these every day." She looked me up and down as if I were being auctioned. *"You should hydrate more. Kidneys."* She squinted at the label. *"It's got vitamins."*

I smiled. *"At least you won't get scurvy."* I didn't interrupt her train of thought.

"You should eat more blueberries. I have three pints every day."

She nodded approvingly to herself.

"Antioxidants."

"I'd like to ask some questions about your history," I said.

She shook her head decisively and placed a thick stack of photographs in front of me.

"No. I'll tell my story. I'm unique. Ask your questions later."

Early photographs showed a beautifully proportioned nose. She admitted to one facelift, four cosmetic eyelid surgeries, and five rhinoplasties followed by silicone injections into her nose. Not much time wasted, and she wasn't yet 40. Contact lenses colored her eyes an iridescent green. Her lower lids were so tight that the sclera showed below her irises. Her eyes were dry and bloodshot. She blinked repeatedly to moisten them. Each operation had made her worse.

"You need an expert to repair your lower lids," I said. *"They are so tight that your eyes don't close."*

She bridled, as if she weren't used to being interrupted.

"I did already, in California, but his surgery got infected, so I went to Florida, and he operated twice. That result wasn't perfect, so I went to another surgeon. It's still not perfect. I'm going to have more eyelid surgery next month."

"*Suppose you have another problem,*" I said.

She shrugged. "*Then I'll have another surgery. That's what I always do.*"

I decided to leave that alone, but I was concerned that she didn't fear surgery, even when the consequences had been uniformly bad. I described my surgical plan. Nothing seemed to alarm her. Sometimes I wasn't even sure she heard me. I followed up with a letter that detailed each procedure. Soon she called.

"*I want my surgery on Thanksgiving.*"

My nurse paused. "*Ma'am, Thanksgiving is a holiday.*"

"*I have lots of money,*" she said.

"*That's nice, but Thanksgiving will still be a holiday,*" my nurse said.

"*All right then, Christmas.*"

"*Christmas is also a holiday.*"

"*He will make an exception for me,*" she said.

"*I'm sorry, he won't.*"

"*You aren't even going to ask him?*"

"*The operating room is closed for elective surgery on Christmas,*" my nurse said.

"*That doesn't matter. I run a studio. You know who I am. I'm famous. My students are famous.*"

This was 14 years ago. Today I might not operate, but her deformity was obvious and her breathing was obstructed. Besides, I was sympathetic.

At her next visit, she paced in the room, holding a sheaf of papers. Her ideas jumped out randomly like corn popping in a pan. I concentrated on following the thread, but finally realized that there might not be any.

"*I researched everything you told me on the Internet and I stayed up very late last night typing out my questions. I'm not sure I want the bridge raised. Will my columella be at a right angle or perpendicular with my face? Can you make the rib incision right underneath my breast so I can wear two-piece costumes? Can you add fat under the skin on the left tip right above the left nostril? Then we can make the left nostril match my right.*"

She caught herself, as if she knew she should add something. She gave her cutest smile, the one that was supposed to make her look like Mary Poppins.

"*This is of course your judgment. I trust you completely. I'm so lucky to have you as my surgeon.*"

She stopped to catch her breath. She paused, looking down at the pages as if to approve them, nodded decisively to herself, and handed me four pages, single-spaced, with seven headings: "Breathing/Functionality, Tip of Nose, Nostrils, Columella, Asymmetrical Nose, 'Knot' on the Nostril, and Nose Recessed Into Face."

I had just read that scientists had now identified 180 distinct brain areas, up from the previous 83. Unquestionably I was outnumbered.

"I answered these questions when you were here and in my letters," I said.

She smiled, but it looked painful. "I know, honey, but I'd like to hear your ideas in person." More questions were implied by her tone. I didn't answer any of them.

I read from page 3 of her notes. Evidently she didn't believe in caesurœ.

"How do you know that you will have enough cartilage? How much will the angle of my nose increase? Can you remove the liquid silicone? Will we be transplanting cartilage to make the columella stronger, transplanting cartilage to make the tip longer, or opening my nostrils? The right side of my nose is 'convex'; you are the only doctor in the world who has noticed. Is the septum crooked on the inside or outside? I like my lips to project so they are bigger than most. My face is asymmetrical; how can you fix that? What will be the hardest thing to correct? What will be the easiest? Will I need a second surgery? How long do I have to wait?"

"That's a lot of questions," I said. "Which ones are most important?"

She sorted her pages, squinting. Most of the edges were dog-eared.

"I don't know. . . . They're all important."

"Go ahead. I'm pretty tough," I said.

She stared at me, allowing the drama to heighten. She sighed.

"I've traveled such a long way see you." She looked around the room. "Me, in the middle of nowhere. But 'even the weariest river winds somewhere safe to sea.'"

She raised her chin. "I majored in nineteenth century Victorian poetry."

"So I guessed," I said. "Swinburne's great-grandson was my co-resident."

Her eyes rested on me for a moment. "You're more cultured than I thought." She stared past me out the window. It was November and already almost dark. An east wind funneled across the parking lot, scattering leaves over the cars. Her voice got softer.

"Look at me, marooned in the sticks."

"It's not really so bad," I said.

Virtue is not, I decided, always its own reward.

Commonalities of Addictions

Children raised in neglectful or abusive households are unconsciously assigned one of three roles by their parents. Each role fills a parental need and in turn determines how their children manifest or distort the five core issues (Self-esteem, Boundaries, Reality, Moderation, and Self-care) and how they will relate to others (Table 3.3). Enmeshment, in which the child/parent boundaries disappear, creates the Hero or Scapegoat. Abandonment, in which the child/parent boundary is a wall, creates the Lost Child.

As the children adapt to these roles and learn to survive in what may be chaotic and sometimes dangerous environments, they develop common characteristics that become unifying patterns for whatever addiction results. Claudia Black calls them "process addictions."[2] Notice how many have already appeared in our surgical vignettes, and how well they also apply to borderline patients, and body dysmorphic patients, and to other addictions and seemingly compulsive behaviors, including plastic surgery:

- Uncontrolled actions when engaged in the addictive substance or behavior
- Negative consequences that directly result from these actions
- Inability and unwillingness to stop, despite negative outcomes
- A progressive increase in tolerance and frequency, requiring larger amounts to achieve the same effect
- Preoccupation with the addictive behavior
- Denial, minimalization, and rationalization, even to the point of delusional thinking

Family members and others surrounding the addict share common maladaptive traits. In the earlier literature, they were called "co-alcoholics," but the broader "codependents" term applies better. Common to both is diminution or loss of the sense of self as the codependent loses his or her individuality trying to cope with the addict:

- Loss of identity, feelings, and needs
- Obsession with the addict
- Living in constant reaction to the addict instead of the codependent's own needs and wants
- Loss of personal priorities
- Assuming responsibility for the actions of others
- Living in denial

This adaptive codependent behavior pattern produces its own casualties. The addictive home creates a sense of unexplainable loneliness, depression, and separation from the rest of the world. Fear and anxiety occur from unidentifiable causes. Relationships become difficult to maintain. Alcohol and drug abuse become parts of the codependents' lives, who themselves may self-medicate with other addictions: work, gambling, sex, excessive spending, food, or obsessions with personal appearance and plastic surgery. Don't talk. Don't trust your own senses. Don't trust your own judgment. Don't feel. Don't think. Don't question. Don't ask. Don't play. Don't make mistakes. Don't trust others.[2] We see each of these traits and associations in compulsive plastic surgery and body dysmorphic patients.

Roles in the Addictive Household

In Black's model, adaptive roles simulate the Hero, Scapegoat, and Lost Child, and the interpersonal roles of Love Avoidant or Love Addict. The co-dependent "Adjuster" avoids, compensates, and disappears, loses his or her sense of life direction, and becomes fearful of making decisions. The co-dependent "Placater" becomes a universal caretaker and empathetic listener, but leaves behind his or her ability to receive help or generate goals. The "Acting-Out Child," similar to the Scapegoat, may be more creative, humorous, independent, and self-aware but remains angry and rebellious, always in trouble.[2]

The literature supports Black's model. Data from a series of 280 treatment-seeking alcoholics* compared to 177 healthy controls indicates that childhood trauma of all types was significantly more common in alcohol-dependent patients than in controls (emotional abuse: 48% vs. 7%; sexual abuse: 21% vs. 6%; physical abuse: 39% vs. 15%; emotional neglect 57% vs. 21%; and physical neglect 28% vs. 10%, respectively—these prevalences are strikingly similar to those in our plastic surgery patients [Chapter 9]).[3] Alcohol-dependent patients were more than ten times likelier than controls to have experienced emotional abuse. Neuroticism traits (particularly impulsiveness) were the mediators between emotional abuse and the amount of childhood trauma. These responses are understandable in terms of Mellody's child development model: grandiosity, poorly defined boundaries, and the inability to live in moderation manifest as impulsiveness and neuroticism.

In a group of 131 men with alcoholic fathers, antisocial behavior was not more common than in 70 control subjects.[4] However, compared to men who were not physically abused, men who were abused were less likely to disagree verbally but more likely to have been violent or to have engaged in criminal acts for which they may never have been arrested (60% vs. 100%, respectively).[5] Even genetic differences on chromosome 4 have been identified in alcoholics who indulge in high-risk behavior, supported by concordance behavior in monozygotic twins.[6, 7] Impulsivity, anxiety, social isolation, violent behavior, and suicidality have also been documented in alcohol and drug abusers.[8] These authors note that such aggressive and tendencies "cluster within families," but speculate that the cause might be neurotransmitter dysfunction. A 2007–2015 closed claims review from The Doctors Company indicates that one of eight factors contributing to poor patient outcomes related to opioid abuse was failure to take a psychiatric and/or abuse history.[9]

★★★★★

The Big Blue Book of Alcoholics Anonymous is full of clues that are not often acknowledged in the search for genetic or neurotransmitter abnormalities.[10]

"Self-esteem" is cited repeatedly. Childhood is often referenced. The bottle is only a symbol. Like the trauma victim and the body dysmorphic patient, the face of the alcoholic changes: "There was something about his eyes ..."[10]

Read the following and substitute opiates, self-injury, work, gambling, sex addiction, or compulsive plastic surgery for "drink" or "alcohol":

> *There is the type of man who was unwilling to admit that he cannot take a drink. . . . He changes his brand or his environment. There is the type who always believes that after being entirely free from alcohol for a period of time he can take a drink without danger. There is the manic-depressive type, who is perhaps the least understood. . . . Then there are types entirely normal in every respect except in the effect alcohol has upon them.*[10]

The Protean Consequences of Abuse and Neglect

The unifying experience of childhood abuse or neglect is toxic shame: inadequacy, insufficiency, vulnerability, and damage. The causes can be physical abandonment, which teaches the child that the world is unsafe, that people cannot be trusted, and that they are unworthy of attention and care; or emotional abandonment, in which parental indifference or neglect discounts the child's feelings and need for nurturing and acknowledgment. The latter is traditionally considered to be the most destructive. I can support that opinion: in our study of Adverse Childhood Events in 175 patients, emotional abuse and neglect co-existed with more other simultaneous types of abuse or neglect than any other varieties questioned (Chapter 9). A study of 155 alcoholics in treatment demonstrated that the severity of childhood abuse correlated directly with posttraumatic stress disorder (PTSD) and suicide attempts in women; and with PTSD, social phobia, agoraphobia, and dysthymia in males.[11] In particular, childhood sexual abuse predicted social phobia, agoraphobia, and PTSD. Of all the variables examined (marital status, educational level, employment, other mental health disorders, suicide attempts, childhood physical or sexual abuse, parental loss, witnessing parental violence, alcoholism and the parents, physical or sexual assault in adulthood), the variable with the largest effect was "maternal dysfunction" (recurrent illness, nervousness, depression, sedative use, and hospitalizations). Each maternal affliction creates an atmosphere of emotional and physical neglect, often more destructive than physical or sexual abuse.[12–16]

In a similar study in 77 women with PTSD and substance dependence, women who were the most dissociated had the worst trauma-related symptoms and histories of childhood emotional abuse and physical neglect.[17] A closer look at the data indicates that self-blame was the most common coping strategy. This is the carried shame that I have often observed in patients who needlessly hold themselves responsible for poor previous surgical results—not having asked enough questions, done enough research, or given the last surgeon enough instructions.

We too often select partners that resemble our parents. We tend to parent as we have been parented, punish as we have been punished, and resolve our differences in the ways that we observed as children. It is not hard to imagine how difficult functional adulthood becomes for someone who has no sense of individual value, and how immature behavior may propagate from generation to generation. This is the legacy of trauma. How it is manifested depends on the limitless ways that abuse or neglect can be individually processed, which emotions dominate, whether these desperate people are shaped by events and supportive acquaintances outside the home, and how well he or she generates that precious skill that we call "resilience."

★★★★★

Reflecting on his alcohol addiction, Errol Flynn writes, "My own confusion became my trademark. . . . How does a man become what he becomes? . . . I do not know. . . . One day I asked Ann Sheridan . . . what she was drinking. It looked like tomato juice. It was, but it had vodka in it. I took up vodka drinking. . . . Nobody need know you have had it, that's the theory. Of course alcoholism is one of the slowest though most certain forms of suicide. . . . It gets your brain, your liver. It destroys your morals, destroys your vitality. . . . And you become sluggish. It is a great pity that Prohibition failed."[18]

Pathologic Eating as Self-Medication

Nearly all physicians have obese patients. The global weight loss and weight management fitness market, surgical equipment (adjustable gastric band, gastric bypass surgery), diet (weight-loss meals, diet soft drinks), and weight-loss services are expected to reach $206.4 billion by 2019 from $148.1 billion in 2014, growing annually at 6.9% (Source: *Weight Loss Magazine*, February, 2015).

Why is the market so large? One might just as equally ask, why isn't there one diet that always works, or one exercise regime that produces slimness and fitness?

An important answer came from a supplemented starvation program begun as part of the Southern California Permanente Medical Group's Positive Choice Weight Loss Program, which began in 1982. Eventually a diet was developed in which morbidly obese patients were given essential amino acids, essential fatty acids, vitamins, and water; their fat stores supplied calorie intake; in theory, these patients could lose up to 300 pounds in a single year. A thoroughly successful program would have had enormous implications for health in this country.[19]

Instead, the program was a weight-loss failure (Chapter 9). From refocusing the study from the consequences of obesity to its causes, the group made several critical observations:

Obesity was emotionally protective, a marker for underlying problems; that is, it was a solution for the patient.

The program removed food as a coping device but exposed underlying issues for which food was the psychoactive key.

Modifying nutritional or eating habits was not the answer: most obese patients knew enough about calories and diet to be healthy; ignorance didn't cause obesity.

Therefore, teaching patients to "eat right" was irrelevant to treating obesity.

Most obese patients were not born obese, but rather gained their weight abruptly, episodically, usually following major life events.

The provocative events underlying weight gain were often easy for interested providers to discover.

Many patients could date their weight gains to sexual abuse or parental loss (divorce, abandonment, or death).

Obesity was therefore physically, sexually, socially, or emotionally protective. Weight loss became threatening.

Some patients immediately recalled the causes of their weight gain, but some were amnesic and dissociated from their traumas.

Good experiences did not produce amnesia, and joy did not produce obesity.

Obesity, therefore, like fever or jaundice, was a physical manifestation of another problem, not a disease in itself.[19]

The two major predictors of weight regain were a history of childhood sexual abuse and current marriage to an alcoholic—in other words, a currently traumatic relationship.[20]

In a group of 190 patients who each lost more than 100 pounds on the program, only half maintained more than 50% of their weight loss for at least 18 months. All but 4 of the 190 patients regained at least some weight.

Thirty-nine percent of the patients had been sexually abused, 11% physically abused. Sixty-six percent were chronically depressed. Therefore, when bariatric surgery fails, there is some factor in the patient's history that has not been addressed.

Group treatment that addressed the reasons for initial weight gain was the most effective type.

★★★★★

There is ample support elsewhere for these conclusions. Early in the literature women were identified for their vulnerability to obesity, particularly those who believed that beauty and goodness were connected and who sought constant approval and perfection. "Many researchers have identified one substantial group of bulimic women . . . who report problems with alcohol or drug abuse. . . . Some experts conclude that bulimia is basically a substance abuse disorder."[21]

Childhood emotional abuse is associated with both alexithymia and disordered eating[22] and mediated by "general distress"[23] or depression.[24, 25] In a group of 290 women from ages 45 to 69, body image dissatisfaction, "social pressures to be thin," and perfectionism predicted eating disorders in middle-aged women.[26] Cementing familial pathology is evidence that the mothers' degree of perfectionism paralleled that of their college-aged daughters.[27]

Abusive and demeaning behavior, threatened abandonment, or an intrusive, overprotective, chaotic, or emotionally cold environment create boundary violations and a sense of betrayal, distrust, and vulnerability in the child;[25, 28] recall how these same factors parallel both BPD and cutters' childhoods. The authors were unable to demonstrate that depression was the mediator between emotional abuse and disordered eating—the proximate mediator was body dissatisfaction. Even the anticipation of body shame predicted eating disorder symptoms in sensitized patients.[29, 30] In two populations of obese African women, physical and emotional neglect and physical and sexual abuse prevalences were high. Divided by BMI and race, those who were black and poor were obese, whereas those who were black and middle-class or white and middle-class were not.[31]

In a group of 383 undergraduates, the impact of weight-related verbal abuse (64% in this group) mediated the relationship between the verbal abuse and resultant disordered eating and predicted binge eating, emotional eating, night eating, and unhealthy weight control.[32] Adults with histories of childhood abuse were more than twice as likely to eat or overeat when stressed than adults who had not been abused.[33]

★★★★★

Her paperwork said that she was 59, but the overall effect was different. She was very thin, dressed thoughtfully in a white top and flowered smock with a short skirt and shoulder straps. Her large-brimmed straw hat tipped back to show bright blonde bangs that she must trim every day. Except for her high-heeled boots, she might have come from Sunnybrook Farm. She looked tired. Still, the effect was good. We shook hands gravely.

She had already undergone three rhinoplasties, two facelifts, cheek implants placed and revised, a lip lift, a neck lift, fat grafts to her lower lids, and facial fillers injected only the day before seeing me. Her rhinoplasty result was not bad, but her airway was impaired and her tip was unnaturally flat. I said hello, and waited. She nodded to herself and searched her purse.

"Please look at this." In her palm she held a yellowing black-and-white photograph of a woman wearing the same straw hat.

"This is my mother. She isn't alive anymore. We used to look exactly the same. She was very beautiful. All my life, people thought we were twins."

They didn't look the same to me. I smiled as if I believed every word.

"How can I help you?"

She made a sound like the tiny sigh of a sleeping child.

"I need to look like my mother again. That's why I had these surgeries. Do you think I can ever be as pretty as my mother?"

"Let's start at the beginning," I said. "What did your nose look like before surgery?"

Some impenetrable barrier slid into place between us. She looked at her hands. I waited. Then her head came up.

"I don't remember."

She was musing.

"I know I was an ugly baby."

"How," I said.

"My father told me. He said so all the time."

I have subsequently realized that for patients like this, the nose is not an organ: it is a contaminated symbol. Maybe changing the subject would help. I paused and measured my words.

"I'm concerned that you are measuring yourself against unattainable goals," I said. I looked at her dog-eared photo again.

"And I don't think your mother had as many operations as you."

She spoke so softly that I had to lean toward her. "Oh, no you have to do it. You just need to make me as pretty as her."

She tipped her chin and pointed at her face.

"See? I've already had implants to make her apple cheeks."

She looked past me to the window and continued.

"And now my bulimia is better. I know it is. My mother never had to worry about her weight. She loved her figure."

She looked at me. The fatigue seemed to be swallowing her.

"I am almost there, except for my nose."

Apparently she had told the story so often that she believed it.

She brushed a strand of hair from her eyes. "Don't you think so? Don't you think I look just like her, except for my nose?" Her voice softened again even though there was no one around.

I didn't have an answer, which was all right because she wasn't really asking me.

It was my usual dilemma. The surgical correction was not complex and likely to succeed. Her airway was poor. I could improve her tip safely, despite the prior scarring. It was not my job to judge her motivation, but rather whether I could achieve what she wanted and ease her discomfort.

Surgery was easy and successful, from my standpoint. During the first few postoperative days and still bandaged, the patient became extremely anxious, calling repeatedly for reassurance. Is my nose too short? Will it be all right? And when can we schedule my next operation?

The day I removed her bandages she wouldn't look at herself, but I could see that the result should be what she wanted. At her visit a few days later, she seemed content and flew home.

Soon she returned. Her lips and cheeks were ballooned and distorted and her eyelids were distractingly tight. Her hands shook as she tried to make noncommittal gestures.

"I went back to the doctor in New York and he did laser and Botox and fillers." She spoke in short, passionate bursts.

"You've done something since I saw you a few months ago," I said.

She blinked repeatedly. Eventually she answered.

"A little."

"How much is that?" I said.

She paused, trying to decide if she had to answer.

"Well, ten procedures—but only fillers."

I took a deep breath. I could see that wasn't true.

"You've had eyelid surgery," I said.

She shook her head unconvincingly

"Oh, no. Never. Just fillers."

"It's only been four months," I said. "You must give your tissues a rest or you'll have problems that no one can fix." I was bothered by her urgency.

Her eyes widened. "No, no I need more fillers. You have to do it. The muscle in my lip is sticking up and it is painful all the time. I am really suffering. The pain is making the muscles separate and causing a dip in my cheek." Her thoughts scattered in almost too many directions for me to follow.

"Oh, and my teeth don't show anymore."

Then her voice dropped in secrecy. "Please help me. When I have surgery, my husband even likes me for a while."

Her trauma history was significant. She was the lost child in a neglectful household. Her mother, whom she idolized, was often slapped repeatedly and was threatened with a firearm by her husband. The patient said that her previous surgeons had added procedures that she had never authorized. Both she and her mother had a large physical trauma wound labeled, "without my permission." She had become Lot's wife, caught in the past.

We talked for a long time about trauma therapy, not surgery. I still hear from her occasionally. Her husband selects her surgeons and buys her airline tickets. Her mother's ghost still chases her. The more I thought about her life, the less I understood. Perhaps that was true for both of us.

The Complexities of Researching and Treating
Obesity and Feeding Disorders

Unrelenting verbal and emotional abuse create depression, anxiety, suicidality, alcohol and drug abuse, disordered eating, and body shame. Why? Why doesn't the child ignore the criticism? There are a variety of reasons. Emotional abuse poisons self-worth, erodes boundaries, and distorts reality. Children who hear constant criticism and teasing "make up" that they deserve it, which only reinforces the lack of self-esteem, body shame, depression, and self-medication by eating or starvation. Reality processing is distorted: the child reconfigures sensory input so that the messages are always unfavorable. "I am being called fat" becomes "I am fat." The implication is the trigger. This process is not conscious, but transmitted by neural pathways created at an early, often preverbal, age. Emotionally cold parents can "wire" a separation between the cerebral hemispheres, sequestering rational thought and feelings. Binge eaters feel out of control when they binge. The antidote, therefore, has nothing to do with willpower. Because traumatized, immature adults live at the extremes, narcissism and grandiosity are associated with both alexithymia and eating disorders.[34]

★★★★★

Treatment failures are instructive. The combination of group, individual, and pharmacologic therapy decreased eating disorder prevalence by 50% in six months in one series, though dissociation and alexithymia were not affected.[35, 36] A study in 654 college students followed 20 years later indicated that 25% of those who had eating disorders in college were still bulimic. Sadly, even at ages 41–43, 4.5% still reported eating disorders, 68% of whom had sustained them since college. The authors interpret this data to indicate that "that women remain vulnerable . . . throughout midlife. . . . One possible explanation . . . may be society's emphasis on maintaining a youthful appearance."[37] Another reasonable explanation is that traumatic childhood imprinting is often permanent unless treated. Fortunately, a recent paper indicates that childhood trauma is not associated with suicide attempts in a study of 204 bulimic patients.[38]

Sexual orientation appears to affect some parameters, but not others: a study of 173 women indicated that lesbians had a higher esteem of their bodies' sexual attractiveness than heterosexual women, though both groups had equal eating disorder prevalences.[39] Childhood trauma was not assessed.

One multicenter study of 139 adolescents, however, demonstrates the complexity of researching childhood trauma. Zeller, Noll, Sarwer, et al.[22] compared multiple-parameter data on 139 adolescents scheduled for weight-loss surgery with 83 adolescents enrolled in nonsurgical weight-loss programs. Assessed were the prevalences of childhood trauma, associated psychopathology, quality of life, self-esteem, body image, high-risk behavior, and family dysfunction.[40] Participants completed self-administered questionnaires. The entire group had a mean BMI of 49.77; mean age was 16.6 years; 81% were young women, 62% white, 26% black, 7% Hispanic, 5% mixed race. Noteworthy to me was that their caregivers' BMI averaged 38.1 kg/m². Despite what ought to be an at-risk population, trauma scores for adolescent men fell within the "none/minimal range" (emotional abuse: 7%; sexual abuse: 5%; emotional neglect: 8%; physical neglect: 6%). Young women scored higher than the men: 29% had histories of childhood trauma, but the numbers were not as high as anticipated. Prevalences were as follows: emotional abuse, 9%; physical abuse, 7%; sexual abuse, 6%; emotional neglect, 9%; and physical neglect, 6%. Patients undergoing nonsurgical weight loss described more abuse than those scheduled for bariatric surgery—except for sexual abuse. These are lower numbers than in the Kaiser Permanente study,[15, 20, 41–46] and much lower than my patient population (Chapter 9).

Higher scores for emotional abuse, emotional neglect, and physical abuse paralleled greater psychopathology, greater family dysfunction, lower weight-related quality of life, less self-esteem, and higher body dissatisfaction.[47] Physical and sexual abuse correlated with more high-risk sexual behavior (e.g., oral sex, unprotected sex, sex under the influence of drugs or alcohol). These data corroborate the ACE study findings[45] as well as the BDD and addiction literature.

Close examination of individual tabulated correlations reveals unexpected findings, at least to me. Emotional abuse was the most common type (as it was in my own patients) and was associated with the most severe internalizing and externalizing symptoms, the lowest quality of life, the least self-worth, the lowest weight-related body esteem, the highest alcohol use, and the greatest family dysfunction compared to other forms of interpersonal trauma. Physical abuse and emotional neglect in combination correlated with internalizing and externalizing symptoms, self-worth, weight-related body esteem, and alcohol abuse. This makes sense. Emotional abuse can be consistent and continuous, unlike physical or sexual abuse. Its biological difference is borne out in treatment successes: At six months, adults treated for single incident trauma had an 83% cure rate. Children with continuous, "complex" trauma had a 30% cure rate. The difference is brain development.[48]

★★★★★

Most surprising was the data from sexually abused patients, who scored lowest in psychopathology, quality of life, self-esteem, and body image parameters, the least destructed global self-worth, the least effect on weight-related body esteem and body shape, and the least alcohol abuse. Sexually abused patients scored highest in risky sexual behavior, the age at which sexual activity began, and the number of sexual partners. These findings parallel those in the Adverse Childhood Events study.[19, 42, 45] Family dysfunction prevalence was inexplicably lower than for any other abuse or neglect inventoried. The authors conclude that young women with childhood trauma histories appeared to be "a significant minority who carry [a great] psychosocial burden ... more likely to be depressed, anxious, oppositional or defiant, and more likely to use psychiatric medications compared to those without trauma histories."

How do we reconcile these seemingly aberrant findings? I can suggest several possibilities. First, much of the data was self-reported. Were inhibiting caregivers present when these adolescents were divulging their intimate information? Surgical candidates might be disqualified if they reported abuse, a strong motive for lying. Patients and their caregivers also knew that abuse would trigger referrals to child protective services. Finally, what percent of teenagers who denied abuse were just dissociated from this terrible trauma? We do not know if these factors influenced the data. Nevertheless, the findings in broad strokes confirm the connection of childhood trauma to morbid obesity.

★★★★★

Other research has validated the relationship. In a study of 340 morbidly obese gastric bypass candidates with mean BMIs of 51 kg/m^2,[49] the prevalence of childhood trauma was 69%. Once again, emotional abuse (46%) and neglect (48.8%) were not only the most common but also the most associated with higher eating concerns, body dissatisfaction, depression, low self-esteem, and binge eating. These prevalences are similar in my own patients, many of whom are driven by perfectionism, low self-esteem, and body shame (Chapter 9).

Overall prevalences of emotional, physical, and sexual abuse and emotional and physical neglect were twice as high as those in a 1,125-woman historical control.[50, 51] The authors caution that histories of childhood maltreatment may be deliberately underreported, which is my own experience as well.

Like soldiers more likely to develop PTSD in combat if they have suffered childhood abuse or neglect[52–54] or to commit suicide if they have been dishonorably discharged,[55] developmental trauma increased the likelihood of psychiatric hospitalization after bariatric surgery.[56]

★★★★★

There were more ramifications. Twenty-two percent of patients with histories of childhood sexual abuse were hospitalized within a two-year follow-up period, compared to 3% of those without abuse histories. All hospitalized patients were women and all had received preoperative mental health treatment. Five had previous psychiatric hospitalizations, five had been physically abused, five had been sexually traumatized as adults, five had been hospitalized for depression, and five indicated that excessive weight was protective for them.[56]

In another study of 230 patients seeking bariatric surgery, 66% had histories of childhood trauma.[57] While there were no significant gender differences in rates of physical abuse or emotional or physical neglect, women were more likely than men to report emotional abuse (52% vs. 26%) and sexual abuse (36% vs. 5%). Each form of maltreatment examined significantly increased the likelihood of an Axis 1 diagnosis (Mood, Anxiety, Substance Use, or Eating Disorders) and substance abuse.[58]

In the same 2008 study, childhood trauma directly corresponded to elevated prevalences of unipolar and bipolar mood disorders compared to patients without trauma histories. While there was no association between childhood trauma and Axis II Personality Disorders, both emotional and sexual abuse accompanied increased prevalences of panic disorder, PTSD, social phobia, obsessive compulsive disorder, generalized anxiety disorder, and agoraphobia without panic.[59] PTSD symptoms were more than six times greater in patients with sexual abuse histories than those without. Too few physicians and surgeons who perform bariatric or body contour surgery are aware of this data or the protean impact of these survivors' childhood experiences.

A Memoir of Childhood Obesity

In 2015 Andie Mitchell wrote a memoir that quickly became a popular weight-loss book and contains many of the themes just discussed.[60] "Self-hatred," "guilt," and "shame" appear often. Shame expressed itself in both parents. Her obese, verbally abusive, raging, alcoholic and mercurial father frightened the family. Unemployed, he ate ceaselessly through the night. Her brother tried to protect his mother from verbal abuse but developed a stutter. Secrecy, walls, loneliness, sadness, and anger permeated the house. Food became the soothing agent when she was bored, after her father had a temper tantrum, when she wanted to forget, when she wanted to binge, when her mother wanted to comfort her, when her father attempted suicide, and after he died. Food was identity: "Until I was 13, I ate with reckless abandon, using food for every reason unbound to hunger. . . . How do you walk away from all you've ever been?" Soon she weighed 300 pounds.

The author successfully lost 135 pounds and substituted compulsive exercise for eating. At the time her book was written, Mitchell had fallen in love with a professional gambler who had also struggled with depression and obesity. The author's story ends happily: she became a successful food blogger. Hers is the story of many young women and men and ties many themes that the literature documents. But the story did not start with an obsession with thin models: it began during childhood, in the home. In so much of the literature, family and self-worth become incidental findings when they should be the core. The personal and societal consequences of obesity balloon healthcare costs.

★★★★★

Nineteen-sixties teen idol Ed Byrnes describes a difficult childhood in his autobiography: poverty, an abusive and alcoholic father (whom he now remembers as "not too bad" [personal communication, 2016]) and a mother struggling to provide for her children. Circumstances forced him to become an adult too early:

"I don't remember very much about my father. . . . What stands out most . . . was all the yelling and screaming. . . . I decided that I better

*become the man of the family. I became the breadwinner. . . . I became
a caretaker. . . . I became my mother's surrogate husband. I told her, 'He
can't take care of you anymore, but I can.' [I wished that] Kirk Douglas,
Robert Mitchell, or Burt Lancaster were my fathers. Then I would be taken
care of. . . . I walked out of that theater pumped up, thinking, I really want
to become an actor!"*[61]

Work Addiction

Work addiction is seductive. It is empowering. Others respect it. They are awed by the addict's prodigious output without recognizing its pain and cost to the addict's life and family. Work addiction creates respect, prestige, income, fame, and self-affirmation.[62] It is self-reinforcing. It triggers euphoria from dopamine release in the limbic system. In patients with histories of childhood trauma, dopamine release correlates with increased alcohol and drug abuse,[63] pathological gambling,[64] psychotic disorders,[65] and "novelty seeking."[66] Executive and inhibitory functions are impaired, facilitating excessive and irresponsibly frenetic activity; motivational centers feed the reward centers, and memory and learning systems coordinate triggers to drive recurrent craving.

Work addiction may be a dopamine vulnerability problem—no one knows yet—but it is surely some kind of vulnerability problem.

Hard work and work addiction are not the same. Hard workers work because they love what they do and need to provide for their families. Work addicts work to generate feelings of self-worth. That is the critical difference.

I can speak best about medicine, where work addiction is common and often obscured to the addict: Who doesn't love the doctor who is always available, who will always accept another committee assignment, another leadership position, author another chapter, textbook, or journal article, and never turns a patient away? The devotion that medicine commands from its physicians blurs the line between absolute integrity and responsibility for their patients' welfare and working beyond exhaustion.[67, 68] For more than three decades work was my own addiction, and once I identified it, my opinion about others' self-medications and addictions changed forever.

★★★★★

Barbara Killinger begins her text—"the respectable addiction"—with a 30-question quiz.[69] Is your work very important to you? Is it important for you to be "right"? Are you overly critical of yourself? Are you afraid of failing? Do you feel uneasy or guilty if there is nothing to do? Do you think that you are special or different? These and other questions point to self-worth, boundaries, reality (in this case, connecting work and self-value), self-care, and living in moderation.

For work addicts, work produces anxiety as well as satisfaction. The workaholic expects perfection from himself or herself and from the rest of the family,[62] but perfectionism denies humanness. Playing is discouraged. Family love becomes conditional upon performance. Guilt, fear, and shaming—all forms of negative control—govern relationships. Killinger stratifies workaholics as "Controllers," "Narcissistic Controllers," and "Pleasers," but they are all forms of boundary failures and immaturity.[69]

Each of these behaviors circles back to the five core symptoms. Every addiction selects people who live at the extremes. Wounded children who have become Adapted Adult Wounded Children still use the boundary systems that their parents taught. The Adapted Adult Wounded Child is quick to use what therapist Terry Real calls "First Consciousness."[70] He distinguishes this type of immature relationality from "Second Consciousness," characteristic of the Functional Adult. Boundaryless individuals either become victims of their environments or become offensive to others. "You made me angry" and "You made me hit you" are each boundary failures. Without boundaries, people are either irresponsible or excessively controlling. Without good senses of reality, workaholics and other addicts don't know who they are. They don't see themselves appropriately; they don't understand their thoughts and can't share them; they don't recognize their own feelings (alexithymia) or they feel overwhelmed; and they are not aware that their actions might be offensive to others. Reality becomes distorted: between the action and the thought a mysterious, deforming metabolic process occurs. Most work addicts become anti-dependent—needless and wantless. They feel "selfish" for having legitimate desires. They lose their personal boundaries and therefore their abilities to maintain relationships, empathy, and ultimately physical and psychological health.[71, 72] Other esteem is learned behavior.

For a moment, drop the word "esteem." Think of it as just "other." Without an internal sense of self-value, power of any kind can only be generated externally, which, like aesthetic surgery for the same reason, inevitably fails. Other esteem, other happiness, other comfort, other reality: each are substitutes for self-worth. The sad truth is that everyone worships something.

★★★★★

Another Remen essay perfectly frames work addiction and other-esteem. Quoting a businessman who had discovered, as we have been seeing, that retaining trauma is swallowing your own energy, she writes:
    "Happiness was 'having the cookie.' . . . Unfortunately, the cookie kept changing. Some of the time it was money, sometimes power, sometimes sex. At other times it was the new car, the biggest contract, the most prestigious address. A year and a half after his diagnosis of prostate

cancer he sits shaking his head ruefully. 'It is like I stopped learning how to live after I was a kid. . . . The minute you have the cookie it starts to crumble. . . . You may not even get a chance to eat it because you are so busy just trying not to lose it.' "[73]

Sexual Addiction

Because we have spent time documenting the victim ravages of sexual abuse,[42, 74-76] it is worth taking a moment to consider the perpetrators. Like other seemingly inexplicable behaviors, sexual addiction has common threads that duplicate the themes that have already emerged in other addictions and in BDD, and whose origin can be traced to childhood.

The core attributes of the sex addict can be outlined as bullet points (adapted from Carnes[77]). Carnes writes about sexual addiction, but note how well the characteristics apply to obesity, alcoholism, work addiction, perfectionism, adult adapted wounded children, and body dysmorphic disorder.

- Addicts judge themselves by society's standards, not by their own internal senses of self-worth and abilities to process reality, self-protect, self-contain, and self-regulate: Think self-worth.
- The addictive process twists and warps creative energy into self-destructive, compulsive behavior. As a result the addict loses personal value and relationships.
- The addict substitutes a sick relationship with the addictive substance for healthy relationships.
- The root cause of all addictions are defective, poisonous carried family messages about the addict's worth, needs, and sexuality (Think reality and boundaries).
- Addicts do not have self-worth but believe themselves to be bad and unlovable. Therefore no one can love them unconditionally: there is always a price to be paid.
- Addicts are untrusting.
- Addicts feel victimized by relationships, by the police, by employers, and by family.
- Sex addicts sense a building internal pressure that requires release [remember identical sensations in cutters] (Chapter 5): Think self-care.
- Addicts rationalize their behavior; their world is delusional. Think reality.
- Addicts are triggered by external stresses: new jobs, promotions, or any high demands for excellence (which can be internally or externally generated).
- Addicts' faulty assumptions, myths, and delusional values insulate them and their addictive cycles from the real world.

- Addicts obsess about their addictions for hours a day. These same delusional thought patterns may also support several addictions: overeating, alcohol, binging behavior. Thirty-eight percent of sex addicts also have eating disorders: Think moderation.
- Other mental health disorders coexist: depression, bipolar disorders, suicidality, obsessive compulsive disorder, posttraumatic stress disorder, and others.
- The addict's behavior and thought processes make life unmanageable.
- The addict feels powerless to change his or her behavior.
- The child molester usually has distortions in sexual development from childhood; "There is a part of the addict that is not any older than the victim."[78]
- Parents who are sexual with their children teach the children that all relationships must be sexual.
- There is pain for the addict at every level of addiction.
- No convincing data exists to generalize about the personalities of sex addicts, not compulsivity, not multiple addictions, not concurrent mental health disorders.
- Compulsive sexual behavior reinforces other concurrent addictions: e.g., overworking to exhaustion.
- Exhibitionists, predatory fathers, and unfaithful spouses share the common link of sexual obsession, complicating data analysis and classification.
- The family is often equally delusional and believes that the addict is like a new mutation who only needs better self-control: "Just stop drinking, don't be depressed, don't obsess about sex, eat normally, spend less money, be responsible, act like an adult."
- Sexual addiction depends on the addict's childlike self-image, interpersonal relationships, and misperception of his or her own sexual feelings and needs. "My needs will never be met if I have to depend upon others." This distorted belief drives the addictive power. Think needless and wantless love avoidants.
- Addicts recall their childhoods as lonely, vulnerable times. Once they are old enough, they self-medicate, which seems to be free, effective, and outside parental control.
- "A young boy who learns never to need anything emotionally from his parents . . . is faced with a dilemma whenever he feels . . . needy or otherwise insecure. If masturbating has been his principal source of good feeling. . . [He may use it] . . . to restore good feelings. . . [even] when he is experiencing needs . . . unrelated to sexuality."[77, 79]
- The "co-addict" copes with denial, rationalization, grandiosity or inadequacy, blame or judgment, protective secrecy, and obsession with the addict's behavior.
- The co-addict often shares the addict's belief that "No one will love me as I am."
- The majority of sex addicts' families have members with drug or alcohol dependence or eating disorders. Core beliefs are shared. Abuse and neglect "run in families."

- Sex addiction, like other addictions and unhealthy behaviors, including body dysmorphic disorder, are family illnesses. There are parallels that cannot be missed. The fundamental driver of each of these addictions is a faulty belief system that generates shame, delusional thought patterns, impaired thinking, and compulsive, self-perpetuating, self-harming behaviors.[77]

★★★★★

Blues great B. B. King grew up too young in the Mississippi Delta. His father deserted the family and "mother whipped me raw." Nevertheless, "I believe my early childhood nourished me." His autobiography is a story of childhood trauma, resilience ("Without Mama or Grandma around, staving off my personal poverty meant depending on myself"), and a series of self-admitted addictions. "I could not impose on anyone else. Mom's death cut me off from the world. . . . As a 10-year-old, I decided to go it alone. . . . My guitar helped me cope. . . . Friends . . . would tell me, 'Man, your daddy's always bragging on you . . . '. He'd tell others, but not me. . . . I enjoy gambling and sex, but they are both pleasures I feel I can control. Work is a different matter. Work controls me. The pattern might go all the way back to the plantation . . . Might go back to wanting to get by . . . and get something better. Might just be in the blood."[80]

Similarities Among Addictions and Self-Harming Behaviors

Each behavior that we have discussed, including body dysmorphic disorder, generates 15 unifying characteristics in its afflicted.[77, 81, 82]

1. The ultimate generator is lack of self-worth and shame: I am unlovable, a fraud, a failure, valueless.
2. I live behind a wall of denial.
3. I have difficulty identifying my feelings (alexithymia).
4. My family and personal life are disrupted.
5. My behavior is compulsive; I will deceive my family and physicians when necessary.
6. There is no relationship between the magnitude of my problem and the anguish that it creates in me.
7. My resources are depleted so I can't meet other needs and wants.
8. I will maintain the addiction to be lovable, acceptable, and not be abandoned— not because of the deformity itself. Only I can know the real meaning of my addiction / deformity.

9. I may have multiple addictions / deformities.
10. I am powerless over my addictions and victimization [by previous surgeons or relevant others]: there is no safe place, just as there wasn't when I was a child.
11. I am isolated from my family, which doesn't understand me; I won't let them control me.
12. My family members suffer in co-dependence. They willingly rationalize, minimize, and conceal my uncontrolled, destructive behavior.
13. I need endless reassurance from my caregivers.
14. I will persist despite bad consequences.
15. I have no exit from the vortex.

Abuse and Neglect Are the Tinder; Shame Is the Fuel

Recovery depends upon replacing defective and damaging beliefs. Addicts must separate themselves from their addictions. They must surround themselves with others who have suffered similarly and whom they trust with their secrets—the healing power of Alcoholics Anonymous and group trauma work. New trust generates new hope. The secret addictive world must be penetrated by new beliefs of self-worth and our addiction language must change. Blame, punishment, and contempt for imagined weakness only intensify the addict's shame and disempowerment, an additive that they cannot afford.[83]

The Unity Among the Afflictions and Their Survivors

Popular culture views deliberate self-injury, alcohol or drug abuse, obesity, and even excessive cosmetic surgery as unrelated oddities, subjects for magazine exposés, or pitiable evidences of weakness and poor self-control. "If she would only stay on a diet . . ." "If she would only recognize that drinking is not the answer to her problems . . ." "If he would only stop sexually harassing his co-workers. . . " "If students would not respond to the stresses of college life with eating disorders, drug addiction, or suicide . . ." "If he were only more self-disciplined . . ." "If she would only stop having cosmetic surgery . . ." In the case of drug addiction, the putative culprit is availability: irresponsible physicians, greedy pharmaceutical companies, or profit-hungry pharmacies.

But availability is not the only issue. People self-medicate for a reason. What each of these well-intentioned opinions misses is that, although food, alcohol, narcotics, school stress, and cosmetic surgery are available to everyone, everyone isn't obese, addicted, or suicidal; and that this self-injurious or addictive behavior is a type of answer, not a problem. Felitti is right: *Virtually every refractory public health issue is a solution: that's what makes it so refractory.*[19, 46]

★★★★★

The disturbing self-injury literature and its astonishing spectrum provides another valuable link between childhood trauma and unconscious, harmful, compulsive, deliberate behavior, a morality play in which the trauma survivor is helpless and everyone else is a threat. It reinforces the unity of these problems as part of a comprehensive whole. While I began as a relative outsider to the mental health and trauma literature, many textbooks and journal papers present the same repeating patterns. At the meta-level it is difficult to miss the similarities. The differences among them are not great, and in some cases it is only the order in which the symptoms manifest and the title of the publication that seems unique. Each compulsive, destructive behavior begins in a setting of intolerable and frightening vulnerability. Only its manifestations differ. If the self-harm is skin injury, we call it cutting. If it is an eating disorder, we call it anorexia—or obesity. If it is vague somatic discomfort and fatigue, we call it fibromyalgia.[84] If it is self-injurious, judgmental, mercurial, and self-damning, we call it Borderline Personality Disorder. If it is a search for amnesia, we call it drug or alcohol abuse. If it is goal-driven anxiety, we call it obsessive-compulsive disorder or work addiction. If it is compulsive sexual activity, we call it sex addiction. If there was an identifiable, overwhelming, life-threatening, provocative event, we call it burnout or posttraumatic stress disorder. If the patient looks normal to the observer, we call it body dysmorphic disorder.

★★★★★

The major distinction among these problems, and others like them, is only its identifying manifestation: the associated symptoms, characteristics, family dynamics, psychological pain, social anxiety, alexithymia, PTSD symptoms, and medicating addictions all overlap and repeat many times, just in different orders.[31] The diagnostic and research emphasis may only depend upon who saw the patient first. The clinical name is an inevitable distraction.

When examined from separate silos, each problem has its own commonality, curious characteristics, neurotransmitter analyses, genetic puzzles, and obscure or debated etiology. But if seen as a single immense group, in which each disorder or compulsive, pathologic behavior becomes just another unique, poisonous bloom of childhood abuse or neglect, the prevalence and size of the human misery and destruction is overwhelming. "Mental illness" is societal and family illness, and these sometimes tormented, sometimes triumphant individuals are its products. It is our job as physicians and caregivers to look deeper and recognize that what happens in the examination room is much larger than a transaction circumscribed by its walls. Each one of us has a past.

What This Information Means

All addictions, even compulsive plastic surgery, are disconnections, grim self-punishments. They are contractions of the self, inevitably secretive, isolating, and solitary. Addictions are not group behavior: they are inwardly directed. Addictions are false substitutes for self-esteem.[85] Addictions build walls. Resilience, alternatively, focuses outward; it is expansive. That is one of the reasons I believe that Alcoholics Anonymous is so successful. Its model breaks the isolation. It forces the organization of traumatic memories when members tell their stories. It fosters supportive social engagement, impedes narcissism, and helps its members look outside themselves instead of contracting inward. The emphasis on a higher power is comforting. And it can be done in small steps.

Addictions have two components: meaning and power. Addictive substances and behaviors have meaning but cannot generate power. Abuse has power, but acts blindly, without meaning. Addicts have both power and meaning: the addiction provides the meaning, but the addict has the power.

Addictions: Meaning Without Power
Abuses: Power Without Meaning
Addicts: Power and Meaning

There is a unity here: Strip any of these addictions or unexplained behaviors of its title and the attributes become almost identical. All have documented connections to toxic or carried shame and absent self-worth.[5] All germinate from the common poisonous root of childhood neglect or abuse, the most important unsolved public health problem we face.[86]

Note

* Opioid addiction is not considered separately from other substance abuses except as it relates to childhood trauma prevalences (Chapter 9).

References

1. Cousins N. *Anatomy of an Illness as Perceived by the Patient: Reflections on Healing and Regeneration.* New York: W W Norton & Company; 1979.
2. Black C. The Adult Child. In: *It Will Never Happen To Me: Growing Up With Addiction as Youngsters, Adolescents, Adults.* 2nd edition. Center City [MN]: Hazelden; 2005:123.
3. Schwandt ML, Heilig M, Hommer DW, et al. Childhood Trauma Exposure and Alcohol Dependence Severity in Adulthood: Mediation by Emotional Abuse Severity and Neuroticism. *Alcohol Clin Exp Res* 2013; 37:6:984–992.
4. Pollock VE, Briere J, Schneider L, et al. Childhood Antecedents of Antisocial Behavior: Parental Alcoholism and Physical Abusiveness. *Am J Psychiatry* 1990; 147:10:1290–1293.
5. Carli V, Jovanovic N, Podlesek A, et al. The Role of Impulsivity in Self-Mutilators, Suicide Ideators and Suicide Attempters: A Study of 1265 Male Incarcerated Individuals. *J Affect Disord* 2010; 123:1–3:116–122.
6. Czerwinski SA, Mahaney MC, Williams JR, et al. Genetic Analysis of Personality Traits and Alcoholism Using a Mixed Discrete Continuous Trait Variance Component Model. *Genet Epidemiol* 1999; 17[suppl 1]:S121–S126.

7. Coccaro EF, Silverman JM, Klar HM, Horvath TB, Siever LJ. Familial Correlates of Reduced Central Serotonergic System Function in Patients with Personality Disorders. *Arch Gen Psychiatry* 1994 Apr 1;51:4:318–324.

8. Goldberg JF, Singer TM, Garno JL. Suicidality and Substance Abuse in Affective Disorders. *J Clin Psychiatry* 2001; 62[suppl 25]:35–43.

9. Marcus H. *Prescribing Opioids Safely*. The Doctor's Advocate. The Doctors Company, Second Quarter 2017:3–10.

10. Alcoholics Anonymous. *The Story of How Many Thousands of Men and Women Have Recovered from Alcoholism*. New York: Alcoholics Anonymous World Services, Inc.; 2001, 9, xxx).

11. Langeland W, Draijer N, van den Brink W. Psychiatric Comorbidity in Treatment-Seeking Alcoholics: The Role of Childhood Trauma and Perceived Parental Dysfunction. *Alcohol Clin Exp Res* 2004; 28:3:441–447.

12. van der Kolk BA, Perry LC, Herman JL. Childhood Origins of Self-Destructive Behavior. *Am J Psychiatry* 1991; 148:12:1665–1671.

13. Carli V, Mandelli L, Zaninotto L, et al. Trait-Aggressiveness and Impulsivity: Role of Psychological Resilience and Childhood Trauma in a Sample of Male Prisoners. *Nord J Psychiatry* 2014; 68:1:8–17.

14. Cuomo C, Sarchiapone M, Giannantonio MD, et al. Aggression, Impulsivity, Personality Traits, and Childhood Trauma of Prisoners With Substance Abuse and Addiction. *Am J Drug Alcohol Abuse* 2008; 34:3:339–345.

15. Lipschitz DS, Winegar RK, Nicolau AL, et al. Perceived Abuse and Neglect as Risk Factors for Suicidal Behavior in Adolescent Inpatients. *J Nerv Ment Dis* 1999; 187:1:32–39.

16. Zhan W, Shaboltas AV, Skochilov RV, et al. History of Childhood Abuse, Sensation Seeking, and Intimate Partner Violence Under/Not Under the Influence of a Substance: A Cross-Sectional Study in Russia. *PLoS One* 2013; 8:7:1–6.

17. Najavits L, Walsh M. Dissociation, PTSD, and Substance Abuse: An Empirical Study. *J Trauma Dissociation* 2012; 13:1:115–126.

18. Flynn E. *My Wicked, Wicked Ways*. New York: Cooper Square Press; 2003:342, 345.

19. Felitti VJ, Jakstis K, Pepper V, et al. Obesity: Problem, Solution, or Both? *Perm J* 2010; 14:1:24–31.

20. Felitti VJ, Williams SA. Long-Term Follow-Up and Analysis of More Than 100 Patients Who Each Lost More Than 100 Pounds. *Perm J* 1998; 2:3:17–21.

21. Striegel-Moore RH, Silberstein LR, Rodin J. Toward an Understanding of Risk Factors for Bulimia. *Am Psychol* 1986; 41:3:246–263.

22. Zeller MH, Noll JG, Sarwer DB, et al. Child Maltreatment and the Adolescent Patient with Severe Obesity: Implications for Clinical Care. *J Pediatr Psychol* 2015; 40:7:640–648.

23. Hund AR, Espelage DL. Childhood Emotional Abuse and Disordered Eating among Undergraduate Females: Mediating Influence of Alexithymia and Distress. *Child Abuse Neglect* 2006; 30:393–407.

24. Gupta MA, Johnson AM. Nonweight-Related Body Image Concerns among Female Eating-Disordered Patients and Nonclinical Controls: Some Preliminary Observations. *Int J Eat Disord* 2000; 27:3:304–309.

25. Mitchell KS, Mazzeo SE. Mediators of the Association between Abuse and Disordered Earing in Undergraduate Men. *Eat Behav* 2005; 6:318–327.

26. Midlarsky E, Nitzburg G. Eating Disorders in Middle-Aged Women. *J Gen Psychol* 2008; 135:4:393–407.

27. Vieth AZ, Trull TJ. Family Patterns of Perfectionism: An Examination of College Students and Their Parents. *J Personal Assess* 1999; 72:1:49–67.
28. Moeller TP, Bachmann GA, Moeller JR. The Combined Effects of Physical, Sexual, and Emotional Abuse During Childhood: Long-Term Health Consequences for Women. *Child Abuse Neglect* 1993; 17:623–640.
29. Troop NA, Redshaw C. General Shame and Bodily Shame in Eating Disorders: A 2.5-Year Longitudinal Study. *Eur Eat Disord* 2012; 20:373–378.
30. Troop NA, Sotrilli S, Serpell L, et al. Establishing a Useful Distinction between Current and Anticipated Bodily Shame in Eating Disorder. *Eat Weight Disord* 2006; 11:2:83–90.
31. Goedecke JH, Forbes J, Stein DJ. Differences in the Association between Childhood Trauma and BMI in Black and White South African Women. *Afr J Psychiatry* 2013; 16:2:1–205.
32. Salwen JK, Hymowitz GF, Bannon SM, et al. Weight-Related Abuse: Perceived Emotional Impact and the Effect on Disordered Eating. *Child Abuse Neglect* 2015; 45:163–171.
33. Rodhe P, Ichikawa L, Simon GE, et al. Associations of Child Sexual Abuse and Physical Abuse with Obesity and Depression in Middle-Aged Women. *Child Abuse Neglect* 2008; 32:9:878–887.
34. Lawson R, Waller G, Sines J, et al. Emotional Awareness among Eating-Disordered Patients: The Role of Narcissistic Traits. *Eur Eat Disord Rev* 2008; 16:44–48.
35. Bagby RM, Parker JDA, Taylor GJ. The Twenty-Item Toronto Alexithymia Scale-I: Item Selection and Cross-Validation of the Factor Structure. *J Psychosom Res* 1994; 38:1:23–32.
36. Iancu I, Cohen E, Yehuda YB, et al. Treatment of Eating Disordered Improves Eating Symptoms but Not Alexithymia and Dissociation Proneness. *Compr Psychiatry* 2006; 47:189–193.
37. Keel PK, Gravener JA, Joiner TE, et al. Twenty-Year Follow-Up of Bulimia Nervosa and Related Eating Disorders Not Otherwise Specified. *Intl J Eat Disord* 2010; 43:492–497.
38. Smith CE, Pisetsky EM, Wonderlich SA, et al. Is Childhood Trauma Associated with Lifetime Suicide Attempts in Women with Bulimia Nervosa? *Eat Weight Disord* 2016; 21:2:199–204.
39. Sharma P, Garg G, Kumar A, et al. Genome Wide DNA Methylation Profiling for Epigenetic Alteration in Coronary Artery Disease Patients. *Gene* 2014; 541:1:31–40.
40. Mullan F. A Founder of Quality Assessment Encounters a Troubled System Firsthand. *Health Aff* 2001; 20:1:137–141.
41. Felitti VJ, Anda RF. The Lifelong Effects of Adverse Childhood Experiences, Chapter 10. In: *Chadwick's Child Maltreatment: Sexual Abuse and Psychological Maltreatment*. 4th edition. Florissant [MO]: STM Learning; 2014.
42. Felitti VJ, Anda RF, Nordenberg D, et al. Relationship of Childhood Abuse and Household Dysfunction to Many of the Leading Causes of Death in Adults. *Am J Prev Med* 1998; 14:4:245–258.
43. Felitti VJ, Anda RF. The Lifelong Effects of Adverse Childhood Experiences. *Chadwick's Child Maltreat: Sex Abuse Psychol Maltreat* 2014; 2:203–215.
44. Felitti VJ. Reverse Alchemy in Childhood: Turning Gold into Lead. *Health Alert* 2001; 8:1:1–11.
45. Felitti VJ, Anda RF. *The Relationship of Adverse Childhood Experiences to Adult Medical Disease, Psychiatric Disorders and Sexual Behavior: Implications for Healthcare. The Hidden*

Epidemic: The Impact of Early Life Trauma on Health and Disease. Edited by Lanius R and Vermetten E. Cambridge, U.K.: Cambridge University Press; 2009: 2–18.

46. Felitti VJ. Origins of Addictive Behavior: Evidence from a Study of Stressful Childhood Experiences. *Praxis der Kinderpsychologie und Kinderpsychiatrie* 2003; 52:8:1–13.

47. Berthelot N, Godbout N, Hebert M, et al. Prevalence and Correlates of Childhood Sexual Abuse in Adults Consulting for Sexual Problems. *J Sex Marit Ther* 2014; 40:5:434–443.

48. van der Kolk BA. Developmental Trauma Disorder toward a Rational Diagnosis for Children with Complex Trauma Histories. *Psychiatric Ann* 2005; 35:5:401–408.

49. Grippo AJ, Trahanas DM, Zimmerman RR, et al. Oxytocin Protects against Negative Behavioral and Autonomic Consequences of Long-Term Social Isolation. *Psychoneuroendocrinol* 2009; 34:10:1542–1553.

50. Ben-Amitay G, Kimchi N, Wolmer L, et al. Psychophysiological Reactivity in Child Sexual Abuse. *J Child Sex Abuse* 2016; 25:2:185–200.

51. Walker EA, Unutzer J, Rutter C, et al. Costs of Healthcare Use by Women HMO Members with a History of Childhood Abuse and Neglect. *Arch Gen Psychiatry* 1999; 56:7:609–613.

52. Fox RP. Narcissistic Rage and the Problem of Combat Aggression. *Arch Gen Psychiatry* 1974; 31:807–811.

53. Hendin H, Haas AP, Singer P, et al. The Influence of Precombat Personality on Posttraumatic Stress Disorder. *Compr Psychiatry* 1983; 24:6:530–534.

54. Wisco BE, Marx BP, Miller MW, et al. Probable Posttraumatic Stress Disorder in the US Veteran Population According to DSM-5: Results from the National Health and Resilience in Veterans Study. *J Clin Psychiatry* 2014; 75:12:1338–1346.

55. Reger MA, Smolenski DJ, Skopp NA, et al. Risk of Suicide among US Military Service Members Following Operation Enduring Freedom or Operation Iraqi Freedom Deployment and Separation from the US Military. *JAMA Psychiatry* 2015; 72:6:561–569.

56. Clark MM, Hanna BK, Mai JL, et al. Sexual Abuse Survivors and Psychiatric Hospitalization after Bariatric Surgery. *Obes Surg* 2007; 17:465–469.

57. Wildes JE, Kalarchian MA, Marcus MD, et al. Childhood Maltreatment and Psychiatric Morbidity in Bariatric Surgery Candidates. *Obes Surg* 2008; 18:3:306–313.

58. King WC, Chen JY, Mitchell JE, et al. Prevalence of Alcohol Use Disorders before and after Bariatric Surgery. *JAMA* 2012; 307:23:2516–2525.

59. Shea MT, Zlotnick C, Dolan R, et al. Personality Disorders, History of Trauma, and Posttraumatic Stress Disorder in Subjects with Anxiety Disorders. *ComprPsychiatry* 2000; 41:5:315–325.

60. Mitchell A. *It Was Me All Along: A Memoir.* New York: Clarkson Potter [Penguin Random House Company]; 2015.

61. Byrnes E, Terrill M. *"Kookie" No More.* New York: Barricade Books, Inc.; 1996:12–20 (and personal communication, 2016).

62. Robinson BE. *Chained to the Desk: A Guidebook for Workaholics, Their Partners and Children, and the Clinicians Who Treat Them.* New York: New York University Press; 1998.

63. Oswald LM, Wand GS, Kuwabara H, et al. History of Childhood Adversity Is Positively Associated with Ventral Striatal Dopamine Responses to Amphetamine. *Psychopharmacol* 2014; 231:2417–2433.

64. Comings DE, Rosenthal RJ, Lesieur HR, et al. A Study of the Dopamine D2 Receptor Gene in Pathological Gambling. *Pharmacogenet* 1996; 6:223–234.

65. Kasanova Z, Hernaus D, Vaessen T, et al. Early-Life Stress Affects Stress-Related Prefrontal Dopamine Activity in Healthy Adults, but Not in Individuals with Psychotic Disorder. *PLoS One* 2016; 11:3:e0150746.

66. Ebstein RP, Novick L, Umansky R, et al. Dopamine D4 Receptor (D4DR) Exon III Polymorphism Associated with the Human Personality Trait of Novelty Seeking. *Nature Genet* 1996; 12:78–80.

67. McCarthy CP, McEvoy JW. Pimping in Medical Education: Lacking Evidence and Under Threat. *JAMA* 2015; 314:22:2347–2348.

68. Stiegler MP. What I Learned about Adverse Events from Captain Sully. *JAMA* 2015; 313:4:361–362.

69. Killinger B. *Workaholics: The Respectable Addicts*. Buffalo [NY]: Firefly Books; 1991.

70. Real, T. *Full Respect Living Tool Kit*, www.terryreal.com, 2016.

71. Khan A. A Death in the Family. *JAMA* 2017: 318:16:1543–1544.

72. Schwenk TL. Resident Depression: The Tip of a Graduate Medical Education Iceberg. *JAMA* 2015; 314:22:2357–2358.

73. Remen RN. *Kitchen Table Wisdom: Stories That Heal*. New York: Riverhead Books; 1996.

74. Briere J. The Long-Term Clinical Correlates of Childhood Sexual Victimization. *Ann NY Acad Sci* 1988; 528:1:327–334.

75. Dorahy MJ, Clearwater K. Shame and Guilt in Men Exposed to Childhood Sexual Abuse: A Qualitative Investigation. *J Child Sex Abuse* 2012; 21:155–175.

76. Hunter JA. A Comparison of the Psychosocial Maladjustment of Adult Males and Females Sexually Molested as Children. *J Interpers Violence* 1991; 6:2:205–217.

77. Carnes P. *Out of The Shadows: Understanding Sexual Addiction*. Center City [MN]: Hazelden; 1983.

78. Groth AN. Sexual Trauma and the Life Histories of Sex Offenders. *Victimology* 1979; 4:6.

79. Kaufman J, Zigler E. Do Abused Children Become Abusive Parents? *Am Orthopsychiat* 1987; 57:2:186–192.

80. King BB. *Blues All Around Me: The Autobiography of B. B. King*. New York: Harper Collins Publishers; 1996, 6, 33, 35, 195, 223

81. Mellody P, Freundlich LS. *The Intimacy Factor the Ground Rules for Overcoming the Obstacles to Truth, Respect, and Lasting Love*. San Francisco: Harper Collins; 2003:7–24.

82. Black C. *It Will Never Happen To Me: Growing Up With Addiction As Youngsters, Adolescents, Adults*. Center City [MN]: Hazelden; 1981.

83. Botticelli MP, Koh HK. Changing the Language of Addiction. *JAMA* 2016; 316:1361.

84. Scaer RC. *The Body Bears the Burden: Trauma, Dissociation, and Disease*. 2nd edition. New York: Routledge; 2007:120–121.

85. Hoffer E. *The Ordeal of Change*. Titusville [NJ]: Hopewell Publications; 2006.

86. van der Kolk BA. *The Body Keeps the Score: Brain, Mind, and Body in the Healing of Trauma*. New York: Viking (Penguin Group); 2014.

How Nature Copes

7

THE EFFECTS OF TRAUMA ON BRAIN AND BODY

Pioneering reconstructive hand surgeon Dr. Paul Brand was the first physician to recognize that leprosy did not directly cause tissue death, but rather that the damage arose secondary to sensory loss caused by the disease: patients did not recognize that the repeated trauma was irreversibly injuring their tissues. He proposed, therefore, that pain could be a paradoxical blessing—a warning sign of potential damage—and detailed his ideas in a wonderfully humanistic book, *The Gift Nobody Wants.*

"I was not sure what contribution I could offer leprosy patients, but the more time I spent among them, the more confirmed I felt in my calling. . . . I had listened to hundreds of stories of rejection and despair. . . . The patients went to Chingleput [in British India, now known as Chengalpattu] because they literally had nowhere else to go. They had become social outcasts simply because of their misfortune and contracting a feared and misunderstood disease. For the first time I grasped the human tragedy of leprosy."

Early in his career, Dr. Brand was heavily influenced by a lecture from anthropologist Margaret Mead, whose theory emphasizes the primacy of human connection:

"What would you say is the earliest sign of civilization? A clay pot? Tools made of iron? . . . These are all early signs. . . . But here is what I believe to be evidence of the earliest civilization." High above her head she held a human femur . . . and pointed to a grossly thickened area

DOI: 10.4324/9781315657721-11

where the bone . . . had . . . healed. "Such signs of healing are never found . . . [in] the earliest, fiercest societies. In their skeletons we find clues of violence. . . . But this healed bone shows that someone must have cared for the injured person—hunted on his behalf, brought him food, served him at personal sacrifice."[1]

Dr. Brand, whom I was privileged to meet in 1978, also first established the correct pediatric penicillin doses when the drug was newly discovered and precious (personal communication, 1998). He impressed upon me that shared pain was central to the human experience. Loneliness, he believed, came in the same package: neither can be shared. Pain and loneliness are blood brothers to trauma.

First Themes

Trauma impairs brain development and attachment, prejudices memory and experience, deforms the personality, and disables the ability to be fully relational.[2-5] At a completely unconscious level, the past becomes the present. The limbic system—part of "the emotional brain"—persistently overrides the prefrontal cortex. The "felt sense," the visceral, skeletal, and autonomic perception of ourselves and our surroundings, largely mediated by afferent vagus nerve fibers, becomes corrupted and unreliable.[6] In a familial or caregiving environment of totalitarian control, abandonment, or enmeshed helplessness, violence or betrayal, children can develop pathologic attachments to their abusers that propel into adulthood and unfavorably color their lives. Instead of feeling precious, they feel toxic shame. Self-regulation becomes impaired and drives secrecy, perfectionism, hypervigilance, risky or addictive behavior, self-injury, or trauma reenactment. Stable adult relationships, nurturing marriages, and loving parenting become highly challenging or impossible. Trauma triggers that may be unconscious to the individual and seemingly irrational to friends and family distort daily interactions and complicate physician/patient relationships. We have seen these phenomena repeatedly in the previous chapters. How do they happen?

Lessons From L'hôpital de la Pitié-Salpêtrière

You are a refined member of late 19th century Parisian high society. Today you have decided to be totally *au courant* and become an observer in the L'hôpital de la Pitié-Salpêtrière in Paris, a former gunpowder factory ("salpêtre" translates "saltpeter") that was converted to a hospital for the poor and mentally ill in 1694, and by 1887 has become a prestigious teaching hospital. You are observing the famous neurologist Jean-Marie Charcot examine a woman with "hysteria," a disease believed to be peculiar to women and presumably originating in the uterus (from the Greek *hysterikos*, womb). Because the hospital is a refuge for the poor and for prostitutes, many of the patients display hysteria, believed to be simple malingering or attention-getting. However, Charcot is not satisfied with that prevailing bias and has begun to document these women's symptoms. His examinations are public, so you are accompanied by friends, who, like you, are chic professionals and curious Parisian aristocrats. The following is what you hear that afternoon. As you take your seat, Dr. Charcot has already produced a hysterical attack in a hypnotized young woman:

CHARCOT: Let us press again on the hysterogenic point. (A male intern touches the patient in the ovarian region). . . . Occasionally subjects even bite their tongues. . . . Look at the arched back, which is so well described in textbooks.

PATIENT: Mother, I am frightened.

CHARCOT: Note the emotional outburst. If we let things go unabated we will soon return to the epileptoid behavior.

PATIENT: Oh! Mother!

CHARCOT: Again, note these screams. You could say it is a lot of noise over nothing.[7]

Neurologists subsequent to Charcot, Janet, Freud, and Breuer continued to investigate and ultimately recognized dissociation, subconscious ideas, and the somatic symptoms that they produced and realized that hysteria symptoms diminished when the traumatic memories could be relived and expressed in words. That's still true and termed *abreaction*, "the talking cure." One salutary upshot of the Adverse Childhood Events study was that outpatient visits dropped by 35% after patients were encouraged to discuss their traumas with their physicians.[8]

By 1896, in an 18-case report entitled *The Aetiology of Hysteria*, Freud had declared that "at the bottom of every case of hysteria there are one or more occurrences of premature sexual experiences, occurrences which belong to the earliest years of childhood. . . . I believe that this is an important finding."[9]

Unfortunately, the implications of his published theory were exceedingly troubling. If Freud were right, the prevalence of hysteria in both Paris and Vienna indicated that childhood sexual abuse was endemic, even within "the respectable classes." Under tremendous peer and societal pressure, Freud repudiated his own thesis: "I was at last obliged to recognize that these scenes of seduction had never taken place, and that they were only fantasies which my patients had made up."

★★★★★

This little vignette is not just an archaic aberrance: it is still the prototype for the way unconventional etiologies are accepted: Assume that it is nothing, or assert that it is really something else. Disregard or minimize accompanying signs and symptoms that do not fit established ideologies. Formulate obscure explanations when more obvious ones present themselves, even when there is accumulating evidence to the contrary.

Probably no area of human interaction is exempt. I have practiced long enough to see this phenomenon occur and recur in medicine and in plastic surgery. "Common knowledge" that was accepted dogma in the 1970's has been replaced by different but still sometimes unsubstantiated common knowledge today. In both cases, grand conclusions and fervent partisan stances develop from often incomplete, untested information. Unproven beliefs became axiomatic. Facts that do not easily fit are disregarded. Science then becomes religion with its faithful followers—maybe a human trait, but one that does not benefit patients.

How Believable Are Trauma Histories?

Complicating trauma research further is continuing societal and professional reluctance to acknowledge that childhood abuse and neglect are so distressingly common, despite demographic data (89.7% in the National Stressful Events Survey).[10, 11]

Yet some of the most sophisticated experts refer to patient stories of developmental trauma (in body dysmorphic disorder patients and others) as "perceived": the authors defend their caution by explaining that the alleged maltreatment has not often been confirmed.[12, 13]

Their caution is responsible and understandable: Without independent corroboration by photographs, videos, witnesses, or biological evidence, can we really know what happened?

But how might reliable verification be obtained? Abusing parents or caregivers could deny it, or might simply believe that what their children called emotional or physical abuse was simply not appreciated as the best way to raise virtuous youngsters. Victims themselves may deny, repress, or dissociate—we know that this happens—or wonder if their memories were generated or real; fewer deliberately fabricate. Even false allegations are really "perceived" without supportive evidence.

★★★★★

There is also a societal paradox here: At the time of this writing, public figures have been attacked and lost their careers after allegations of sexual impropriety, some of which have little or no evidence behind them. If we are willing to punish adults without conclusive proof, how can we also doubt childhood memories without conclusive proof?

Perhaps this dilemma is most germane when litigation is involved. Among my patients, there are no such stakes. Trauma is just part of their past medical histories and is relevant to their behavior, personality characteristics, and their resilience. In my own limited experience, I have seen more patients whose self-esteem, reality processing, addictions, somatic symptoms, depression, and poor self-care implicate developmental trauma, but who deny it in their A.C.E. survey. I cannot remember a patient who alleged trauma whom I did not believe. If I trust patients' histories of hypertension, asthma, or airway obstruction, why shouldn't I also trust their childhood experiences?

How can we make more progress in understanding addictions, self-destructive behavior, and body dysmorphic disorder? First remove the question marks from "perceived abuse." It starts there.

Psychologist Alan Schore, some of whose concepts we shall explore presently, describes the effect of culture upon childhood maturation as follows: *"Individual development arises out of the relationship between the brain, mind, and body of both infant and caregiver held within a culture and environment that either supports, inhibits, or even threatens it. . . . These relational origins are forged and expressed in nonverbal attachment communications in the first year and influenced by the cultural surroundings. They indelibly shape the individual's way of experiencing the world."*[14]

A Brain Model and Anatomy Relevant to Trauma

If childhood abuse and neglect alter the brain, where and how does this occur and what does it mean for its survivors?

In 1990, neuroscientist Paul McLean described a model first developed in 1960 in which brain function was conceptualized in three layers: the reptilian brain, functional at birth and responsible for brainstem and autonomic functions; the mammalian brain (or limbic system) responsible for emotions and monitoring the environment for safety; and the neocortex, the thinking brain (Figure 7.1).[15]

Although in some ways insufficiently complex, the Triune Brain model conceptualizes the evolution and development of human behavior. At birth, only our brainstems are fully functional. During infancy, our midbrains, limbic systems, thalamus and amygdala come fully online, responding to emotions and learning to recognize danger—the most primitive survival instinct.[16] It is not until age two that children's frontal lobes begin to develop, and not till first grade that they can plan and think abstractly, or plan purposeful activity. Remember what it was like to dress your two-year-old: you put on one sock, and as you put on the second sock, the child pulls off the first. To the child, this is not purposeful activity: it's just a game.

Normal Nervous System Responses to the Environment

Next to develop and based on experience, the limbic system learns to identify and control responses to external stimuli, both dangerous and pleasurable. Its primary components are ordinarily identified as the amygdala (van der Kolk's "smoke detector"),[17] hippocampus, thalamus, hypothalamus, basal ganglia, and cingulate gyrus. Think of the limbic system as a safety and danger center that processes the environment, controls the conscious brain, and body, and determines subjective

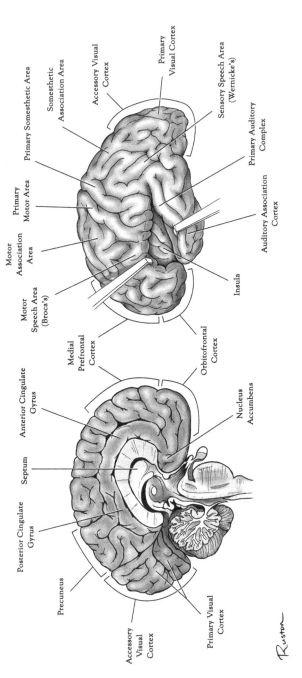

FIGURE 7.1 Schematic of Brain Areas Relevant to Trauma Processing

feelings and emotional reactions to external stimuli and then the body's physiologic responses to them.

Sensory information through touch, vision, and sound transports to the *thalamus*, which routes the information either instantaneously to the amygdala, or slightly more slowly to the pre-frontal cortex. The single exception to this schema is the sense of smell, which transmits directly to the amygdala. The amygdala affects our abilities to be social, to sense fear, pleasure, and respond to pheromones. A woman whose right amygdala was resected to treat refractory temporal lobe epilepsy could express fear but lost had her ability to recognize facial expressions, suggesting an additional role for the amygdala.

Sensory input also travels to the locus ceruleus in the brainstem, our most primitive alarm system, which in turn routes messages to the right amygdala. When the system functions perfectly, the amygdala incorporates information from the right hippocampus and transmits it instantaneously to the right orbitofrontal cortex for interpretation and to the hypothalamus and brainstem, recruiting the hormones that belong to the hypothalamic-pituitary axis and the autonomic nervous system. The hypothalamus plays a key role in short and long-term memory, interprets emotions, and remembers prior or cause and effect—therefore connecting actions and consequences.

This process is fast and unconscious unless the frontal lobes are involved. The medial pre-frontal cortex (MPFC), van der Kolk's "watchtower," adds context and executive control, modulating our reptilian responses: the classical example is deciding whether the long, straight object on the ground is a stick or a rattlesnake. You jump before you know.

★★★★★

The hypothalamus forms the core of the mind/body connection, and can engage the autonomic nervous system, immune and endocrine function, as well as learning and memory through hippocampal connections. The cingulate cortex also modulates incoming data and is responsible for cognitive flexibility, adaptation, and interpreting emotions, and mediates stress—evoked cardiovascular activity.[18, 19] The cingulate gyrus can inhibit the amygdalar response for minor threats. Otherwise, the autonomic nervous system activates, and epinephrine is released by the adrenal cortex, which increases blood glucose, shunts blood from abdominal viscera to skeletal muscle, and increases pulse, blood pressure, and cardiac output. Pupils dilate and muscles become ready to respond.

Simultaneously, the hypothalamus triggers activity in the hypothalamic/pituitary/adrenal (HPA) axis, therefore releasing corticotrophic releasing hormone (CRH) and adrenal corticotrophic hormone (ACTH) from the anterior pituitary and provoking cortisol release from the adrenal cortices. Endogenous opioid release blunts fear and pain perception. The entire body activates. The amygdala receives information from the thalamus faster than the cortex and so may preempt the decision of whether incoming information is threatening even before we consciously recognize what is happening. Cortisol modulates the stimulatory effect of norepinephrine and inhibits the HPA axis, therefore slowing the brain's stress response. However, long term, sustained arousal modulated by cortisol creates significant health problems including diabetes, hypertension, gastric ulcers, and atherosclerosis.[20]

Fight and flight are always in context: the buck and the hunter each have the same sympathetic nervous system arousal, the same dilated pupils, the same cardiac and muscle activity, the same diminished pain sensitivity, and the same heightened vigilance: but to the buck the goal is survival; to the hunter it is only lunch.

★★★★★

The freeze response is the last-resort survival mechanism and can be replicated in the laboratory by exposing animals to inescapable shock. Even when escape later becomes possible, the animals still freeze when shocked instead of fleeing. The same phenomenon occurs in the "learned helplessness" of chronic trauma.[21] However, deliberate, "top-down" conscious calming behavior—e.g., recognizing situations as controllable—can decrease amygdalar sensitivity.[22] We can still manage our brains.[23, 24]

The near death freeze experience is uniformly described by those who have experienced it as peaceful. Margaret Mackworth, a passenger on the Lusitania when it sank in 1915 and terrified of the water before the trip, wrote after she survived, "I had got [sic] through this test without disgracing myself. . . . The only explanation I can give is that when I was lying back in that sunlit water I was, and I knew it, very near to death. . . . Somehow, one had a protected feeling, as if it were a kindly thing."[25]

Similarly, we have this account from a Civil War battle:

> There had been nothing in their lives before to prepare these young men for [the battle at Henry Hill.] . . . Gunner William Thomas Proague described a strange calm feeling. . . "A most novel sensation. . . . Hard to describe, a sort of warm, pleasing glow enveloping the chest and head with an effect something like entrancing music in a dream. [But] my observing, thinking, and reasoning faculties were normal."[26]

Higher Centers

The orbitofrontal cortex (OFC) is the center of much of this trauma processing, including the adaptive and non-adaptive states that follow developmental trauma. The OFC, our "core self," starts to mature in the middle of the second year of life, when it is essentially preverbal and unconscious. In a nurturing environment, its development creates an internal sense of security and resilience and the capacity to temper emotions. Thus it is also easy to understand how traumatic environments at young ages can create self-regulatory deficits and the inability to modulate emotions or sense one's own body.[27]

The orbitofrontal cortex is the only cortical structure that directly connects with the hypothalamus, the amygdala, and the brainstem reticular formation that regulates arousal. The OFC processes face and voice information, appraises the external environment, and integrates subcortical data from the viscera, critical functional adult processes.[28]

In young childhood, the pre-frontal cortex/amygdalar circuit is strong and quick to respond, making young children properly wary of strangers. During adolescence, this fear-learning normally extinguishes. Early life adversity impairs fluid frontal cortex development: myelination is delayed, cortical volumes are smaller, the HPA axis is more active, and inflammatory levels are much higher. Women seem to show more dramatic differences than men.[29] Similar abnormalities are found in adults with histories of childhood maltreatment, who have smaller gray matter volumes in their medial pre-frontal cortices and anterior cingulates and insulae.[30–32] Even destructive but pleasurable stimuli (e.g., drug abuse or excessive eating) disrupt homeostasis by conditioning the HPA axis and the autonomic nervous system.[33] Fortunately, these affected areas are plastic and recover significantly when the provocative stimulation stops (See Figure 7.2).[34, 35]

★★★★★

In Chapter 9 we will consider strong evidence that childhood abuse and neglect correlate precisely with body dysmorphic disorder and many common adult diseases. The latter observation was presaged by physician and essayist Lewis Thomas, former medical school dean at Yale and New York universities and president of Memorial Sloan-Kettering Institute:

> *I thought of [inflammation], and still do, as an example of largely self-induced real disease rather than pure defense, with all sorts of mutually incompatible, combative mechanisms turned loose at once, frequently resulting in more damage to the host than to the invader, a biological accident analogous to a multicar accident involving fire engines, ambulances, police cars, and tow trucks all colliding on a bridge. "*[36]

Self-monitoring is critical to self-regulation, but only a few midline structures (the orbitofrontal cortex, medial pre-frontal cortex, anterior and posterior cingulate, precuneus, and insula) form the centralized strip of brain tissue that performs this function and are the only areas that have contact with the midbrain. During functional MRIs, resting non-traumatized individuals monitor themselves—their bodies, their sensations, and their thoughts. In traumatized patients, the same midline strip remains dark: these survivors do not introspect.[37] As clinicians, we see patients who don't know what they want and can't make up their minds; the most severely affected don't recognize their appearances. When you lose your body awareness, you lose your sense of self (See Figure 7.3).

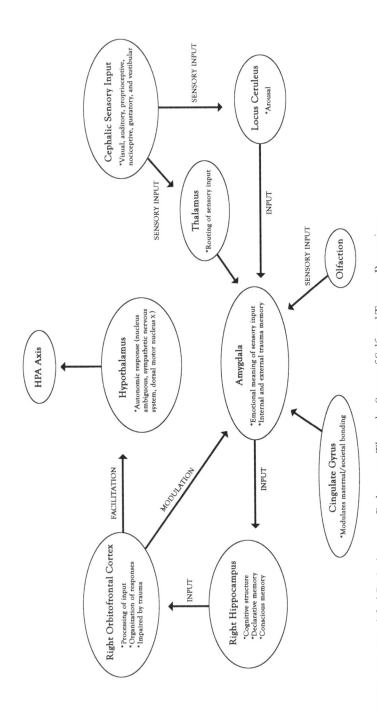

FIGURE 7.2 Simplified Brain Anatomy Relevant to Thought, Sense of Self, and Trauma Processing

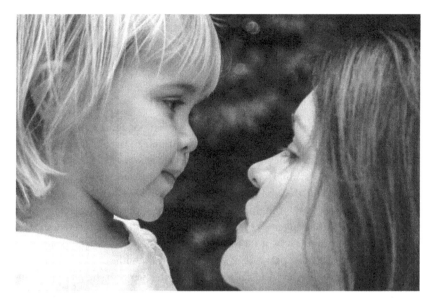

FIGURE 7.3   Photo of Mother and Child

Early Development, Attachment, and Attunement

We are hardwired to be relational and intimate. "Attachment," the outcome of the child's genetically determined biological predisposition as modified and "attuned" by his or her caregivers and by the home environment—even brain-to-brain interaction with the mother or intimate caregiver—determines how we self-regulate and manage our relationships.[38, 39]

The first year of life requires a reliable attachment between the infant and the primary caregiver. Through "empathic mirroring,"[40] the nurturing mother tunes her child's sensory and emotional processing so that the infant eventually becomes able to perform these processes alone (Figure 7.3). Skin to skin contact between mother and child tunes the social engagement system as measured by improvement in respiratory sinus arrhythmia (RSA).[41, 42] Recent functional magnetic resonance imaging establishes right hemisphere dominance in this process. Facial processing, auditory perception, attention, tactile information, prosody, and social experiences all create right-brain systems that function properly for the child. "From infancy throughout all later stages of the lifespan, the right hemisphere is dominant for the nonconscious reception, expression, and communication of emotion, as well as the cognitive and physiological components of emotional processing. . . . Self-awareness, empathy, identification with others . . . are largely dependent upon . . . right hemisphere resources."[43, 44]

A curious frontal lobe phenomenon is "mirroring," one of several processes by which we feel empathy. Through "mirror neurons" we imitate each other's vocal rhythms and prosody, sitting or standing positions, and sense hostility, depression, or elation even though it is not verbalized. We can sense anger or warm connection. As we sit with friends, we often adopt identical postures: the same hands on chins, hands in laps, and crossed legs duplicated. Watch for it—it's surprisingly common.

Relational Trauma and Brain Development

Childhood trauma disrupts this normal maturation sequence, affecting brain growth, the development of the hypothalamic-pituitary axis and the autonomic nervous system and how they function, the development of the midbrain and cortex, and therefore a child's memory, thinking processes, ability to relate to and "read" others, and the abilities to trust and sense danger.[45-47] Accordingly, patients traumatized early in life misread facial expressions and voice tones; they either don't recognize danger or they see it everywhere. The limbic system does not process in an orderly way: it jumps to conclusions based on sights, sounds, or emotions. This disordered physiology continues into adulthood, so when some trigger—an event, voice, even facial expression—invokes fear, helplessness, vulnerability, or learned self-hatred, their rational brains go offline. Chronic stress produces catecholamine release levels that rapidly impair cognitive function in the pre-frontal cortex while strengthening the emotional and habitual responses generated by the amygdala and basal ganglia. Chronic stress also provokes dendritic atrophy in the pre-frontal cortex and dendritic growth in the amygdala and strengthens the sympathetic response.[48, 49] Traumatized individuals have lower thresholds (or "kindling") for arousal, avoidance, and re-experiencing, apparently from permanent changes in neuronal network excitability.[50, 51] Consequently even apparently neutral stimuli can trigger fear responses when paired with traumatic events—or something that simulates them. *Feeling becomes fact.* Trauma survivors may not be aware that they are re-experiencing the past—they become enraged, ashamed, or frozen.[52] They feel the distress but don't know where it comes from, so they look for someone to blame for these awful feelings: And there sits the spouse, the employer, or the physician.

Memory and Conditioning

Declarative, explicit memory of facts and events is conscious and modifiable: it's what we use to tell our stories. Declarative memory appears around three years of age and is mediated by the hippocampus and pre-frontal cortex; it is lost in post-traumatic amnesia and during flashbacks. Non-declarative or implicit memory, on the other hand, is nonverbal and unconscious: the skills and habits that we have developed—procedural memories—like riding bicycles or playing guitars. Implicit memory is stored in the motor cortex, amygdala, brainstem, cerebellum, and basal ganglia. The right brain appears to process not only conscious but also unconscious emotions and is home to procedural memory.

Conditioned responses are also forms of non-declarative memory and largely disappear over time, unlike other types of non-declarative memory.[53–56] However, if the conditioned response is learned at a time of perceived life-threatening danger, the association between trigger and action can become deeply embedded in one traumatic episode, which explains why sounds, smells, body positions, prosody, and facial expressions can trigger such strong and unexplainably disproportionate emotions.[57] Past interpersonal trauma increases the chance of misinterpreting incoming information just as it alters time and perspective. Highly disturbing past events are more likely to be stored in long-term memory, and with time they can become more distorted by subsequent experiences.

★★★★★

Fear memories are encoded by the amygdala according to their sensory features.[58, 59] A study of combat veterans with and without PTSD demonstrated that the odor of diesel fuel increased regional blood flow in the amygdala, insula, medial pre-frontal cortex, and anterior cingulate, supporting the powerful neural circuitry stimulation that olfactory triggers can produce.[60] Traumatic events store more easily in implicit memory because the amygdala does not succumb to the stress hormones that suppress hippocampal activity.[61–63] Repeated childhood ("complex") trauma resets the patient's baseline, so that these vestigial symptoms, like my own prosody sensitivity or exaggerated startle response, remain even though other, more obvious signs have disappeared. In this way, childhood trauma encodes meaning into subsequent lifetime events, which is why triggers are so hard to anticipate or explain—to the observer or even those experiencing them.[64] In the same fashion, the terrific effects of wartime on soldiers' brains was long misunderstood: "Cushing saw survivors of Messina and other engagements who were so "shell-shocked" that they fell into uncontrollable convulsing at the sound of artillery."[65]

Right Brain Dominance in Trauma Processing

The right brain develops first in the fetus and appears to carry nonverbal communication between mothers and infants. The left brain, which remembers words and facts, becomes functional when children begin to speak and understand language. The right brain stores sensory memories and their related emotions, voice responses, facial features, and gestures. It creates what we loosely call "intuition." Interestingly, Broca's area, the speech center, is in the left frontal cortex; nevertheless, it also responds to trauma and goes dark on functional MRI, which explains why we feel "speechless terror."[66–69]

Sight, prosody, and touch are three of the skills that facilitate relational behavior. Touch is influenced early. There is evidence that the emotional impact of mother/infant body contact is more profound when the infant is held on the left side of the mother's body, allegedly because the mother's heart and left breast makes direct contact with the child's developing right brain.[70, 71] Curiously, depressed mothers and those with histories of domestic violence naturally cradle on the right side instead.[72, 73] Cardinal elements of the ability to be relational appear to be dominantly right-brain phenomena.

★★★★★

High-resolution structural MRI scans in 42 adolescents with psychiatric disorders demonstrate that childhood trauma reduces volumes in their right prefrontal and dorsolateral pre-frontal cortices; physical abuse reduces insular volume; physical and emotional neglect decrease cerebellar volume; emotional neglect decreases volume in the orbitofrontal complex, the pre-frontal cortex, ventral striatum, amygdala, and hippocampus; physical abuse, physical neglect, and emotional neglect are associated with reductions in the pre-frontal cortical volumes.[74, 75] These are just observed gross volumetric deficits; one can only hypothesize the neurobiological changes. Age is important: women traumatized before the age of 12 are more likely to develop major depression, whereas women who were traumatized between ages 12 and 18 more frequently develope PTSD.[76, 77]

Compared to the left hemisphere, the right brain is densely connected with the limbic system and with subcortical areas throughout the brain that generate both arousal and autonomic responses to emotional stimuli. The sympathetic nervous system produces high-energy responses to trauma (so you run), whereas the parasympathetic system disengages the individual from the external environment and is energy-conserving (so you space out).[78] The infant's response to trauma is massive and disturbs critical right cortical and subcortical development. Early abuse deeply impacts healthy limbic system maturation and creates a child with affective instability, abnormal pain tolerance, poor stress response, memory disturbances, and tendencies toward hyperactivity or dissociation.[79, 80] It is no wonder that childhood trauma can generate foreboding before surgery and unmanageable stress afterward, and will profoundly test the patient's equilibrium when complications or even minor imperfections occur.

The right cortical deficits described in children have observable adulthood ramifications. Individuals with poor attachment display diminished capacities for empathy and for reading the subtleties of facial expression—and therefore interpret emotions inaccurately. Body dysmorphic patients struggle similarly.[81, 82] As a result, they cannot read their own body cues, an impairment called "desomatization."[83]

Right hemispheric coping deficits limit anyone's ability to modulate emotions, especially the more primitive ones (e.g., shame, rage, excitement, elation, disgust, and fear). When stressed, traumatized people experience diffuse, inchoate, chaotic sensations with overwhelming somatic and visceral components—the basis of alexithymia. If you lose the ability to interpret others' emotions and to understand your own, you lose the ability to be fully relational. These phenomena contribute to the inarticulate and apparently irrational patient responses in our vignettes. My most difficult patients have been the most dissociated, disengaged, and unreachable.

★★★★★

A recent patient dispassionately recounted a violent snowmobile accident in which she broke numerous bones and was hospitalized for four months, undergoing some 11 surgeries. Despite my expressions of amazement and questions about flashbacks or PTSD symptoms she smiled and said, "I'm fine."

That is what van der Kolk calls "a cover story" and what psychologist Denise Gelinas has termed "a disguised presentation." The patient's unconscious memory is probably closer to this: "I was on my snowmobile and suddenly there was a tree. I froze. I couldn't stop. I saw faces and felt awful pain. People yelled. Someone was screaming. Was it me? Everything hurt. I was strapped and smothered. I had to run away. I was powerless and terrified. Where was my daughter? *I knew I was going to die*." That's closer to her real experience; the cover story is the public-consumption version. Adult recollections of a powerless, vulnerable childhood can sound the same, or else disappear altogether.

The space between the real experience and the cover story is where the fear hides.

★★★★★

Our paperwork insisted that she was 22, but when I saw her reclining on the examination table, legs outstretched and arms folded across her chest, she appeared closer to 12. She wore a sort of Sound of Music milkmaid dress with a blue top and flowered skirt and with laced over-the ankle boots.

She stared at me gravely. Her parents looked out the window. Her younger sister sat in the corner mugging selfies into her phone. Light snow had begun to fall and the forecasters were dizzily apocalyptic about the possibilities.

"Well," I said. "You hold today's record for traveling the farthest to see me." I smiled. No one else did.

"We were referred," Mother said soberly. "They thought you might have some ideas about her nose."

The patient had been born with an unusual craniofacial cleft treated by a team at an excellent medical center. Still many things were left undone. The residual deformity was obvious. Half of her nose had grown normally, but the other half was only two-thirds its size. There was more. Her teeth didn't fit. Her lower jaw receded. Ideas began to form in my head about what I could do for the nose, but I needed to focus on the patient first.

"What don't you like about your nose?"

Shrug. Her voice was small. "I guess I can't breathe too well."

In fact that was the only reason for referral. I wondered why her referring surgeon hadn't mentioned her other anomalies. Why didn't the patient mention them? Why hadn't she come earlier? Most patients and their parents are motivated to schedule reconstructions at younger ages. It is human and healthy to want to look normal.

I smiled again. "Let me examine you so I know what I am talking about. Nothing I'm going to do will hurt."

It didn't matter. The patient stiffened, holding her arms rigidly at her sides with her fists clenched. She squeezed her eyes shut and set her jaw.

I minimized my examination. It was difficult to see into her right nostril, which barely admitted the tip of a cotton applicator. The whole lower nose on that side was too small, too short, and too high on her cheek. A bigger, staged operation, like a paramedian forehead flap, would provide a dramatic improvement, but I couldn't even imagine mentioning it. I decided on a simple airway plan. But I needed to know more.

"The right side of your nose is a little small," I said in my gentlest voice. "Your nostril is tiny, which is part of the reason you can't breathe on that side. I think you are also blocked on the inside, but I can't see very well." I paused. "What do you think about the shape of your nose?"

She played with a strand of her hair. "The right side of my nose is small?" She looked at her mother. Her father was absorbed in a book of poems by Langston Hughes.

I gave my patient a mirror. She started to say something, then put the mirror on her lap and settled back in a lump.

"I just hate my face."

There was something else to learn but one of them had to tell me what it was. Maybe the big picture would help. I turned to her parents and smiled.

"What do your other doctors plan? It might influence our timing."

Her father put down his book and stared out the window. The snow was falling heavier. It was Christmas day for the forecasters. Her sister constructed new selfie poses. It's good to have a life purpose.

"That's undecided," her mother said slowly. Her face contained no emotion. "They've talked about braces, maybe surgery. The dentists said it, I think." Her voice trailed off.

I could feel the young woman starting to wall up. Her shoulders lifted and began to move in a small, circular motion. Her lower lip jutted into a *pout. Her legs slid back and forth as if she were beginning to run in place. The table paper crumpled. She stared at her parents and began to breathe in short gasps, then looked toward the floor, defocused. Her mother sat quietly, turning a water bottle in her hands. I waited. Priming the pump wasn't working. I felt I should say something.*

"If you want to breathe better, the simplest solution is to take a small amount of skin and cartilage from one of your ears and use it to open your nostril," I said. "That will also bring the nostril down, and help your nose look more normal. It's a pretty simple operation. We can always do more in the future." I smiled again and waited.

Her father continued to look out the window. Perhaps he was staring at nothing. Perhaps he was waiting for baseball season. Perhaps he was thinking about driving in the snow. It wouldn't matter if the forecasters were right.

"I don't know," her mother said aimlessly, staring at her daughter. "There's so much to do."

"When is your next appointment," I said.

"I'm not sure. Two years. I don't know. Maybe she'll get braces."

I looked at the patient. She didn't seem bored anymore. Her shoulders had tightened as she wrapped her arms around her chest, cold and collapsing into herself, like an orphan in a hurricane. It took her a minute to come back to me. Her eyes flashed around. Her face constricted. She began talking in the piercing whine that a child uses when she doesn't want to take a bath.

"You're creeping me out. I can't stand it. You want to do surgery and break my bones and cut my face and saw my jaws. I feel sick. I don't want pain again. You can't do this to me."

She ran from the office without shutting the door. Her mother sighed.

"She's like the Road Runner when she gets upset," her mother said.

"So I can see," I said.

Her mother looked at me for a long time, then she and her husband stood and left without speaking. Her sister reluctantly pocketed her phone and followed.

The snow had gotten heavier and started to compress the branches. The forecasters had been right about the weather. For a few days the city will look clean again.

*****

What had happened here? No one had mentioned bone surgery or jaws or causing pain. But to the patient, that formed the entire conversation. An appointment that she herself had requested became a frightening conspiracy about painful procedures. This was disordered information processing, perhaps triggering PTSD lying in her cell structure. My only emotion was compassion; the patient's was terror.

The Ravages of Trauma: Brain

The lifetime prevalence of PTSD is approximately 7.8%, though women are at higher risk (lifetime risk for women 10%, 4% for men).[84–89] Those with higher intelligence appear to be at lower risk.[90] Other predisposing factors are a family history of mental disorders, lower education, trauma severity, poor social support, and current life stressors.[91] Dissociation, avoidance, and re-experiencing (all right-brain phenomena) are the hallmarks of chronic, unrelenting trauma.

If, instead of nurturing, the child's early experiences are separation, neglect, abandonment, fear, rage, physical pain, or inconsistency, both psychological and neurological pathways develop differently than in attentive, supportive environments.[92, 93] Personality is not just superficially learned; it is encoded. It is likely that epigenetic changes (see below) influenced by social history recalibrate the production and expression of oxytocin, vasopressin, physiology, and behavior.[94] Maternal scents alone trigger oxytocin and norepinephrine release,[95] which stimulate physical bonding and nurturing. Higher oxytocin levels are associated with better health, better stress management, lower cortisol levels during stressful exposure, less depression,[96] less anxiety, better accuracy at facial recognition, an improved ability to assess trustworthiness, betrayal, and altruistic behavior[97]—just like stress and trauma are conversely associated with illness.[98] Maternal depression, hostility, or verbal abuse create "disorganized attachment" (in which the child perceives the mother is the source of both comfort and fear) and predict depression in the affected children.[99, 100]

In a collection of essays published in 1946 and still relevant today, Harry Emerson Fosdick, the Protestant minister whom we met earlier, reinforces what the evidence shows: that traumatic acts affect the abuser in the same way that they affect the abused:

> *But then the day comes when the evil passes from anticipation, through committal into memory, and something momentous happens, as the sense of guilt takes hold, settles down, will not let go. . . . We either pay dust for diamonds, or diamonds for dust, one or the other. . . . Stop being fooled by the idea that you can choose between self-indulgence and self-sacrifice. . . . All we can really choose between is two kinds of self-sacrifice. Take what you want, the good with the evil, take it and pay for it.[101]*

The Ravages of Trauma: Growth and Development

Children separated or isolated by neglect, abandonment, or inconsistent, inattentive caregiving have delayed motor development, growth, and cognition as well as more health problems and impaired social and emotional behaviors.[102–105] A three year follow-up of Romanian orphans adopted after at least eight months in institutional care showed more behavioral problems, poorer attachment, and lower IQ scores than never-adopted or earlier-adopted children, and that parenting them was understandably more stressful.[106, 107] It is not hard to imagine how caregiving in shifts—love and attention regularly given and withdrawn—can create such profound attachment and behavioral problems and fuel higher prevalences of criminality, sexual promiscuity, and suicide as these orphans grow up. Neither is it difficult to see why other survivors of childhood neglect or abuse and impaired social engagement systems turn to addictive substances or behaviors to calm themselves. In the most severe cases, those children who prefer to interact with objects instead of people have the most refractory mental health conditions (e.g., autism spectrum disorders, borderline personality disorder, or violent antisocial behavior).

These same Romanian orphans developed functional and structural brain changes in their corpus callosa, fusiform, and lingual gyri.[108–110] Such brain changes manifest in children as learning deficits and in adults as uncontrollable fear.[111] Peer bullying and parental verbal abuse create similar brain changes, particularly dissociation, limbic irritability, depression, and anxiety. Chronic stress impairs memory and hippocampal atrophy, probably from cumulative exposure to high glucocorticoid levels.[112] The right amygdala is preferentially stimulated in depression, particularly among patients who have sustained physical abuse in childhood (though not as adults).[113] Stress and glucocorticoids (which promote the conversion of proteins and lipids to carbohydrates and provide good short-term energy) appear to speed the atrophy that occurs under stress. However, hippocampal neurons demonstrate remarkable plasticity and can recover by remodeling dendrites and replacing synapses.[114, 115] Similarly, high plasma neuropeptide Y (a transmitter produced in sympathetic nervous system neurons and in the hippocampus) levels in combat veterans with PTSD correlated with resilience and recovery.[116] EMDR may increase hippocampal volume in trauma survivors.[117]

People cope with trauma by switching off the tools that they use to interact with the environment till all systems collapse and the individual finally dissociates. Trauma induces wall and inhibits resilience. Early traumatic attachments generate the most severe types of pathologic dissociation, including PTSD and borderline personality disorder.[118, 119] Dissociation detaches us from our environments and from our bodies, actions, and identities.[120, 121] In PTSD and borderline personality disorder, right-brain development, the ability to monitor emotions and bodily sensations, sense the self, and preserve one's identity are impaired; and it is therefore reasonable to speculate that other, as yet unidentified, conditions with similar clinical presentations, like substance addictions and body dysmorphic disorder, may share common familial and central nervous system attributes, as the literature implies.

The Ravages of Trauma: Social Interaction

Mental illness is isolating: think of depression. For tribal animals like humans, disconnection creates suffering. Conversely, close, even casual relationships depend on the ability to "read" others. Being relational and appropriately intimate requires the characteristics of functional adults.[122, 123] We respond to facial expressions as others do to ours. How does this happen? How do body and facial movement control what we think and how we feel? Why do our best relationships calm us? And why is misattunement so painful?

Good answers come from Stephen Porges' "Polyvagal Theory," the result of his and his co-authors' decades of neurophysiological and neuroanatomical observations.

The Polyvagal Model

The tenth cranial nerve, the vagus, is not solitary but rather a small family: it is "polyvagal" and originates in two primary and one lesser nucleus: the best known are the dorsal motor nucleus of the vagus (DMNX) in the dorsomedial medulla and the nucleus ambiguus (NA) in the ventrolateral reticular formation. A third nucleus, located near the DMNX, the nucleus tractus solitarius (NTS) receives afferent fibers from peripheral organs—stretch receptors and chemoreceptors in the walls of the cardiovascular, respiratory, and intestinal tracts; taste fibers from cranial nerves VII, IX, and X, and general visceral sensory fibers; and even fibers from the ear's cymba concha, perhaps not coincidentally acupuncture point CO15, which slows heart rate and lowers blood pressure in experimental animals.[124]

The vagus is long and busy. Nerve branches originating in the DMNX are unmyelinated and constitute the more primitive system that we share with reptiles. This so-called vegetative vagus modulates digestion and respiration. The left dorsal motor nucleus innervates the cardiac and body portions of the stomach that secrete gastric fluid. The right dorsal motor nucleus innervates the lower stomach and pyloric sphincter; and these two dorsal motor nuclei-originating nerves supply the trachea, lungs, intestines, pancreas, and colon. The DMNX branches are largely *subdiaphragmatic* and energy-conserving, restorative, and reparative: they are a metabolic brake, dramatically slowing the heart and mediating the freeze response. Often not recognized is that the vagus nerve is 80–90% afferent, which means that most of its fibers run toward the brain, not away from it. Those troubling "gut feelings," the dry throat when nervous, the "butterflies" when speaking in public, and the "broken heart" on prom night—are the DMNX vagus nerve talking (See Figure 7.4).

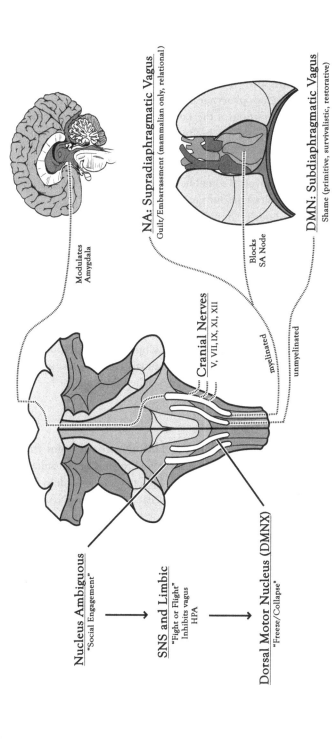

FIGURE 7.4 Brainstem Anatomy Relevant to Porges' Polyvagal Theory

An evolutionary and phylogenetic shift unique to mammals added the myelinated vagus, which originates in the nucleus ambiguus (NA). This so called "smart vagus" facilitates attention, motion, emotion, and communication because of a key anatomic point: the NA vagus has special (visceral efferent) branches to the muscles and structures that also receive (general visceral afferent) nerves from the trigeminal, facial, glossopharyngeal, hypoglossal, and accessory cranial nerves. Thus, only the rostral portion of the nucleus ambiguus innervates subdiaphragmatic structures; most of its branches innervate *supradiaphragmatic* structures (larynx, pharynx, salivary glands, soft palate, esophagus, bronchi, and heart), and these body parts talk back to it. We experience them differently: we feel guilt, which is always relational—i.e., involves someone else—in our chests, faces, and heads; we feel shame, which is solitary, in our guts.

Why the two vagal nuclei should serve the body so differently stems from their embryonic origins. Whereas skeletal muscles of the trunk and extremities develop from somites, the striated muscles of the face develop from branchial arches. Thus the nerves that innervate the facial muscles do not arise from the anterior horns of the spinal cord but from nuclei of five cranial nerves (trigeminal, facial, glossopharyngeal, vagus, and accessory—V, VII, IX, X, and XII, respectively), and all share the same medullary nucleus ambiguus. It should not be surprising that these cranial nerves might be linked. Thus branches from the nucleus ambiguus control not only the earliest functions of infants (sucking, swallowing, and breathing) but also the unique social behaviors found in mammals: facial expression, vocalization, orienting, and hearing—even "mother's ears" when listening for her children.

Cardiac Vagal Innervation

The heart receives dual innervation. The DMNX-derived vagus facilitates the freeze response in reptiles and creates a severe neurogenic bradycardia in humans, a clear sign of distress in neonates and a lethal phenomenon in adults (also thought to facilitate "voodoo death"[125]). The mammalian, myelinated, NA-derived smart vagus, on the other hand, acts like a "brake" on heart, slowing the sinoatrial node substantially below its intrinsic rate. When the vagal brake releases, heart rate immediately accelerates and readies the individual for action. The right nucleus ambiguus provides the primary vagal input to the sinoatrial node that regulates atrial rate, whereas the left nucleus ambiguus provides primary vagal input to the atrioventricular node, which regulates ventricular rate. Consequently, right-sided brain damage is associated with heart rate deficits during attention-demanding tasks.[126]

The vagal brake can therefore stimulate or calm an individual by its tonic effect on the sinoatrial node. The "health" of this vagal brake can be monitored by respiratory sinus arrhythmia (RSA), the normal heart rate variability that accompanies spontaneous breathing: heart rate normally increases with inhalation, decreases with exhalation. Abused individuals, orphaned children, patients with borderline personality disorder, and preterm infants have impaired vagal brakes and more chaotic HRV, just like patients who maintain stable heart rate variability while recalling prior traumatic experiences are less likely to suffer PTSD than those patients whose heart rate variability is impaired.[127]

★★★★★

The health of the paired vagal systems links physiologically to the individual's ability to modulate emotions, calm fear, and engage socially.[128] Abnormal or interrupted development is costly: Premature infants and children raised in deprived or traumatic circumstances have more limited abilities to regulate the functions that the nucleus ambiguus supplies, and rely instead on their sympathetic nervous systems and their older, unmyelinated DMNX. This means that they become vulnerable to the bradycardia that the DMNX causes and susceptible to periods of hypotension and hypoxemia. Patients with abuse or neglect histories exhibit fight-or-flight behavior more quickly and have more difficulty calming themselves and becoming fully relational after the stress disappears.[129] Even our popular terminology recognizes this phenomenon: the most severe psychological reactions to extreme threats, such as panic or fury, have virtually no NA vagal control but high primitive DMNX system arousal:[130] we recognize one of them as "reptilian rage."

The Intermediate Sympathetic Nervous System

Sandwiched functionally between the two vagal systems is the sympathetic nervous system. Both sympathetic and parasympathetic systems regulate a large number of organs, including the eyes; lacrimal, salivary, and sweat glands; blood vessels; heart, larynx, trachea, and bronchial tree; lungs, stomach, adrenal glands; kidney, pancreas, intestines, bladder, and external genitalia. In broad terms, the vagal parasympathetic nervous system modulates these target organs at times of growth and restoration; the sympathetic nervous system increases metabolic output to deal with environmental challenges and prepare the organism for "fight or flight." The sympathetic and parasympathetic systems are antagonistic: whereas the sympathetic system dilates the pupils, accelerates heart rate, inhibits intestinal function and dilates musculoskeletal vasculature, the parasympathetic system constricts the pupil, slows the heart, facilitates peristalsis, and decreases peripheral blood flow. We shiver with fear but don't cry; this parasympathetic crying response only triggers during recovery.

The autonomic system does not just work during emergencies; it continuously modulates to maintain homeostasis. Stress can disrupt this balance—for example hypertension decreases parasympathetic tone while increasing sympathetic tone. Homeostasis, therefore, is dynamic (See Table 7.1).

TABLE 7.1 Polyvagal Theory: Phylogenetic Stages of Neural Control

Autonomic Nervous System Component	Origin of Motor Neurons	Behavioral Functions	Autonomic Function	Observed Effect
Myelinated vagus (*ventral vagal complex*)	Nucleus ambiguous (NA) *Functional Focus*: Primarily Above the Diaphragm	Social engagement and caregiving. Expressed as a coordinated face–heart connection and observed as enhanced regulation of striated muscles in the face and head, increased calming of the viscera, dampening of sympathetic/adrenal functions, and reducing fear.	Neuroprotection. Stabilization of autonomic processes, including respiratory sinus arrhythmia (RSA), which protects the heart and enhances oxygenation of the brain. By regulation state and calming the individual, these functions of the autonomic nervous system permit sociality and provide resources necessary for symbiotic and reciprocal social interactions.	Eye contact Smiling, calm Actively engaged face + voice Alert hearing Prosody sensitivity *Feels Guilt*
Sympathetic–Adrenal System (*sympathetic nervous system*)	Spinal cord	Mobilization. Active adaptations including flight-or-fight responses	Activation. Increased heart rate, release of glucocorticoids and catecholamines. Production of energy, including glucose, and conversion of norepinephrine to epinephrine.	Fear Fight/Flight Sweating Dilated pupils Can't hear
Unmyelinated vagus (*dorsal vagal complex*)	Dorsal nucleus of the vagus (DMNX) *Functional Focus*: Primarily Below the Diaphragm	Immobilization. Passive adaptations including death-feigning and loss of consciousness.	Conservation. Prevalence of bradycardia (slowing the heart) and Apnea (cessation of breathing). Reduced energy production.	Freezing Fainting Shaking Sweating Pallor *Feels Shame*

Adapted from Porges SW. *The Polyvagal Theory: Neurophysiological Foundations of Emotions Attachment Communication Self-Regulation*. New York: W W Norton & Company; 2011.

"I think we ought to get married. When are you going to leave your wife?"

Lying on the operating room table and pre-medicated for anesthesia, she grinned at me, perky as a chickadee. Then she fell asleep.

This was going to be her 12th rhinoplasty, the first by me. Her deformities were real but subtle. Her nose lacked shape and her nostrils had been nearly sutured shut, collapsing her airway.

Surgery proceeded successfully. Recovery was uneventful, but there were daily, sometimes twice daily, phone calls to the office. Can I brush my teeth? Can I get out of bed? Can I go to a theme park? Do I need more lab work? If I cry will it ruin my nose? Can laughing affect my nostril symmetry? Why does my nose look different in bright light? I think there is a lump in my left nostril. Can I take my bandage off for a few hours? Can you wake me for my appointment; I don't get up till noon. Am I still swollen?

Her 80 year-old father always drove her, not quite understanding why she needed more surgery. During the consultation, he cleaned his nails with a file. She ignored him. When he started to talk, she spoke over him.

"I know you don't think I'm smart enough to have a job. But look at my ugly eyebrows. And my nose is still crooked." She looked at her father and began to cry. *"And I can't breathe."*

He looked up but didn't seem to have anything to add. He returned to his nails.

Then her eyes clouded over. She turned toward him.

"Freddie, wait outside." He shuffled out. The atmosphere tightened. She was silent. I waited. Her hands were large and had too many rings. Her perfume was heavy. She crossed her legs, then crossed them the other way. That covered the obvious options.

"Men like me, you know." I was silent. She didn't need encouragement. She began to swing one foot up and down.

"Look at me. Why wouldn't they? If they don't, they have a hormone problem."

Then she leaned forward. Now we were getting serious.

"I want more surgery. You still haven't fixed my nose."

"I'm sorry you feel that way," I said. *"Last time you said you were thrilled."*

Her mouth turned into a crooked half-smile.

"I'll fight the impulse to applaud. It's a lousy result." She held the mirror and studied her face.

"And now my eyes are getting baggy. And I need another brow lift." She spread her palm across her forehead and pushed.

"See how it's come down? It's disgusting. It's supposed to be higher, like this. Just like the movies."

"You don't need those operations," I said. "Besides, you've already spent too much money on plastic surgery."

Her head swung back and forth. "That doesn't matter. Charge whatever you want." She looked toward the waiting room. "He'll pay."

She nodded as if to congratulate herself. Her eyes had narrowed. Her speech quieted to a whisper and slowed for emphasis.

"I hate him. He could have protected me from my mother."

I waited. She wasn't being cute anymore.

"So now you are getting even?"

She smiled and looked away. As far as I could tell, she was talking to herself.

"I always get even."

Suddenly she rose as if she had lost all interest. As she passed my wife's desk she turned her head and smiled brightly. "I've got my Charlotte clothes on. Don't I look 'Charlotte-y' today?"

I thought about what I'd seen. As isolated behavior, it seems bizarre and boundaryless. But her mother had subjected her to diets and daily enemas starting at age three so that she wouldn't gain weight; now she exercised four hours a day. Educated but shame-filled, she had never worked, dressed like a mature cheerleader, spent her days in psychotherapy, and had undergone numerous cosmetic operations on her breasts, abdomen, and face. Imagine the shaming messages that she had received: You'll always be a failure. You're flawed. You need constant surgery to make you acceptable. Meanwhile, her father looked on and did nothing.

How the Vagal and Autonomic Nervous Systems Affect Relationality

This vagal/SNS response system is conditioned during childhood and responds strategically to threats in phylogenetic order. The newest system (myelinated vagus from the nucleus ambiguus) is used first. If highest-order relationality fails, the older circuits are used in order—fight, flight (SNS), and finally freeze (DMNX).

Equilibrated and relaxed, most people engage and respond appropriately with their voices, faces, and emotions (NA system). As stress increases, relationality decreases, and fight or flight becomes dominant (SNS); and when stress becomes intolerable, the primitive survival mechanism (DMNX) dominates until the organism is overwhelmed and the system collapses. When these system transitions occur—how much stress we can tolerate and how well—and in what form they manifest depends largely on our childhood wiring and tuning. We experience kind faces and soothing voices mentally and physically very differently than we respond to expressionless eyes, monotonic speech, or behavior that signals danger. But danger to one is not necessarily danger to all: during routine felt-pen skin markings for breast reduction, a teenage patient suddenly vomited and fainted. My thought was only preoperative planning; hers was, "I am going to die."

We all observe the ways in which muscles from these five cranial nerves synchronize: soothing voices alter facial expression; laryngeal and pharyngeal muscles coordinate prosody and intonation with head turning. The neural mechanisms for eye contact are shared with those that modulate voice. As a trauma patient's stress load increases, the social engagement system drops out and the autonomic system takes over. Alarmed patients cannot hear what I am saying; they have impaired abilities to discriminate emotions. Their eyes defocus and begin to disengage and resemble the "thousand yard stare" of PTSD. Compare the eyes in Figures 7.5 and 7.6. They are not posed: they are the patients' facial expressions when taking routine preoperative photographs. The differences, which are measurable, can connote trust, confidence, self-worth, and appreciation just as they display shame, fear, disempowerment, profound sadness, and other powerful, revealing emotions. There are associations between these expressions and the likelihood of satisfaction after plastic surgery.[131, 132]

There is evidence that altered comprehension of prosody is present in women with PTSD, who are slow to identify happy, sad, and fearful prosody, but not anger. These abnormalities appear to be transgenerational—but so is family behavior.[133]

Maltreatment creates heightened sensitivity to angry sounds, not habituation, which helps us anticipate hazardous encounters. Even here there is an anatomical explanation: in safe environments, the trigeminal nerve-innervated stapedius muscle tenses the middle ear ossicular chain so that mammals can hear higher-pitched, airborne sounds inaudible to reptiles—by which we melt at our loved one's praise

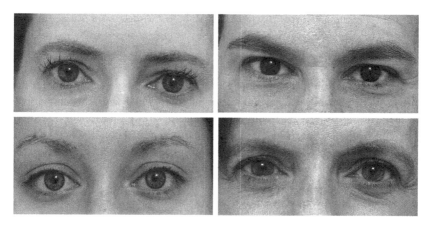

FIGURE 7.5 Eyes of Patients in Varying Stages of Social Engagement, Part 1

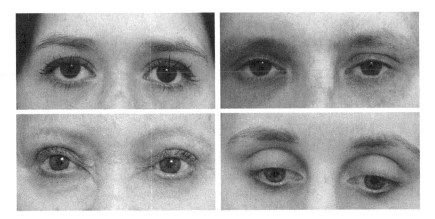

FIGURE 7.6   Eyes of Patients in Varying Stages of Social Engagement, Part 2

or thrill to operatic voices. As the sympathetic nervous system takes over and the social engagement system drops out, hearing becomes impaired. When stress increases further, even the autonomic system doesn't suffice. Patients become diaphoretic, pale, nauseated, shaky, and may faint. The dorsal motor nucleus vagus system has prevailed.

How the Polyvagal Theory Explains Healthy and Unhealthy Behavior

A fully functional nucleus ambiguus circuit allows us to down-regulate defense systems when appropriate and remove the vagal brake for fight or flight when appropriate. Both healthy transitions are impaired by abuse, which stimulates hypervigilance and hypersensitivity and dampens the abilities to socially engage and trust. Porges speculates that PTSD may be a manifestation that the unmyelinated, lower brainstem primitive defense system has been triggered and has become the dominant physiologic regulator. Like borderline personality disorder patients, those suffering from PTSD appear to have misattuned relational systems that impede trust and facilitate fight or flight defensive strategies and mood disturbances. The default state becomes a patient controlled by a barely compensated sympathetic nervous system who cannot tolerate stressful information without disequilibrating.[134] I speculate that Postural Orthostatic Tachycardia Syndrome,[135] a disabling affliction where blood pressure drops and heart rate accelerates when patients change from supine to upright positions, is not only vagal-generated but will eventually be associated with childhood trauma. Similar connections with chronic fatigue syndrome, whiplash, spasmodic torticollis, vague somatic complaints, complex regional pain syndromes, fibromyalgia, myofascial syndrome, and diabetes mellitus have already been established.[136–140]

Context is critical: any stimulus can be neutral, pleasant, or terrifying. Consider, for example, the basketball player struck in the face by an opponent's elbow. If the opponent immediately shows concern through voice, facial expression, and behavior, the injured player's response will be very different than if the opponent turns and walks away. Play requires social engagement; at the other extreme, autism, borderline personality disorder, addictions, PTSD, and body dysmorphic disorder are characterized by isolation and impaired interpersonal responses.

$$\star\star\star\star\star$$

By definition, neglect and abuse impair neuroception; autonomic system transitions become blurred or abrupt or occur too soon or too late. How this occurs is influenced by what happens in early development. "Sinking," "aching," "wrenching," or feeling hungry, crampy, sleepy, or fatigued are all *subdiaphragmatic* DMNX responses to external stimuli. Conversely, infatuation and love manifest as blushing, a fluttering heart (regulated by the myelinated vagus), vocal tone, sharper hearing, a sense of breathlessness, and heightened awareness to surroundings: all are regulated by the "social engagement" system controlled by the *supradiaphragmatic* NA vagus nerve branches and connecting to cranial nerves that control facial expression, prosody, hearing acuity, sensitivity to pitch, head movement, breathing, and vocalization.[141]

Patients with borderline personality disorder, in whom abuse histories are so common, whose emotional attachments are insecure, and who fear abandonment have impaired respiratory sinus arrhythmia (RSA) and poorly operative vagal brakes. Porges measured RSA in a group of borderline personality disorder patients by monitoring their reactions to film clips in which conflict occurred. The BPD patients had impaired baseline RSA and exhibited withdrawal of the vagal brake (indicating transition to fight or flight behavior) in comparison to the controls, who were better able to self-regulate and who increased their cardiac vagal control instead. The BPD patients saw danger instead of dramatic conflict. They became defensive, whereas the control group became more relational. The same findings were evident in a group of 27 patients who reported childhood abuse. Abuse miscues the autonomic nervous system so that fight or flight strategies mobilize sooner and recover more slowly.

$$\star\star\star\star\star$$

The vignettes in this text demonstrate similar relational impairment in patients with distorted body image. BDD patients share many characteristics in brain morphology and activity and in social behavior with PTSD patients. Our research indicates that some patients severely disturbed by unsuccessful rhinoplasties will screen positive for PTSD (Chapter 8), especially if they have abuse histories. As clinicians have observed, these patients do not trust normally, modulate their emotions poorly, have impaired abilities to socially engage, misread facial and vocal cues, cannot manage disappointment, and become immobilized or

aggressive without apparent justification. These are the manifestations of a dysregulated autonomic system. The insula, which monitors and interprets bodily states'
visceral feelings, is among the brain structures that do not function normally in
traumatized patients.[142, 143]

Before surgery I always sit beside my patients lying in the operating table. If
it is a woman, I hold one hand and put my other hand on her forehead. If it is
a man, I place my hand on his shoulder. I emphasize care and safety. We look at
each other. Maintaining eye contact helps patients stay socially engaged when
they might otherwise drop into fight or flight: the "reward (dopamine) and caregiving (oxytocin) systems activate and the amygdala quiets."[144] I am surprised
by how often patients remember and appreciate that small gesture of humanness.
Peter Levine describes a similar circumstance after being struck by a car, when
the comforting words and touch of a passing pediatrician kept him from developing PTSD. Other physicians have recounted similar phenomena.[145] "Before every
session I take a moment to remember my humanity. . . . There is no experience
that this man has that I cannot share with him. . . . No suffering that I cannot care
about, because I too am human. . . . He does not need to be ashamed in front of
me. And because of this, I am enough."[146]

★★★★★

In practice, the behaviors explained by the Polyvagal Theory and Mellody's
developmental model behave as a continuum, not in discrete stages. As long as
patients remain relational, maintain responsive eye contact, animated faces, appropriate interpretation of vocal tone and modulate their voices, the "data flow"
between patient and physician works. But if some trigger, often hard to recognize,
plunges patients into old wounds, their survival systems activate. They stop listening. They don't look at me when they talk. When I take photographs, they close
their eyes. Their voices are unexpressive. These physiologic reactions, of course,
apply in all human encounters. van der Kolk has produced evidence that patients
with PTSD do not activate their pre-frontal cortices and mirror neurons when
they see faces; only the midbrain periaqueductal gray area (involved in pain modulation, hypervigilance, startling, and cowering) lights up. They dissociate, have
flashbacks, and describe terrifying childhood experiences without expression or
apparent feeling. PTSD avoidance, arousal, and re-experiencing symptoms can last
for decades after unsuccessful surgeries, particularly in patients who have trauma
histories (Chapter 8).[147–150]

No one lives free from experiences that are intensely emotional, pleasurable or
not; but whether any prior event is "traumatic" depends partially on its meaning
to the individual who experienced it and the sense of powerlessness and overwhelming life threat that it evokes.[151, 152] Immobilization is always a component
of trauma and the basis of the speechless terror that patients feel. Posttraumatic
stress is not a phobia: in PTSD the original life-threatening experience was real.
Recently I was about to perform a minor procedure on a man who weighed

450 pounds. The morning of surgery he was pale, sweating heavily, and shaky; his dorsal vagal complex and SNS were clearly in control. "I can't go through surgery. I won't lie on my back." He couldn't describe his feelings or identify his physical sensations. He substituted actions for emotions. "What are you feeling?" I asked. "I'm feeling that I want to run away." The prospect of lying on his back triggered some inaccessible and terrible survival response. This large, powerful man felt helpless in a dangerous universe. "All trauma," van der Kolk writes, "is preverbal."

★★★★★

The physiologic responses to trauma were not designed to be the default setting.[153, 154] Combat veteran studies responding to visual or auditory reminders of war consistently show exaggerated heart rates, blood pressures, EMG changes, and elevated plasma epinephrine and urinary norepinephrine.[155, 156] Core physiology changes. Hippocampal volumes are reduced in children subject to early trauma; glucocorticoids remain elevated; Broca's area may be dark. The cingulate gyrus shows reduced activities in PTSD victims (as it does in patients with body dysmorphic disorder).[157, 158] Combat veterans without PTSD do not display these physiologic and serologic abnormalities.[159, 160] The same changes occur in victims of sexual abuse or vehicular accident survivors with PTSD.[161] These arousal symptoms are only triggered by stimuli that simulate the original PTSD source. Thus patients who are high-functioning in one area of their lives can still be triggered into disempowerment by reminders of childhood trauma, e.g., those that provoke body shame.

Epigenetics: The Mediator Between Our Genes and the Environment

To help understand epigenetics a few terms must be defined. The chromosomal DNA winds around proteins called *histones*. The DNA in each human cell is about 1.2 m long, but wound and condensed around the histone, becomes only 120 μm long. The DNA/histone complex is termed *chromatin*. An organism's total chromatin comprises its *genome*, or heritable genetic material. An epigenetic trait or change is a chemical alteration of the DNA or its associated histones that change the structure of the chromatin product but do not alter the DNA sequence. Epigenetics, therefore, determines which genes are expressed and which are suppressed; these modifications are heritable. The genes that you express now aren't necessarily those that you expressed at birth. Epigenetics have modified them, which must stimulate us to modify concepts of "genetic" addictions and other psychopathologies.[162]

Epigenetic changes have ramifications. Histone modifications, RNA "silencing" (or non-expression of short RNA segments), and DNA "methylation"—adding a methyl groups (CH_3-) to susceptible cytosine nucleotides at their phosphate/guanine nucleotide connection ("CpG" site)—have been varyingly associated with colorectal and prostate cancer development. Both methylation and demethylation are associated with coronary artery disease, schizophrenia, depression,[163, 164] and with congenital anomalies attributable to nutritional deficiencies.[165] Cytokines, growth factors, stress hormone and neurotrophic factor levels all modulate according to stresses placed on the organism through epigenetic modifiers.

★★★★★

Epigenetic disruption of fetal development by the maternal environment can create congenital anomalies. Maternal health, maternal diet, smoking,[166] caesarean section, domestic or societal violence,[167] and even paternal obesity or alcohol consumption alter gene expression in offspring.[168, 169] Following birth, maternal bonding (or separation) and other early life positive and negative family experiences—poverty, neglect, sexual abuse, vitamins-poor diet, exercise, heavy metal exposure, recreational drugs (especially cocaine, as well as opiates, amphetamines, alcohol, and nicotine) contribute to epigenetic modifications like DNA methylation that alter neuronal circuits in developing brains and therefore its behavior.[170–177] Genetic modifications may predict PTSD in soldiers.[178] Suicide victims with childhood abuse histories demonstrate increased DNA methylation leading to increased HPA activity and elevated stress levels: in some cases suicide appears to have a genetic origin. As we age, become menopausal, or develop age-related diseases, epigenetic changes continue and may contribute to osteoarthritis and Alzheimer's or cardiovascular disease.[179–182] A recent study comparing 96 maltreated children with 96 demographically age-matched controls indicated that the maltreated children had significantly different methylation values at 2,868 CpG sites. This gene set contained numerous markers of diseases now documented to vary with the prevalence of early childhood trauma: neuropsychiatric disorders; cardiovascular disease, and obesity; respiratory disease; diabetes; addictions; risky behavior; lung, prostate, and breast cancers; and many others.[183, 184]

★★★★★

Thus we adapt and evolve based on our environments. "Genetic" can signify an environmental response as well as an inherited trait. The optimal physiologic state would be consistent nucleus ambiguus vagal complex dominance: social engagement and the interpersonal harmony that it facilitates.[185] But when the autonomic nervous system, built for fight or flight, and the dorsal vagal complex, which controls the freeze response, are persistently activated, the organism suffers. The trauma survivor may become controlled by a vagal/autonomic/endocrine system genetically modified by an environment that operates almost independent of his or her cerebral cortex, a self-perpetuating arrangement that does not improve even if the external stimulus disappears.[186] The result is what we call somatic or psychosomatic disease, complicated by implicit childhood memories, shame, body image disorders, and obscured by addictions.

What This Information Means

It is easy to be distracted by the poisonous blossoms and miss the roots. The evidence is overwhelming that our environment and experiences can modify our genetic complex (chromatin) and in turn affect our health and behavior. That's the micro view. The increasing body of data that links the childhood environment with adult health is the macro view and will be the next piece of our puzzle.

No matter how it is expressed, trauma is always somatic. Abuse and neglect are felt first in the body.[187, 188] Infants regulate first through their bodies, not their minds; body shame is thus easy to understand. Patients may seem fully compensated and functional when we meet them, but the physical and psychological stresses and uncertainties of surgery magnify the potential for problems: even surgery limited to one area can affect the rest of the body. Extreme emotional states become the default setting for trauma survivors. They are adapted wounded children thinking in Manichean absolutes, which explains their hyperbolic, victim language. Whatever the issue, it's a wildly operatic, never-ending, fever dream catastrophe that encapsulates their shame and attacks the surgeon personally: "I'm ugly." "I'm hideous." "My face is disgusting." "My nose is huge." "You ruined me forever." "You abandoned me." "I can't live like this." "What you have done to me borders on the criminal." "You have destroyed my family, my friends, and my joy in living."

Complicating both the patient's emotions and the physician's reaction are triggers and implicit memories. Physiologic responses, numbness, trembling, muscular tension, nausea, and shivering that seem incongruous to the physician and perhaps unexplainable even to the patient can be the vestigial manifestations of nonverbal, implicit memories. These incongruous behaviors were provoked, imprinted, and permitted by caregivers—reactions that might have been protective for the child but now disrupt their adult lives. This conduct is rooted in observable gross and microscopic brain changes and provides a biologic basis for the addictions and behaviors described in earlier chapters.[189] Is childhood trauma just an occasional oddity in plastic surgery patients? Our story unfolds further.

References

1. Brand P, Yancey P. *The Gift Nobody Wants: The Inspiring Story of A Surgeon Who Discovers Why We Hurt and What We Can Do About It*. New York: Harper Collins; 1993.
2. Herman JL. *Trauma And Recovery: The Aftermath Of Violence: From Domestic Abuse To Political Terror*. New York: Basic Books (Perseus Books Group); 1992.
3. Herringa RJ, Birn RM, Ruttle PL, et al. Childhood Maltreatment Is Associated with Altered Fear Circuitry and Increased Internalizing Symptoms by Late Adolescence. *Proc Natl Acad Sci* 2013; 110:47:19119–19124.
4. Cloninger CR, Svrakic DM, Przybeck TR. A Psychobiological Model of Temperament and Character. *Arch Gen Psychiatry* 1993; 50:975–990.
5. Hengartner MP, Cohen LJ, Rodgers S, et al. Association between Childhood Maltreatment and Normal Adult Personality Traits: Exploration of an Understudied Field. *J Personal Disord* 2015; 29:1:1–14.

6. Gendlin, E, *Focusing*. New York: Bantam, 1981.
7. Herman JL. *Trauma And Recovery: The Aftermath Of Violence: From Domestic Abuse To Political Terror*. New York: Basic Books (Perseus Books Group); 1992:11.
8. Felitti VJ, Anda RF, Nordenberg D, et al. Relationship of Childhood Abuse and Household Dysfunction to Many of the Leading Causes of Death in Adults. *Am J Prev Med* 1998; 14:4:245–258.
9. Herman JL. *Trauma And Recovery: The Aftermath Of Violence: From Domestic Abuse To Political Terror*. New York: Basic Books (Perseus Books Group); 1992:13.
10. Kilpatrick DG, Resnick HS, Milanak ME, et al. National Estimates of Exposure to Traumatic Events and PTSD Using DSM-IV and DSM-5 Criteria. *J Traumatic Stress* 2013; 26:5:537–547.
11. Olff M, Langeland W, Draijer N, et al. Gender Differences in Posttraumatic Stress Disorder. *Psychol Bull* 2007; 133:2:183–204.
12. Neziroglu F, Barile N. Environmental Factors in Body Dysmorphic Disorder. In: Phillips KA, ed. *Body Dysmorphic Disorder: Advances in Research and Clinical Practice*. New York: Oxford University Press; 2017:277–284.
13 Lipschitz DS, Winegar RK, Nicolau AL, et al. Perceived Abuse and Neglect as Risk Factors for Suicidal Behavior in Adolescent Inpatients. *J Nerv Ment Dis* 1999; 187:1:32–39.
14. Schore AN. *The Science of the Art of Psychotherapy*. New York: W W Norton & Company; 2012:28.
15. McLean PD. *The Triune Brain In Evolution: Role In Paleocerebral Functions*. New York: Springer; 1990.
16. Anderson AK, Phelps EA. Expression without Recognition: Contributions of the Human Amygdala to Emotional Communication. *Psychol Sci* 2000; 11:2:106–111.
17. van der Kolk BA. *The Body Keeps The Score: Brain, Mind, And Body In The Healing Of Trauma*. New York: Viking (Penguin Group); 2014.
18. Boscarino JA. Post-Traumatic Stress Disorder and Cardiovascular Disease Link: Time to Identify Specific Pathways and Interventions. *Am J Cardiol* 2011; 108:1052–1053.
19. McEwen BS. Sex, Stress and the Hippocampus: Allostasis, Allostatic Load and the Aging Process. *Neurobiol Aging* 2002; 23:921–939.
20. Buchmann AF, Holz N, Boecker R, et al. Moderating Role of FKBP5 Genotype in the Impact of Childhood Adversity on Cortisol Stress Response during Adulthood. *Eur Neuropsychopharmacol* 2014; 24:6:837–845.
21. Scaer RC. *The Body Bears The Burden: Trauma, Dissociation, And Disease*. 3rd edition. New York: Routledge; 2014.
22. Maier SF. Behavioral Control Blunts Reactions to Contemporaneous and Future Adverse Events: Medial Prefrontal Cortex Plasticity and a Corticostriatal Network. *Neurobiol Stress* 2015; 1:12–22.
23. Shalev AY. Stress Versus Traumatic Stress. In: van der Kolk B, McFarlane AC, Weisaeth L, eds. *Traumatic Stress*. New York: The Guilford Press; 2007:77–101.
24. Stoddard FJ Jr. Outcomes of Traumatic Exposure. *Child Adolesc Psychiatr Clin N Am* 2014; 23:2:243–256, viii.
25. Larson E. *Dead Wake*. New York: Crown; 2015:351, 92,
26. Gwynne SC. *Rebel Yell: The Violence, Passion And Redemption Of Stonewall Jackson*. New York: Scribner; 2014, p. 126.
27. Gaon A, Kaplan Z, Dwolatzky T, et al. Dissociative Symptoms as a Consequence of Traumatic Experiences: The Long-Term Effects of Childhood Sexual Abuse. *Isr J Psychiatry Relat Sci* 2013; 50:1:17–23.
28. Schore AN. *Affect Regulation and The Repair Of The Self*. New York: W W Norton & Company; 2003.

29. DeSantis SM, Baker NL, Back SE, et al. Gender Differences in the Effect of Early Life Trauma on Hypothalamic-Pituitary-Adrenal Axis Functioning. *Depress Anxiety* 2011; 28:5:383–392.

30. de Brito SA, Viding E, Sebastian CL, et al. Reduced Orbitofrontal and Temporal Grey Matter in a Community Sample of Maltreated Children. *J Child Psychol Psychiatry* 2013; 54:1:105–112.

31. Gouin J, Glaser R, Malarkey WB, et al. Childhood Abuse and Inflammatory Responses to Daily Stressors. *Ann Behav Med* 2012; 44:2:287–292.

32. Kelly PA, Viding E, Wallace GL, et al. Cortical Thickness, Surface Area, and Gyrification Abnormalities in Children Exposed to Maltreatment: Neural Markers of Vulnerability? *Biol Psychiatry* 2013; 74:845–852.

33. Ulrich-Lai YM, Herman JP. Neural Regulation of Endocrine and Autonomic Stress Responses. *Neuroscience* 2009; 10:397–408.

34. McEwen BS, Morrison JH. The Brain on Stress: Vulnerability and Plasticity of the Prefrontal Cortex over the Life Course. *Neuron* 2013; 79:16–29.

35. Christoffel DJ, Golden SA, Russo SJ. Structural and Synaptic Plasticity in Stress-Related Disorders. *Rev Neurosci* 2011; 22:5:535–549.

36. Thomas, L. *The Youngest Science, Notes of a Biology Watcher*. New York: Viking Press, 1983:240.

37. van der Kolk BA. Developmental Trauma Disorder toward a Rational Diagnosis for Children with Complex Trauma Histories. *Psychiatric Ann* 2005; 35:5:401–408.

38. Schore AN. *The Science Of The Art Of Psychotherapy*. New York: W W Norton & Company; 2012:32.

39. DiGangi J, Guffanti G, McLaughlin KA, et al. Considering Trauma Exposure in the Context of Genetics Studies of Posttraumatic Stress Disorder: A Systematic Review. *Biol Mood Anxiety Disord* 2013; 3:2:1–12.

40. Kohut, H. *The Analysis of the Self*. New York: International Universities Press; 1971.

41. Porges SW. *The Polyvagal Theory: Neurophysiological Foundations Of Emotions Attachment Communication Self-Regulation*. New York: W W Norton & Company; 2011.

42. Porges SW. A Phylogenetic Journey Through the Vague and Ambiguous 10th Cranial Nerve: A Commentary on Contemporary Heart Rate Variability Research. *Biol Psychol* 2007; 74:2:301–307.

43. Schore AN. *The Science Of The Art Of Psychotherapy*. New York: W W Norton & Company; 2012.

44. Decety J, Chaminade T. When the Self Represents the Other: A New Cognitive Neuroscience View on Psychological Identification. *Conscious Cog* 2003; 12:4:577–596.

45. Hauger RL, Olivares-Reyes JA, Dautzenberg FM, et al. Molecular and Cell Signaling Targets for PTSD Pathophysiology and Pharmacotherapy. *Neuropharmacology* 2012; 62:2:705–714.

46. Kuhlman KR, Geis EG, Vargas I, et al. Differential Associations between Childhood Trauma Subtypes and Adolescent HPA-Axis Functioning. *Psychoneuroendocrinol* 2015; 54: 103–114.

47. Siegel DJ. *The Mindful Therapist: A Clinician's Guide To Mindsight And Neural Integration*. New York: W W Norton & Company; 2010.

48. Arnsten AFT, Raskind MA, Taylor FB, et al. The Effects of Stress Exposure on Prefrontal Cortex: Translating Basic Research into Successful Treatments for Post-Traumatic Stress Disorder. *Neurobiol Stress* 2015; 1:89–99.

49. Cunningham CL, Martinez-Cerdeno V, Noctor SC. Microglia Regulate the Number of Neural Precursor Cells in the Developing Cerebral Cortex. *J Neurosci* 2013; 33:10:4216–4233.

50. Scaer RC. *8 Keys To Brain-Body Balance*. New York: W W Norton & Company; 2012.

51. Scaer RC. *The Body Bears the Burden: Trauma, Dissociation, and Disease*. 2nd edition. New York: Routledge; 2007:34, 85,180–181.

52. Francis M. *Diary Of A Stage Mother's Daughter: A Memoir*. New York: Weinstein Books; 2012.

53. Levine PA. *Trauma and Memory: Brain And Body In A Search For The Living Past: A Practical Guide For Understanding And Working With Traumatic Memory*. Berkeley [CA]: North Atlantic Books; 2015.

54. Levine PA, Frederick A. *Waking The Tiger: Healing Trauma*. Berkeley [CA]: North Atlantic Books; 1997.

55. Levine PA. *In An Unspoken Voice: How The Body Releases Trauma And Restores Goodness*. Berkeley [CA]: North Atlantic Books; 2010.

56. Levine PA, Kline M. *Trauma-Proofing Your Kids: A Parents' Guide For Instilling Confidence, Joy And Resilience*. Berkeley [CA]: North Atlantic Books; 2008.

57. Scaer RC. *The Body Bears the Burden: Trauma, Dissociation, and Disease*. 2nd edition. New York: Routledge; 2007:34, 85,180–181.

58. Debiec J, Diaz-Mataiz L, Bush DEA, et al. The Amygdala Encodes Specific Sensory Features of an Aversive Reinforcer. *Nat Neurosci* 2010; 13:5:536–537.

59. Taylor DJ, Pruiksma KE, Hale WJ, et al. Prevalence, Correlates, and Predictors of Insomnia in the US Army Prior to Deployment. *Sleep* 2016; 39:10:1795–1806.

60. Vermetten E, Schmahl C, Southwick SM, et al. A Positron Tomographic Emission Study of Olfactory Induced Emotional Recall in Veterans with and without Combat-Related Posttraumatic Stress Disorder. *Psychopharmacol Bull* 2007; 40:1:8–30.

61. Lanius R, Lanius U, Fisher J, et al. Processing Traumatic Memory and Restoring Acts of Triumph. In: Ogden P, Minton K, Pain C, eds. *Trauma and the Body*. New York: W W Norton & Company; 2006:236–238.

62. Rothschild B. *8 Keys To Safe Trauma Recovery: Take-Charge Strategies To Empower Your Healing*. New York: W W Norton & Company; 2010.

63. Rothschild B. *The Body Remembers: The Psychophysiology Of Trauma And Trauma Treatment*. New York: W W Norton & Company; 2000:31.

64. Scaer RC. *Eight Keys to Brain-Body Balance*. New York: W W Norton & Company; 2012:12–13, 120–121.

65. Bliss, M. *Harvey Cushing, a Life in Surgery*. New York: Oxford University Press; 2005:317.

66. van der Kolk B. Trauma and Memory. In: van der Kolk B, McFarlane AC, Weisaeth L, eds. *Traumatic Stress*. New York: The Guilford Press; 2007:3289–3296.

67. Saar-Ashkenazy R, Cohen JE, Guez J, et al. Reduced Corpus-Callosum Volume in Posttraumatic Stress Disorder Highlights the Importance of Inter-Hemispheric Connectivity for Associative Memory. *J Traumatic Stress* 2014; 27:1:18–26.

68. van der Kolk B, van der Hart O. The Intrusive Past: The Flexibility of Memory and the Engraving of Trauma. *American Imago* 1991; 48:425–454.

69. Brown DW, Anda RF, Edwards VJ, et al. Adverse Childhood Experiences and Childhood Autobiographical Memory Disturbance. *Child Abuse Neglect* 2007; 31:9:961–969.

70. Schore AN. Early Superego Development: The Emergence of Shame and Narcissistic Affect Regulation in the Practicing Period. *Psychoanalysis and Contemporary Thought* 1991; 14:187.

71. Bourne V J, Todd BK. When Left Means Right: An Explanation of the Left Cradling Bias in Terms of Right Hemisphere Specialization. *Development Sci* 2004; 7:1:19–24.

72. Schore AN. Early Superego Development: The Emergence of Shame and Narcissistic Affect Regulation in the Practicing Period. *Psychoanalysis and Contemporary Thought* 1991; 14:187.

73. Weatherill RP, Almerigi JB, Bogat GA, et al. Is Maternal Depression Related to Side of Infant Holding? *Internat J Behav Develop* 2004; 28:5:421–427.

74. Edmiston EE, Wang F, Mazure CM, et al. Corticostriatal-Limbic Gray Matter Morphology in Adolescents with Self-Reported Exposure to Childhood Maltreatment. *Arch Pediatr Adolesc Med* 2011; 165:12:1069–1077.

75. Jaworska N, MacMaster FP, Gaxiola I, et al. A Preliminary Study of the Influence of Age of Onset and Childhood Trauma on Cortical Thickness in Major Depressive Disorder. *BioMed Research International* 2014;2014:1–9.

76. Carballedo A, Lisiecka D, Fagan A, et al. Early Life Adversity Is Associated with Brain Changes in Subjects at Family Risk for Depression. *World Journal of Biological Psychiatry* 2012; 13:569–578.

77. Lupien SJ, McEwen BS, Gunnar MR, et al. Effects of Stress Throughout the Lifespan on the Brain, Behaviour and Cognition. *Neuroscience* 2009; 10:434–445.

78. Recordati G. A Thermodynamic Model of the Sympathetic and Parasympathetic Nervous Systems. *Autonom Neurosci: Basic Clin* 2003; 103:1.

79. Schore AN. Early Superego Development: The Emergence of Shame and Narcissistic Affect Regulation in the Practicing Period. *Psychoanal Contemp Thought* 1991; 14:187.

80. Schore AN. *Affect Regulation and The Repair Of The Self*. New York: W W Norton & Company; 2003.

81. Buhlmann U, Wilhelm S, McNally RJ, et al. Interpretive Biases for Ambiguous Information in Body Dysmorphic Disorder. *CNS Spectrums* 2002; 7:6:435–443.

82. Buhlmann U, McNally RJ, Wilhelm S, et al. Selective Processing of Emotional Information in Body Dysmorphic Disorder. *Anxiety Disord* 2002; 16:289–298.

83. Schore AN. *Affect Regulation and The Repair Of The Self*. New York: W W Norton & Company; 2003.

84. Davidson JRT, Hughes D, Blazer DG, et al. Post-Traumatic Stress Disorder in the Community: An Epidemiological Study. *Psychol Med* 1991; 21:713–721.

85. Kessler RC, Sonnega A, Bromet E, et al. Posttraumatic Stress Disorder in the National Comorbidity Survey. *Arch Gen Psychiatry* 1995; 52:12:1048–1060.

86. Luthra R, Abramovitz R, Greenberg R, et al. Relationship between Type of Trauma Exposure and Posttraumatic Stress Disorder among Urban Children and Adolescents. *J Interpers Violence* 2009; 24:11:1919–1927.

87. Luz MP, Coutinho ES, Berger W, et al. Conditional Risk for Posttraumatic Stress Disorder in an Epidemiological Study of a Brazilian Urban Population. *J Psychiatr Res* 2016; 72:51–57.

88. Osofsky HJ, Osofsky JD. Hurricane Katrina and the Gulf Oil Spill: Lessons Learned. *Psychiatr Clin N Am* 2013; 36:3:371–383.

89. Spoont MR, Williams Jr JW, Kehle-Forbes S, et al. Does This Patient Have Posttraumatic Stress Disorder? Rational Clinical Examination Systematic Review. *JAMA* 2015; 314:5:501–510.

90. Breslau N, Lucia VC, Alvarado GF. Intelligence and Other Predisposing Factors in Exposure to Trauma and Posttraumatic Stress Disorder. *Arch Gen Psychiatry* 2006; 63:1238–1245.

91. Brewin CR, Andrews B, Valentine JD. Meta-Analysis of Risk Factors for Posttraumatic Stress Disorder in Trauma-Exposed Adults. *J Consult Clin Psychol* 2000; 68:5:748–766.

92. Schore AN. *Affect Regulation and The Repair Of The Self.* New York: W W Norton & Company; 2003.

93. Jasarevic E, Rodgers AB, Bale TL. A Novel Role for Maternal Stress and Microbial Transmission in Early Life Programming and Neurodevelopment. *Neurobiol Stress* 2015; 1:81–88.

94. Landgraf R, Neumann ID. Vasopressin and Oxytocin Release within the Brain: A Dynamic Concept of Multiple and Variable Modes of Neuropeptide Communication. *Front Neuroendocrinol* 2004; 25:150–176.

95. Insel TR, Young LJ. The Neurobiology of Attachment. *Neuroscience* 2001; 2:129–136.

96. Grippo AJ, Trahanas DM, Zimmerman RR, et al. Oxytocin Protects against Negative Behavioral and Autonomic Consequences of Long-Term Social Isolation. *Psychoneuroendocrinol* 2009; 34:10:1542–1553.

97. Heinrichs M, von Dawans B, Domes G. Oxytocin, Vasopressin, and Human Social Behavior. *Front Neuroendocrinol* 2009; 30:548–557.

98. Green BL, Chung JY, Daroowalla A, et al. Evaluating the Cultural Validity of the Stressful Life Events Screening Questionnaire. *Viol Women* 2006; 12:12:1191–1213.

99. Main M. The Organized Categories of Infant, Child, and Adult Attachment: Flexible vs. Inflexible Attention under Attachment-Related Stress. *J Am Psychoanalytic Assoc* 2000; 48:4:1055–1096.

100. Bureau JF, Martin J, Lyons-Ruth K. Attachment Dysregulation as Hidden Trauma in Infancy: Early Stress, Maternal Buffering and Psychiatric Morbidity in Young Adulthood. In: Lanius RA, Vermette E, Pain C, eds. *The Impact of Early Life Trauma On Health And Disease: The Hidden Epidemic.* Cambridge [UK]: Cambridge University Press; 2010, 48–56.

101. Fosdick HE. *On Being Fit To Live With.* New York and London: Harper & Brothers; 1946:54, 201.

102. Andersson P. Post-Traumatic Stress Symptoms Linked to Hidden Holocaust Trauma Among Adult Finnish Evacuees Separated from their Parents as Children in World War II, 1939–1945: A Case-Control Study. *Int Psychogeriatr* 2011; 23:4:654–661.

103. Heilala C, Kalland M, Komulainen E, et al. Effects of Evacuation in Late Adulthood: Analyzing Psychosocial Well-Being in Three Cluster Groups of Finnish Evacuees and Non-Evacuees. *Aging Ment Health* 2014;18:7:869–878.

104. Heilman KM, Van Den Abell T. Right Hemisphere Dominance for Attention: The Mechanism Underlying Hemispheric Asymmetries of Inattention (Neglect). *Neurology* 1980; 30:327–330.

105. Ventevogel P, Spiegel P. Psychological Treatments for Orphans and Vulnerable Children Affected by Traumatic Events and Chronic Adversity in Sub-Saharan Africa. *JAMA* 2015; 314:5:511–514.

106. Chisholm K. A Three Year Follow-Up of Attachment and Indiscriminate Friendliness in Children Adopted from Romanian Orphanages. *Child Develop* 1998; 69:4:1092–1106.

107. Forkey H, Szilagyi M. Foster Care and Healing from Complex Childhood Trauma. *Pediatr Clin N Am* 2014; 61:5:1059–1072.

108. Chugani HT, Behen ME, Muzik O, et al. Brain Functional Activity Following Early Deprivation: A Study of Post-Institutionalized Romanian Orphans. *Neuroimage* 2001; 14:6:1290–1301.

109. Eluvanthingal TJ, Chugani HT, Behen ME, et al. Abnormal Brain Connectivity in Children after Early Severe Socio-Emotional Deprivation: A Diffusion Tensor Imaging Study. *Pediatrics* 2006; 117:6:2093–2100.

110. Teicher MH, Rabi K, Sheu Y, et al. Neuobiology of Childhood Trauma and Adversity. In: Lanius RA, Vermette E, Pain C, eds. *The Impact of Early Life Trauma On Health And Disease: The Hidden Epidemic*. Cambridge [UK]: Cambridge University Press; 2010, 112–122.

111. Heilala C, Kalland M, Komulainen E, et al. Effects of Evacuation in Late Adulthood: Analyzing Psychosocial Well-Being in Three Cluster Groups of Finnish Evacuees and Non-Evacuees. *Aging Ment Health* 2014;18:7:869–878.

112. McGowan PO, Sasaki A, D'alessio AC, et al. Epigenetic Regulation of the Glucocorticoid Receptor in Human Brain Associates with Childhood Abuse. *Nat Neurosci*, 2009; 12:3:342–348.

113. Grant MM, Cannistraci C, Hollon SD, et al. Childhood Trauma History Differentiates Amygdala Response to Sad Faces Within MDD. *J Psychiatr Res* 2011; 45:7:886–895.

114. Levone BR, Cryan JF, O'Leary OF. Role of Adult Hippocampal Neurogenesis in Stress Resilience. *Neurobiol Stress* 2015; 1:147–155.

115. Sierra A, Beccari S, Diaz-Aparicio I, et al. Surveillance, Phagocytosis, and Inflammation: How Never-Resting Microglia Influence Adult Hippocampal Neurogenesis. *Neural Plast* 2014; 1–15.

116. Yehuda R, Brand S, Yang R. Plasma Neuropeptide Y Concentrations in Combat Exposed Veterans: Relationship to Trauma Exposure, Recovery from PTSD, and Coping. *Biol Psychiatry* 2006; 59:660–663.

117. Nakazawa DJ. *Childhood Disrupted: How Your Biography Becomes Your Biology, And How You Can Heal*. New York: Atria Books; 2015.

118. Melges FT, Swartz MS. Oscillations of Attachment in Borderline Personality Disorder. *Am J Psychiatry* 1989; 146:9:1115–1120.

119. Brady KT, Killeen TK, Brewerton T, et al. Comorbidity of Psychiatric Disorders and Posttraumatic Stress Disorder. *J Clin Psychiatry* 2000; 61:7:22–32.

120. Ensink K, Bégin M, Normandin L, et al. Mentalization and Dissociation in the Context of Trauma: Implications for Child Psychopathology. *J Trauma Dissociation* 2016; 1–20.

121. Lanius RA, Williamson PC, Bluhm RL, et al. Functional Connectivity of Dissociative Responses in Posttraumatic Stress Disorder: A Functional Magnetic Resonance Imaging Investigation. *Biol Psychiatry* 2005; 57:8:873–884.

122. Adler A. Course and Outcome of Visual Agnosia. *J Nerv Ment Dis* 1950; 111:1:41–51.

123. Hamilton JL, Stange JP, Abramson LY, et al. Stress and the Development of Cognitive Vulnerabilities to Depression Explain Sex Differences in Depressive Symptoms during Adolescence. *Clin Psychol Sci* 2015; 3:5:702–714.

124. Briggs, JP, Shurtleff, D. Acupuncture and the Complex Connections between the Mind and the Body. *JAMA* 2017;317:2489–2490.

125. Scaer RC. *The Body Bears The Burden: Trauma, Dissociation, And Disease*. 2nd edition. New York: Routledge; 2007.

126. Yokoyama K, Jennings R, Ackles P, et al. Lack of Heart Rate Changes During an Attention—Demanding Task after Right Hemisphere Lesions. *Neurology* 1987; 37:4:624.

127. Richards JE. Infant Visual Sustained Attention and Respiratory Sinus Arrhythmia. *Child Develop* 1987; 58:488–496.

128. Marangell LB, Rush AJ, George MS, et al. Vagus Nerve Stimulation (VNS) for Major Depressive Episodes: One Year Outcomes. *Biol Psychiatry* 2002; 51:280–287.

129. Gilbert P, Miles J, eds. *Body Shame: Conceptualization, Research And Treatment*. East Sussex [UK]: Routledge; 2002.

130. George DT, Nutt DJ, Walker WV, et al. Lactate and Hyperventilation Substantially Attenuate Vagal Tone in Normal Volunteers: A Possible Mechanism of Panic Provocation? *Arch Gen Psychiatry* 1989; 46:2:153–156.

131. Constantin MB, Lin CP. Why Some Patients Are Unhappy: Part 1: Relationship of Preoperative Nasal Deformity to Number of Operations and a History of Abuse or Neglect. *Plast Reconstr Surg* 2014; 134:4: 823–835.

132. Constantin MB, Lin CP. Why Some Patients Are Unhappy: Part 2. Relationship of Nasal Shape and Trauma History to Surgical Success. *Plast Reconstr Surg* 2014; 134:4:836–851.

133. Nazarov A, Frewen P, Oremus C, et al. Comprehension of Affective Prosody in Women with Post-Traumatic Stress Disorder Related to Childhood Abuse. *Acta Psychiatr Scand* 2015; 131:342–349.

134. Hopper JW, Spinazzola J, Simpson WB, et al. Preliminary Evidence of Parasympathetic Influence on Basal Heart Rate in Posttraumatic Stress Disorder. *J Psychosom Res* 2006; 60:83–90.

135. Grubb BP. Postural Tachycardia Syndrome. *Circulation* 2008; 117:21:2814–2817.

136. Phillips KA, Quinn G, Stout RL. Functional Impairment in Body Dysmorphic Disorder: Prospective, Follow-Up Study. *J Psychiatry Res* 2008; 42:701–707.

137. Sack M, Boroske-Leiner K, Lahmann C. Association of Nonsexual and Sexual Traumatizations with Body Image and Psychosomatic Symptoms in Psychosomatic Outpatients. *Gen Hosp Psychiatry* 2010; 32:315–320.

138. Margalit D, Har LB, Brill S, et al. Complex Regional Pain Syndrome, Alexithymia, and Psychological Distress. *J Psychosom Res* 2014; 77:273–277.

139. Freeman R, Wieling W, Axelrod FB, et al. Consensus Statement on the Definition of Orthostatic Hypotension, Neurally Mediated Syncope and the Postural Tachycardia Syndrome. *Clin Autonom Res* 2011; 21:2:69–72.

140. Harth W, Hermes B. Psychosomatic Disturbances and Cosmetic Surgery. *JDDG: Journal der Deutschen Dermatologischen Gesellschaft* 2007; 5:9:736–744.

141. Ardiç FN, Topaloğlu I, Öncel S, et al. Does the Stapes Reflex Remain the Same after Bell's Palsy? *Am J Otology* 1997; 18:6:761–765.

142. Critchley HD, Wiens S, Rotshtein P, et al. Neural Systems Supporting Interoceptive Awareness. *Nat Neurosci* 2004; 7:2:189–195.

143. Marusak HA, Etkin A, Thomason ME. Disrupted Insula-Based Neural Circuit Organization and Conflict Interference in Trauma-Exposed Youth. *Neuroimage Clin* 2015; 8:516–525.

144. McGonigal K. *The Upside Of Stress: Why Stress Is Good For You, And How To Get Good At It*. New York: Avery [Penguin Random House]; 2015.

145. Markwalter DW. In the Hands of Another. *JAMA* 2015; 313:9:899–900.

146. Remen RN. *Kitchen Table Wisdom: Stories That Heal*. New York: Riverhead Books; 1996.

147. van der Kolk B, McFarlane AC, van der Hart O. A General Approach to Treatment of Posttraumatic Stress Disorder. In: van der Kolk B, McFarlane AC, Weisaeth L, eds. *Traumatic Stress*. New York: The Guilford Press; 2007:428–429.

148. Foa EB, Ehlers A, Clark DM, et al. The Posttraumatic Cognitions Inventory (PTCI): Development and Validation. *Psychol Assess* 1999; 11:2:303–314.

149. Cobb S, Lindemann E. Neuropsychiatric Observations after the Coconut Grove Fire. *Ann Surg* 1943; 117:814–824.

150. Forbes D, Phelps A, McHugh T. Treatment of Combat-Related Nightmares Using Imagery Rehearsal: A Pilot Study. *J Traumatic Stress* 2001; 14:2:433–442.

151. Barnum T. *Boston's Infamous Cocoanut Grove Fire of 1942*. http://safetymatters.aonfpe.com/2011/3rd-quarter/historical-events.aspx.

152. Lindemann E. Symptomatology and Management of Acute Grief. *Am J Psychiatry* 1994; 151:6:155–160.
153. Brady KT. Posttraumatic Stress Disorder and Comorbidity: Recognizing the Many Faces of PTSD. *J Clin Psychiatry* 1997;58:12–15.
154. Brett EA. The Classification of Posttraumatic Stress Disorder. In: van der Kolk B, McFarlane AC, Weisaeth L, eds. *Traumatic Stress*. New York: 'The Guilford Press; 2007:121–123.
155. Youssef NA, Green KT, Dedert EA, et al. Exploration of the Influence of Childhood Trauma, Combat Exposure, and the Resilience Construct on Depression and Suicidal Ideation Among U.S. Iraq/Afghanistan Era Military Personnel and Veterans. *Arch Suicide Res* 2013; 17:2:106–122.
156. Beebe GW. Follow-Up Studies of World War II and Korean War Prisoners: II: Morbidity, Disability, and Maladjustments. *Am J Epidemiol* 1975; 101:400–422.
157. Phillips KA. *The Broken Mirror: Understanding and Treating Body Dysmorphic Disorder*. Revised and expanded edition. New York: Oxford University Press; 2005.
158. McCurdy-McKinnon D, Feusner J. Neurobiology of Body Dysmorphic Disorder: Heritability / Genetics, Brain Circuitry, and Visual Processing. In: Phillips KA, ed. *Body Dysmorphic Disorder: Advances in Research and Clinical Practice*. New York: Oxford University; 2017:253–256.
159. Hendin H, Haas AP, Singer P, et al. The Influence of Precombat Personality on Posttraumatic Stress Disorder. *Compr Psychiatry* 1983; 24:6:530–534.
160. Wolfe J, Schnurr PP, Brown PJ, et al. Posttraumatic Stress Disorder and War-Zone Exposure as Correlates of Perceived Health in Female Vietnam War Veterans. *J Consul Clin Psychol* 1994; 62:6:1235–1240.
161. Scaer RC. *The Body Bears the Burden: Trauma, Dissociation, and Disease*. 2nd edition. New York: Routledge; 2007:138–140.
162. Liberzon I, King AP, Ressler KJ, et al. Interaction of the ADRB2 Gene Polymorphism with Childhood Trauma in Predicting Adult Symptoms of Posttraumatic Stress Disorder. *JAMA Psychiatry* 2014; 71:10:1174–1182.
163. Aguilera M, Arias B, Wichers M, et al. Early Adversity and 5-HTT/BDNF Genes: New Evidence of Gene—Environment Interactions on Depressive Symptoms in a General Population. *Psychol Med* 2009; 39:9:1425–1432.
164. Heim C, Bradley B, Mletzko TC, et al. Effect of Childhood Trauma on Adult Depression and Neuroendocrine Function: Sex-Specific Moderation by CRH Receptor 1 Gene. *Front Behav Neurosci* 2009; 3:1–9.
165. Rivera RM, Bennett LB. Epigenetics in Humans: An Overview. *Curr Opin Endocrinol, Diabetes Obes* 2010;17:6:493–499.
166. Sabol SZ, Nelson ML, Fisher C, et al. A Genetic Association for Cigarette Smoking Behavior. *Health Psychol* 1999; 18:1:7–13.
167. Murthy RS. Mass Violence and Mental Health—Recent Epidemiological Findings. *Int Rev Psychiatry* 2007; 19:3:183–192.
168. Jang KL, Livesley WJ. Why Do Measures of Normal and Disordered Personality Correlate? A Study of Genetic Comorbidity. *J Personal Disord* 1999; 13:1:10–17.
169. Kanherkar RR, Bhatia-Dey N, Csoka AB. Epigenetics Across the Human Lifespan. *Front Cell Development Biol* 2014; 2:1–49.
170. Pollock VE, Briere J, Schneider L, et al. Childhood Antecedents of Antisocial Behavior: Parental Alcoholism and Physical Abusiveness. *Am J Psychiatry* 1990; 147:10:1290–1293.
171. Cloninger CR, Van Eerdewegh P, Goate A, et al. Anxiety Proneness Linked to Epistatic Loci in Genome Scan of Human Personality Traits. *Am J Med Genet Neuropsychiatr Genet* 1998; 81:313–317.

172. Deater-Deckard K, Fulker DW, Plomin R. A Genetic Study of the Family Environment in the Transition to Early Adolescence. *J Child Psychol Psychiat* 1999, 40:5:769–775.

173. Enoch MA, Albaugh BJ. Genetic and Environmental Risk Factors for Alcohol Use Disorders in American Indians and Alaskan Natives. *Am J Addict* 2016 Sep 6. doi:10.1111/ajad.12420. PubMed PMID: 27599369.

174. Hemmings SMJ, Lochner C, van der Merwe L, et al. BDNF Val66Met Modifies the Risk of Childhood Trauma on Obsessive-Compulsive Disorder. *J Psychiatric Res* 2013; 47:1857–1863.

175. Meaney MJ. Maternal Care, Gene Expression, and the Transmission of Individual Differences in Stress Reactivity across Generations. *Ann Rev Neurosci* 2001; 24:1:1161–1192.

176. Reif A, Lesch K. Toward a Molecular Architecture of Personality. *Behav Brain Res* 2003; 139:1–20.

177. Weaver ICG, Cervoni N, Champagne FA, et al. Epigenetic Programming by Maternal Behavior. *Nat Neurosci* 2004; 7:8:847–854.

178. Nievergelt CM, Maihofer AX, Mustapic M, et al. Genomic Predictors of Combat Stress Vulnerability and Resilience in U.S. Marines: A Genome-Wide Association Study across Multiple Ancestries Implicates PRTFDC1 as a Potential PTSD Gene. *Psychoneuroendocrinology* 2015; 51:459–471.

179. Sharma P, Garg G, Kumar A, et al. Genome Wide DNA Methylation Profiling for Epigenetic Alteration in Coronary Artery Disease Patients. *Gene* 2014; 541:1:31–40.

180. Maes M, Berk M, Goehler L, et al. Depression and Sickness Behavior Are Janus-Faced Responses to Shared Inflammatory Pathways. *BMC Med* 2012; 10:66:1–19.

181. Pavlov VA, Tracey KJ. The Vagus Nerve and the Inflammatory Reflex: Linking Immunity and Metabolism. *Nat Rev Endocrinol* 2012; 8:12:743–754.

182. Xu Z, Taylor JA. Genome-Wide Age-Related DNA Methylation Changes in Blood and Other Tissues Relate to Histone Modification, Expression and Cancer. *Carcinogenesis* 2014; 35:2:356–364.

183. Yang B, Zhang H, Ge W, et al. Child Abuse and Epigenetic Mechanisms of Disease Risk. *Am J Prev Med* 2013; 44:2:101–107.

184. Yang J, Li W, Liu X, et al. Enriched Environment Treatment Counteracts Enhanced Addictive and Depressive-Like Behavior Induced by Prenatal Chronic Stress. *Brain Res* 2006; 1125:132–137.

185. Jaycox LH, Foa EB, Morral AR. Influence of Emotional Engagement and Habituation of Exposure Therapy for PTSD. *J Consult Clin Psychol* 1998; 66:1:185–192.

186. Voellmin A, Winzeler K, Hug E, et al. Blunted Endocrine and Cardiovascular Reactivity in Young Healthy Women Reporting a History of Childhood Adversity. *Psychoneuroendocrinol* 2015; 51:58–67.

187. Ogden P, Fisher J. *Sensorimotor Psychotherapy: Interventions for Trauma And Attachment.* New York: W W Norton & Company; 2015.

188. Roberts AL, Rosario M, Corliss HL, et al. Sexual Orientation and Functional Pain in U.S. Young Adults: The Mediating Role of Childhood Abuse. *PLoS One* 2013; 8:1:1–7.

189. Ryan NP, Catroppa C, Godfrey C, et al. Social Dysfunction after Pediatric Traumatic Brain Injury: A Translational Perspective. *Neurosci Biobehav Rev* 2016; 64:196–214.

8

BEHAVIOR, PTSD, AND SURGICAL COMPULSION IN PLASTIC SURGERY PATIENTS

Trailing the Trauma Prevalence

"I want a smaller nose that is much thinner, and no bump, and tipped up, and pointed on the end, like this. You know, the same nose but smaller."

The young woman spread a sheaf of magazine photographs on the examination table. She was slender with blonde hair, cut and sprayed into a perfect pageboy. She wore a shirtwaist dress in a small blue flowered print with a matching headband and low, patent leather heels. Except for the sadness in her face, she could have been Betty Crocker. Her boyfriend sat on a chair next to her, his forearms on his thighs and hands clasped, leaning forward over her photographs. He wore headphones with his cap brim facing backward. His head moved rhythmically. He had short cropped blond hair, a narrow waist, and a tight sleeveless shirt that showed how often he worked out. I tried to be brave.

The patient's nose already resembled what she wanted, except that it had a very small bump. Some of the longest, saddest rhinoplasty histories I have seen started like hers. Patients with straight profiles, good airways, and symmetrical noses asked for the same nose in a smaller size. Too often that was not possible because nasal skin volume and distribution ultimately limited what the surgeon could do without creating distortion. Noses with straight bridges have only small tolerances for change. There is no big bump to be removed, no significant shortening or narrowing necessary. But innocent suggestions made by family, fashion photographers, or

DOI: 10.4324/9781315657721-12

the patients themselves can set into action a descending cascade of almost inevitable new problems.

Today I would be thinking beyond the surgical request. Why would an attractive woman with a normal nose want surgery? Today I would recognize that a significant percentage of patients who seek perfection in features that are already normal are motivated by body shame, not body dissatisfaction.[1]

When I first met her I had not yet drawn those conclusions and so overlooked the obvious signs.

"Your nose could be a little shorter and perhaps a little narrower, but I don't really see a bump. Show me," I said.

She sighed operatically and held the hand mirror to her face. She slid her index finger along her bridge.

"It's right here."

She shook her head as if she were already tired of speaking.

"Look—it's so obvious. My whole family tells me how bad it is. They call me 'pig nose.'"

Her boyfriend gave me a challenging stare. I began to feel like the boy with the five loaves and two fishes.

"The bump you see is very small," I said. "That means I can't make big changes because it will throw off nasal proportion. I do not want to promise more than I can safely do."

"Look at this selfie. See all these views? In this one my nose is so fat but in this one it's a beak," she said.

"That picture is distorted," I said. "When it's taken that close, your nose never looks right."

She shook her head and frowned, so I continued.

"I'm looking at you. That phone picture is not accurate."

"What are you talking about?" she said. I could hear her voice trying to decide whether to cry. "My nose is big and very ugly. My mother calls me 'the hook.' That's how bad it is. Don't you get it?" Her gaze was simultaneously defiant and frightened.

I thought about that but decided not to pursue it, so I returned to the easier topic. I discussed surgery. I illustrated results in other patients with similar problems. They couldn't wait to proceed. Surgery should have produced a result she liked. Of course it didn't.

Before she left the hospital she had developed a migraine and excruciating nasal pain. She was sure that she would hemorrhage. Her boyfriend paced in the hallway, telephoning worried relatives. Two days later she was still vomiting.

At six days I removed her splint. Everything looked as it should. Her airway was wide open.

Her shoulders fell.

"The bump is still there. You didn't do anything."

Her boyfriend narrowed his eyes, trying hard to look scary. I spoke as quietly as a fourth grader in study hall.

"It's only six days," I said. "You are healing fine. Everything will look different someday than now. Please be patient."

Her boyfriend concentrated on his mad look, vacillating between contemptuous and overconfident. He interlocked his fingers and worked his hands back and forth. Suddenly the stare gave way to a gratuitous laugh.

"What are you, a wiseass? I'll bet you never even finished the operation. Did you forget?"

The following day he called the office. She was in bed. She was suffering. He was mad. She was depressed. Seven days had passed. Why hadn't she healed? Why was she swollen? She looked worse than before surgery.

Reassuring words felt useless. I imagined him flexing in the mirror.

Eventually she left her sick bed to send emails: Why had I left the bump? Nobody on the Internet has a bump. It's going to stay swollen forever; I just know. My family hates it. They say you have to operate again, right away.

"Can I have cortisone shots? The Internet says cortisone always works."

"I don't think the Internet requires proof," I said.

"At least I can cover my nose with glasses. Maybe I should add a bandage. But can I wear my glasses all the time? What if they make dents? I think the bones are coming out. Doctors on the Internet massage the bones."

Reviewing her chart today, I can count 52 office visits or phone calls in the first postoperative year. Operating under the illusion that I am Sir Gawain is always a mistake. I might have been ready if a dragon showed up, but this was different. A good technical result was irrelevant. What healed this young woman was not me. What healed her were marriage and a baby. She ultimately pulled her own sword from the stone.

A Disease of Emotions

Shame is the biblical mustard seed: "At the time of its sowing . . . the smallest of all the seeds . . . Yet once it is sown it grows into the biggest shrub of them all and becomes and puts out big branches so that the birds of the air can shelter in its shade."[2] When grown, shame creates shelter for mental illness, addictions, and seemingly limitless self-harming behavior.[3–7]

Body dysmorphic disorder, where this thread began, is primarily a disease of emotions, particularly toxic shame—not appearance. An observable deformity creates anguish disproportionate to what others see or understand. Patient life disruption can be extreme, the family consumed in the patient's vortex. If a surgeon operates, the recovery may become a drama that dwarfs the procedure itself. When dressings are removed, the patient may be disconsolately unhappy, sometimes furiously and vindictively so—the child's thinking with the adult's capacity for revenge. Why?

One end of the thread was the observation that many patients who had undergone multiple surgeries—particularly rhinoplasties—originally had normal noses but underwent surgery anyway, to be good enough, or accepted, or loved, they told me. Their overriding emotions were not body dissatisfaction, but rather body shame.

The First Glimpse

In 2009 I had seen 20 patients within a short time with similarities that I could not instantly identify. Comparing this puzzling group to 20 other revision rhinoplasty patients, I found fascinating differences: The test group were all women (compared to 85% in the control group) and were older (50 versus 35 years).[8] Eighty percent had undergone other cosmetic operations (compared to only 10% in the control group), and altogether they had accumulated a stunning 137 rhinoplasties, almost 7 each (compared to 1.5 rhinoplasties for the control group). Compared to 15% of controls, 40% were depressed or unusually demanding of staff or surgeon time—either disempowered or grandiose.

★★★★★

Three observations stood out: Fifty-five percent of these women explicitly recounted histories of childhood abuse or neglect during conversations with me (compared to 30% of the controls). Sixty-eight percent of the childhood trauma group were not satisfied postoperatively and wanted further surgery for perceived imperfections, compared to 35% in the control group. Most incongruous was the recognition that 85% had normal noses before their first surgeries—no deformities and no airway obstructions—no indications for surgery—whereas all of the control group patients had indications for surgery. All of these changes were statistically significant.

If patients had noses that they knew were normal but had surgery anyway, didn't that define body dysmorphic disorder? The numbers of operations, the personalities, and the low surgical success rate all fit. Except for my own textbook chapter,[9] to my knowledge only one paper in the literature had connected childhood trauma to body dysmorphic disorder.[10] Could we uncover the same association in a larger group? The brilliant Bengali polymath, Rabindranath Tagore, hints at the answer: "Who is this who follows me in the silent dark? . . . He is my own little self, my lord, he knows no shame."[11]

The Relationship of Trauma to Surgical History

Paul Lin, then a biostatistician at the University of Wisconsin, and I wanted to answer four questions: If the most common motivation for rhinoplasty was to correct deformities, such as "bumps" on the bridge, why would patients without deformities undergo rhinoplasties and then multiple revisions? Was there any relationship between the absence of a deformity and a childhood trauma history? Did the personality characteristics of patients who had minimal deformities differ from those who had more obvious nasal deformities? Would those traits be congruent with body dysmorphic disorder?[11–18]

We tabulated age, gender, marital status, employment, depressed or demanding behavior, and histories of childhood abuse or neglect on consecutive patients * for whom I had performed secondary rhinoplasties until we had 50 who originally had nasal dorsal humps and wanted smaller noses and 50 who never had deformities but sought surgery anyway.

Though not yet familiar with the Adverse Childhood Events study (Chapter 9), I had empirically observed that body image, body shame, perfectionism, eating disorders, posttraumatic stress disorder, and body dysmorphic disorder influenced patient personality and could impact surgical outcome. When someone's past surfaced during the consultation or whenever I sensed self-esteem difficulties or the patient's behavior demonstrated immaturity, inadequate sense of reality, lack of self-care, or poor boundaries,[19, 20] I would ask, "Tell me about your childhood." My goal was not to perform a mental health examination but only to assess the patient's suitability for surgery.

These were the trauma types for which we were specifically watching:

- Desertion/Death of a parent/friend
- Depression/mental illness in a parent
- Severe childhood illness or loneliness
- Alcohol or drug abuse in a parent
- Poverty
- Adoption
- Being a refugee or raised by refugees
- Raging, threatening, or emotional abuse
- Physical abuse
- Never being "good enough"
- Racial or ethnic discrimination
- Sexual abuse
- Too-rigid or too-lenient parents

We separated these groups in order not to overstate our conclusions. Even with such precautions, some obvious and statistically significant differences were observed. There was nothing unusual about demographics: 86% of the patients were women, 61% were married, and 56% were employed. However, 52% demanded unusual amounts of time from my staff and me, and 42% were depressed—the latter four times the national average.

★★★★★

These 100 patients had undergone an average of 4.17 previous aesthetic surgeries, of which 78% were rhinoplasties. Seventy-one percent had originally wanted noses that were smaller, straighter, or more functional, but 29% had noses that they believed were normal but sought surgery anyway because they were "not perfect enough." Forty-five percent of the entire 100 patient population had trauma histories, consistent with the population at large.[21]

As we had documented in the initial small survey, the 50 patients whose original noses were straight (i.e., without bumps) were older (45 vs. 37 years), more dominantly women (90% vs. 82%), and twice as likely to show demanding behavior (72% vs. 32%) or be depressed (54% vs. 30%). Surgical motivations also differed: All 50 patients with bumps wanted noses that were smaller or more functional. However, 58% of the patients without bumps had wanted surgery only because their noses weren't "perfect enough" ($p < 0.0001^\dagger$).

Patients without bridge bumps had undergone three times more rhinoplasties than patients who originally had bumps (6.3 vs. 2.0 surgeries), as well as more other aesthetic operations such as breast, eyelid, or facelift ($p < 0.05$). Thus these 50 patients with normal noses had more plastic surgery than the 50 patients with deformed noses—a perfect illustration of the common observation that "perceived"—even imaginary—flaws can create significant anguish.[22-25] These women also had three times the trauma histories of the hump nose patients (68% vs. 22%).

★★★★★

When we compared our patients by numbers of cosmetic operations, additional provocative differences appeared. Compared to patients who had undergone fewer than three aesthetic surgeries, those patients who had undergone more than three surgeries were 10 years older, more than three times more likely to have had no visible deformities, twice as likely to be demanding, and seven times more likely to have undergone rhinoplasties to improve noses that weren't "perfect enough." These same patients were also twice as likely to have had trauma histories (66% vs. 31%), and to have undergone three times more rhinoplasties, and four times more other aesthetic surgeries (eight vs. two) than those who had three or fewer surgeries. The more surgeries patients had undergone, the more they wanted—and the more likely they were to have been abused or neglected as children.

This difference was magnified further when we compared patients at the extremes: those who had only one cosmetic operation versus those who had seven or more: Compared to those who had only one surgery, patients who had undergone more than seven surgeries were 93% women; 87% exhibited demanding or depressed behavior; and 73% wanted to correct noses that were subjectively normal. Eight-seven percent had childhood trauma histories.

We concluded the following points.

1. A childhood trauma history was common among the revision rhinoplasty group that we studied—perhaps expected in cosmetic surgery patients, but no more common than in the general population.[26]

2. Trauma prevalence correlated with nasal shape (bump or no bump), and the motivation for the original surgery (i.e., to correct a deformity or to "be more perfect"). Finally, 50 patients who originally had neither deformities nor functional problems but underwent surgery anyway (therefore qualifying for body dysmorphic disorder) had the most surgeries and had the highest trauma prevalences.

Does a Trauma History Impact Surgical Satisfaction?

Energized by the differences we had uncovered, we looked further.[12] Had these patients undergone these surgeries because earlier ones had been unsuccessful or because they might never be satisfied, even with successful outcomes?

We separated the patients according to whether they had been satisfied after only one operation. We found that satisfied patients were twice as likely to be men and to have had dorsal bumps—visible deformities—than normal noses. Satisfied patients were also less likely to be demanding (14% vs 56%) or depressed (10% vs 52%,), had undergone fewer aesthetic operations (17% vs. 78% having had >3 operations), and were almost never motivated to correct noses that weren't "perfect enough" (1 of 34 patients). Only 17% had trauma histories, close to one-third of the 65% prevalence of the whole cohort of 100 patients (all p < 0.01 or greater),[12] well below reported averages in the United States today.[27]

Somewhat sobering was the finding that patients who wanted more surgery were the largest group (62 of 100 patients). Most of these patients were women (65% versus 43% who were satisfied) and 86% originally had straight noses that weren't "perfect enough." The majority (79%) exhibited demanding behavior and 81% were depressed. Seventy-seven percent had trauma histories, which is 2.5 times the 17% prevalence of those patients who were happy with their surgical results after one operation. The success rate after one rhinoplasty for patients with these characteristics was 100%.

Patients who wanted more surgery had already undergone more operations (five vs. three) than the happy patients but were not yet satisfied. As might be expected, those patients who had undergone more than three cosmetic surgeries were more likely to be unhappy than those who had undergone fewer than three surgeries and were almost five times as likely to want more surgery (78% vs. 17%).

It is important to note that most of the patients who wanted more surgery were not totally dissatisfied—my result just wasn't "perfect enough." There were, however, four patients who felt that my surgery was a failure. All were women, 75% were unemployed, all were demanding and depressed, and 75% had originally wanted more perfect noses. All four of my "failure" patients had trauma histories. Thus patients who had undergone the most surgeries had childhood trauma, were most likely to request additional surgery, and least likely to be satisfied.

Predicting Patient Happiness After Surgery

Can we know preoperatively which patients are likely to be happy? In this group, the total number of previous surgeries was the most important variable predicting success, followed by demanding behavior, motivation for perfection instead of removing a bump, a history of abuse/neglect, and depression.[28, 29] Thus, patients with fewer surgeries who were neither demanding nor depressed, not looking for more perfect noses, and without trauma histories were most likely to be satisfied (See Table 8.1).

The odds of making a patient happy in one operation were almost four times higher if the patient had no trauma history. Similarly, patients who originally had deformed noses were 91% more likely to be satisfied after one surgery than those whose noses had been subjectively normal but "not perfect enough."

★★★★★

The success rate—total satisfaction without any desire for revision after one rhinoplasty—for patients with these characteristics was only 3% (See Table 8.2).[12]

These data confirmed what many surgeons already instinctively know and what the body dysmorphic disorder literature reinforces: the smaller the original deformity, the greater the patient distress and life disruption, the more demanding, depressed, or perfectionistic the patient, the more operations they have already had, and the more turbulent their childhoods—the less likely they will be pleased with the operations that that they want so intensely.

The qualities of disempowerment or grandiosity, living at the extremes, and the products of non-nurturing upbringing manifest in patient behavior and can interfere with the physician-patient relationship and the ease with which patients can achieve their goals (See Table 8.3).

TABLE 8.1 Characteristics Associated With Happy Patients in Our Study

1. Being a Man
2. Only One Previous Aesthetic Surgery
3. No Demanding Behavior
4. No Depressive Behavior
5. Original Nose Had a Dorsal Hump—i.e., a Deformity
6. Motivation for Surgery Was a Smaller Nose
7. No History of Abuse or Neglect

TABLE 8.2 Characteristics Associated With Unhappy Patients in Our Study

1. Being a Woman
2. Three or More Previous Aesthetic Surgeries
3. Demanding Behavior
4. Depressive behavior
5. Original Nose Was Straight and Subjectively Normal—i.e., No Indication for Surgery
6. Motivation for Surgery Was Greater Perfection
7. Confirmed History of Neglect or Abuse

TABLE 8.3 Traits of Functional Adults and Examples of How Abuse or Neglect May Alter Their Behavior

Functional Adults	Disempowered Patients	Falsely Empowered Patients
Appropriate Self-esteem	Absent self-esteem False sense of inferiority Unable to make decisions Unsure of themselves or surgeon Require extra time of surgeon and staff Manifest victim behavior	Excessive sense of self-Importance Perennially late Dictate operative plan Request holiday and weekend appointments Demand extra time of surgeon and staff Request special fees and/or discounts
Functioning Boundaries: Self-containment and Self-protection	Overly sensitive to language and advice Take everything as criticism No sense of humor Accompanied by overpowering "protectors" May seek revenge on the Internet	Argue Interrupt May act offensively or manipulatively to staff May seek revenge on the Internet
Sense of Reality	Unable to describe surgical goals Seem inarticulate Exaggerate imperceptible deformities Use disaster language	Impractically precise about surgical expectations Exaggerate or imperfections or deformities Use disaster language Expect perfection
Able to Live in Moderation	Possible histories of alcohol abuse and/or antidepressant use Associated depression, migraines, fibromyalgia, eating disorders or obsessive compulsive behavior History of multiple surgeries without adequately considering risks	Possible histories of stimulant use, risk-taking, gambling, high-risk sports or professions Work or sex addictions High-intensity lives History of multiple surgeries without adequately considering risks

(Continued)

TABLE 8.3 (Continued)

Functional Adults	Disempowered Patients	Falsely Empowered Patients
Capable of Self-care	Dependent on surgeon and staff for every detail of perioperative care	Disregard perioperative instructions
	Forget appointments, unable to make decisions	Alter perioperative instructions to fit personal preferences
	Do not remember or follow written instructions	Act entitled
		Guarded
	Request and need constant advice and reassurance via phone or email	Remote
		May reject routine postoperative care
	May self-injure, become reclusive or threaten suicide	May become aggressive or threatening
Have Body Dissatisfaction	Have Body Shame	Have Body Shame

★★★★★

She held large photographs of a very pretty, smiling woman.

"These are my studio head shots. I'm an actress." Her eyes were big and wide and compassionate.

"That's wonderful," I said. "Are you working?"

"I was . . ." Her voice began to drift. ". . . until the accident."

"This is me in the hospital." Her voice was small. She held a picture of a badly wounded face, recently sutured, eyes swollen, hard to relate to the woman sitting across from me.

"After you fix my nose, I can get more work." She nodded to herself.

She looked down at her stomach and pinched.

"Next I need to get rid of this disgusting roll of fat." She gave a little shudder. All I saw was skin.

"Do you do liposuction? I need liposuction."

"Tell me about your injury first." She ignored me.

"By the way, do you have more happy patients or more unhappy patients?"

I knew she'd eventually get to the point, so I waited.

She smiled self-consciously. "Forget my little conceit. I withdraw the question. But look at this ugly turkey neck. I need you to fix that, too."

"Please tell me about the picture. What happened to you," I said.

She looked over my shoulder as if she were watching her own past. "He beat me. I should know better. He always beats me when I don't do what he wants."

She folded her arms across her stomach as if she felt sick. As she spoke, she squeezed tighter, and began rocking slowly.

"Now he's following me, and last week he broke into my apartment and wrote scary things on the walls."

"Have you told the police?"

She looked up and laughed suddenly at a joke I couldn't hear. "What are you—some kind of Boy Scout? They can't help me. What I need is to have my nose fixed."

"Why do you stay?"

"Because I don't have anywhere to go and because he threatens me if I leave and . . ."

Suddenly she stopped and looked at me for a while. She had caught herself filibustering.

"I guess I don't really know."

"That's a beginning," I said.

As is regrettably so often true in these desperate patients, the surgical reconstruction of her collapsed septum was the easiest part of her management. Six days after surgery she was ecstatic about her airway and appearance—as is so often true, it was short-lived happiness.

"I don't know how you did it. For the first time in years I look like myself again. I'm so happy!"

Two weeks later the emails began. "I'm definitely going to need a revision. There is a chunk missing of my nose. It looks as if someone took a potato peeler or ice cream scoop and ripped something out of that side. I'm frightened. There are ridges that my handyman noticed, and the ball on the end of my nose is getting bigger. Can he take some fat and put it in my face? I think I need crushed cartilage put over the bump and then maybe some fat. I have so much pain but I have a lot of faith. My nose is so bumpy. The camera picks up everything. I'm so scared. But I know the doctor can work miracles. He's a genius. Thank you and hugs."

I looked at my nurse. "Do you think she's flirting with me?"

My nurse gave me a knowing smile. She is expert at knowing smiles.

I continued to read.

"I'm horrified by just how bad my nose looks. I'm having nightmares. I think about the beating even if I don't want to, and then I get all sweaty. My heart pounds. I dislike my face now. The whole bottom half of my nose is too large. The appearance makes me want to cry. I feel very ugly. I'm not looking for perfection. I just want to look like me again. Please reassure me."

"I guess she's not flirting with me," I said.

★★★★★

Can Rhinoplasty Patients Have Posttraumatic Stress Disorder?

Body image disorders, body dysmorphic disorder, and PTSD share common features. Among them are the following:

- Disturbance of body image: appearance
- Disturbance in the sense of oneself: self-esteem, reality processing
- View of oneself as helpless, damaged, victimized
- Intrusive memories of traumatic experiences
- Difficulties with trust, intimacy, self-assertion
- Inability to process stressful information without becoming disequilibriated
- Memory distortion and fragmentation
- Inability to put feelings into words: Alexithymia (Broca's area affected)
- Loss of emotions as reliable signals

It should not be surprising then that many unhappy or body dysmorphic patients spontaneously recount flashbacks, nightmares, and autonomic nervous system responses (sweating, nausea, palpitations) in response to triggers that remind them of their surgeries. Do some unhappy rhinoplasty patients actually manifest the arousal, re-experiencing, and avoidance traits that characterize PTSD?

★★★★★

To answer this question, we screened 35 consecutive secondary (revision) rhinoplasty patients for PTSD using Brewin, Rose, Andrews et al.'s brief 10 question PTSD screening questionnaire,[30–32] which has a sensitivity of 0.84 and a specificity of 0.95. I administered the test personally.

Twenty women and 15 men with a mean age of 42 were interviewed; each had undergone an average of 2.8 previous rhinoplasties. None of these patients would have filled all criteria for body dysmorphic disorder because their deformities were hardly imagined: on a 5-point Likert scale (5 being worst), the patient's view of the deformity was 4.0 and mine was 4.1. The deformities were severe.

Sixty-five percent (23 of 35 patients) had directly admitted stories of childhood abuse or neglect (by history, not survey), somewhat less than our current prevalence of 80%, but identically matching the original ACE study prevalence (Chapter 9).[33–35] Childhood trauma appeared to influence surgical motivation: Among patients without trauma histories, only 8% had normal noses, whereas among patients with childhood trauma, 54% had normal noses, almost 6 times more. Thus these latter patients fulfilled one of the criteria for body dysmorphic disorder when they first had surgery: -perceived deformity.

The Effect of Personality on the PTSD Prevalence and Revision Surgery Outcomes

Personality characteristics also differed: prevalences of depression, demanding personality, and being accompanied by an aggressive "protective" person who tried to override the patient's desires or control the surgical procedure differed significantly between patient groups (all p< 0.05) (See Table 8.4).

I asked: "During the past week, have you experienced any of the following symptoms?"

Tables 8.4 and 8.5 give responses for the 35 patient group.

When patients were stratified by their trauma histories, striking differences were evident (Table 8.6).

Six or more positive answers defined PTSD.[30-32] Among all 35 patients, 51% (18/35) screened positive for PTSD, and 87% (17/18) of those had a trauma history. Among the 12 patients without trauma histories, only one (8%) had PTSD; but of the 23 patients with trauma histories, 17 (73%) had PTSD. This is precisely the phenomenon observed of soldiers going into battle: it is not simply the terror

TABLE 8.4 Characteristics of Rhinoplasty Patients in the PTSD Study

- *20% Were Depressed*
  Non-Trauma Patients: 0%
  Trauma Patients: 69%
- *45% Were Demanding*
  Non-Trauma Patients: 8%
  Trauma Patients: 26%
- *40% Accompanied by a "Protector"*
  Non-Trauma Patients: 8%
  Trauma Patients: 56%

TABLE 8.5 PTSD Screen Results for the Entire Group

I asked: "During the past week, have you experienced any of the following symptoms?"

1. Upsetting thoughts or memories?	74%
2. Upsetting dreams?	34%
3. Sensations of re-experiencing surgery?	28%
4. Upsetting reminders of the surgery?	82%
5. Do you have bodily reactions (sweating, palpitations, or nausea)?	54%
6. Insomnia?	51%
7. Irritability or anger?	51%
8. Difficulty concentrating?	51%
9. Feel like you are a potential danger to yourself or others?	40%
10. Are you easily startled?	48%

TABLE 8.6 PTSD Screen Results Stratified by Trauma History

During the past week, have you experienced:

Question	No Trauma History	Trauma History
1. Upsetting thoughts?	41%	91%
2. Upsetting dreams?	0%	52%
3. Sensations of re-experiencing surgery	0%	43%
4. Upsetting reminders of the surgery?	41%	100%
5. Do you have bodily reactions (sweating, palpitations, or nausea)?	33%	65%
6. Insomnia?	16%	60%
7. Irritability/Anger?	33%	60%
8. Difficulty concentrating?	25%	65%
9. Feel like you are a potential danger to yourself or others?	16%	52%
10. Are you easily startled?	16%	65%

faced that determines PTSD, but rather the soldier's intrinsic sense of self before going to war.[36] The most fragile suffer worst.

Outcomes also differed among the two groups. Overall, 77% (27 patients) were totally happy with their surgical results. Eight patients (23%) wanted additional surgery; all of these patients had trauma histories and 87% of them originally had normal noses. These data precisely fit the prevalences and trends that we found in the group of 100 patients reported above.

Seventeen patients were tested both before and after surgery. Of this group, 11 were happy, but 6 (all of whom had trauma histories) wanted additional surgery.[37] Five of the 6 who wanted revisions originally had normal noses.

Among these 17 patients tested before and after surgery, mean preoperative scores were 6.3 out of 10. Most striking was the fact that postoperative PTSD symptomatology scores decreased to a mean of 0.9, ($p < 0.001$). Gratifyingly, 12 of 17 patients tested positively for PTSD before surgery but only one tested positive after surgery.

★★★★★

Perhaps most disturbing was the finding that these symptoms had persisted for as long as 39 years, (averaging 16 years). Imagine these patients' lives during that period. How did they function? How did they work? How were their families affected? The ravages of unsuccessful surgery on susceptible patients cannot be underestimated.

In this small group of patients operated on by the same surgeon, the data suggest that even long-term symptoms characteristic of PTSD can be improved by a single successful corrective rhinoplasty. This is an encouraging outcome.

★★★★★

Chronically unhappy postoperative rhinoplasty patients can manifest the same psychophysiological signs as PTSD victims, a finding supported by similar functional MRI studies in both groups.[25, 38–42] However, these disquieting physiologic responses can improve with successful surgery in the majority of affected patients.

A trauma history impacts perceived surgical success. Even though these were all rhinoplasty patients, the surgical literature suggests what is intuitively obvious: trauma histories and the personality traits that they engender can influence patient responses—and human responses. The question posed earlier in this book remains, not what makes patients happy, but what makes people happy?

The Nexus Among Trauma, Shame, and Plastic Surgery

Almost all people care about the way they look, some to the extreme. Plastic surgeons are expected to accept this truism and perhaps notice only those at the edges—e.g., patients who are delusional or have body dysmorphic disorder. But all patients have histories,[43] which presumably influences their motivations and the need to seek perfection.[44, 45] What might explain these differences?

We believe that two conclusions can be safely drawn.

1. A history of trauma is common among revision rhinoplasty patients. Human resilience accounts for the fact that most people exposed to trauma do not develop psychiatric disorders.[21, 46] However, some people are unable to integrate their experiences and develop pathologic patterns of behavior that color their lives. Carried shame absorbed from parents or caregivers is the thread that unifies these seemingly disparate but ubiquitous trauma types; and when that sense of shame manifests as body shame, some of those individuals seek plastic surgery.[47, 48]

2. A trauma history impacts behavior and therefore the surgical experience. Trauma can produce a chronic state of physiologic hyperarousal, driving some patients to relive their experiences in thoughts, actions, and images; the Brewin PTSD screen results reinforce this principle.[49] These distressing recollections and the meaning that patients attach to them color their post-traumatic lives,[50, 51] and the patients' choice of defenses depends on the ages at which the trauma occurred.[27, 52, 53] Postoperatively, unhappy patients act as if they are being traumatized all over again, unaware of being dissociated from the original traumatic memory.[25, 54, 55]

★★★★★

These patients are not an unusual revision rhinoplasty population. Even the 45% prevalence of trauma history typifies the United States population at large.[21, 26, 27] Recent data from the National Stressful Events Survey cites a striking trauma prevalence of 89.7% using DSM-5 criteria and a posttraumatic stress disorder prevalence of 8.5%.[27, 56] When that population self-selects as plastic surgery patients and then as unhappy revision rhinoplasty patients, our 45% trauma prevalence seems less surprising. The 42% depression prevalence is also congruent with the literature for patients with body image concerns.[57–62] Women experience traumatic events more commonly than men,[63, 64] also consistent with our findings: 45% of female patients (39/86) but only 28% of the men (4/14) had trauma histories (unpublished data). The common thread is not the fight, flight, or freeze physiological response that trauma can provoke, but rather the sense of helplessness, abandonment, and shame generated by presumably protective caregivers.

We have seen that abuse and neglect heavily influence body image (Chapters 4–6),[47, 58, 65] often contributing to anger,[66, 67] anxiety and distrust,[66] depression,[68–72] and a sense of betrayal, especially when parents impose surgery on their children.[73] "The sad truth is that in every relationship involving love and trust, there exist the seeds of betrayal. . . . Such betrayals can be repaired. However, the new level of trust is different from what existed before. It is built upon the reality of experience rather than on innocent hopes and dreams."[74]

Childhood trauma creates messages of shame, inadequacy, or superiority in children that mercilessly lurch forward into adulthood.[72, 75, 76] The therapeutic relationship with traumatized patients becomes complicated by the way they can replay mistrust, dependency, love, and hate in ways that are irrelevant to the surgical experience.[50] The unifying theme is that some wounded patients do not behave like functional adults. It is not entirely their fault.

Tracing the Body Shame/BDD Associations

The hypothesis that interpersonal trauma can generate body shame and therefore surgical failure can be tested by working in reverse: What evidence is there that BDD patients display signs of neglect or abuse? It is scattered but ample: the study most similar to ours indicated that 78.7% of 75 patients with confirmed BDD had histories of neglect or abuse.[10] We have documented abuse histories in unhappy rhinoplasty patients;[9] Edgerton, Langman, and Pruzinsky did the same.[77] Other reports document associated traits: poor social functioning,[56] social anxiety,[78] depression, anxiety, anger, and somatic symptoms,[79–81] anxiety, depression, and neuroticism,[67] shame, eating disorders, dissociation and posttraumatic stress disorder,[82] obsessive compulsive disorder,[83] alexithymia,[84] eating disorders,[85] hypersensitivity to teasing, distorted memories of childhood trauma,[86, 87] positive family history,[88] sexual abuse,[89, 90] anorexia nervosa,[91] memory dysfunction,[38, 39, 86] hypochondriasis,[59, 85, 92] and characteristic emergence in childhood or adolescence.[93, 94] Plastic surgeon Maxwell Maltz first coined the term "imaginary ugliness" in his 1960 book *Psychocybernetics*[95] and linked the condition to shame, noting that these patients' perceived deformities lingered postoperatively "the same as the phantom limb."[96]

"There are many complaints which are fundamentally not medical. . . . The patient goes to the surgeon, is operated on, recovers from the operation. To the surgeon, it is a cure and so he records it. But to the family doctor it is a failure, because the patient returns to him again and again

with the same complaint as before. . . . This . . . explains why working at the profession is called the practice of medicine. The doctor learns by practice what patients not to operate on. . ."

So Dr. Arthur Hertzler summarizes the art of patient selection, a key theme of this text.[97]

What This Information Means

Aside from its impact on daily life, trauma affects body image and can create the compulsive but unsatisfied drive for plastic surgery. So far we have found associations among childhood trauma, body shame, obsessive plastic surgery, unhappiness with the surgical result, and PTSD symptoms improved by successful surgery.[98] But what type of trauma was this? What additional information can we generate about the lives and personalities of plastic surgery patients? This is where the thread leads next.

Notes

* So that selection bias could not skew results.
† p value indicates the probability that the finding was an accident. In this case ($p < 0.001$) that probability is less than 1 in 1,000.

References

1. Constantian MB, Lin CP. Why Some Patients Are Unhappy: Part 1: Relationship of Preoperative Nasal Deformity to Number of Operations and a History of Abuse or Neglect. *Plast Reconstr Surg* 2014; 134:4:823–835.
2. Mark, 4: 30–33. *The New Jerusalem Bible*, New York, Doubleday, 1985:1666.
3. Mellody P. How The Symptoms Sabotage. In: *Facing Codependence*. New York: Harper Collins; 2003:51–60.
4. Black C. Family Violence. In: *It Will Never Happen To Me: Growing Up With Addiction as Youngsters, Adolescents, Adults*. 2nd edition. Center City, Minn: Hazelden; 2005:102.
5. Black C. *It Will Never Happen To Me: Growing Up With Addiction As Youngsters, Adolescents, Adults*. Center City [MN]: Hazelden; 1981.
6. Black C. Shame Circle. In: *It Will Never Happen To Me: Growing Up With Addiction as Youngsters, Adolescents, Adults*. 2nd edition. Center City, Minn: Hazelden; 2002:65–84.
7. Black C. The Adult Child. In: *It Will Never Happen To Me: Growing Up With Addiction as Youngsters, Adolescents, Adults*. 2nd edition. Center City, Minn: Hazelden; 2005:123.
8. Aarts PGH, Op den Velde W. Prior Traumatization and Aging: Theory and Practical Implications. In: van der Kolk B, McFarlane AC, Weisaeth L, eds. *Traumatic Stress*. New York: The Guilford Press; 2007:371.
9. Constantian MB. Unhappy Patients and Those with Body Dysmorphic Disorder. In: Constantian MB, ed. *Rhinoplasty: Craft and Magic*. St. Louis: Quality Medical Publishing; 2009:1401–1448.
10. Didie ER, Tortolani CC, Pope CG, et al. Childhood Abuse and Neglect in Body Dysmorphic Disorder. *Child Abuse Neglect* 2006; 39:10:1105–1115.

11. Fosdick HE. *The Meaning of Prayer.* New York: Association Press; 1915.
12. Constantian MB, Lin CP. Why Some Patients Are Unhappy: Part 2. Relationship of Nasal Shape and Trauma History to Surgical Success. *Plast Reconstr Surg* 2014; 134:4:836–851.
13. Breiman L. *Manual on Setting Up, Using, and Understanding Random Forests,* Version 3.1. http://oz.berkeley.edu/users/breiman/Using_random_forests_V3.1.pdf. Accessed May 10. 2013.
14. Breiman L. Random Forests. *Mach Learn* 2001; 45:5–32.
15. 325. Jasti S, Dudley WN, Goldwater E. SAS Macros For Testing Statistical Mediation in Data with Binary Mediators or Outcomes. *Nurs Res* 2008; 57:118–122.
16. Kraemer HC. Biserial Correlation. In: Kotz S, Johnson NL, ed. *Encyclopedia of Statistical Sciences.* Vol. 1. New York: Wiley; 1982:276–279.
17. Liaw A, Wiener M. Classification and Regression by Random-Forest. *R News* 2002; 2:18–22.
18. Mackinnon DP, Warsi G, Dwyer JH. A Simulation Study of Mediated Effect Measures. *Multivariate Behav Res* 1995; 30:41.
19. Scaer RC. Concepts of Trauma: The Role of Boundaries. In: *The Body Bears the Burden: Trauma, Dissociation, and Disease.* 2nd edition. New York: Routledge; 2007:1–7.
20. Scaer RC. *Eight Keys to Brain-Body Balance.* New York: W W Norton & Company; 2012:12–13, 120–121.
21. McFarlane AC, De Girolamo G. The Nature of Traumatic Stressors. In: van der Kolk B, McFarlane AC, Weisaeth L, eds. *Traumatic Stress.* New York: The Guilford Press; 2007:129–155.
22. Wilhelm S. *Feeling Good About The Way You Look: A Program For Overcoming Body Image Problems.* New York: The Guilford Press; 2006.
23. Veale D, Kinderman P, Riley S, et al. Self-Discrepancy in Body Dysmorphic Disorder. *Br J Clin Psychol* 2003; 42:157–169.
24. Veale D, Riley S. Mirror, Mirror on the Wall, Who Is The Ugliest of Them All? The Psychopathology of Mirror Gazing in Body Dysmorphic Disorder. *Behav Res Ther* 2001; 39:1381–1393.
25. van der Kolk B, van der Hart O. The Intrusive Past: The Flexibility of Memory and the Engraving of Trauma. *Am Imago* 1991; 48:425–454.
26. van der Kolk B. The Complexity of Adaptation to Trauma: Self-Regulation, Stimulus, Discrimination, and Characterological Development. In: van der Kolk B, McFarlane AC, Weisaeth L, eds. *Traumatic Stress.* New York: The Guilford Press; 2007:182–213.
27. Kilpatrick DG, Resnick HS, Milanak ME, et al. National Estimates of Exposure to Traumatic Events and PTSD Using DSM-IV and DSM-5 Criteria. *J Traumatic Stress* 2013; 26:5:537–547.
28. Baron RM, Kenny DA. The Moderator-Mediator Variable Distinction in Social Psychological Research: Conceptual, Strategic, and Statistical Considerations. *J Pers Soc Psychol* 1986; 51:1173–1182.
29. Benjamini Y, Hochberg Y. Controlling the False Discovery Rate: A Practical and Powerful Approach to Multiple Testing. *J R Stat Soc B* 1995; 57:289–300.
30. Blake DD, Weathers FW, Nagy LM, et al. The Development of a Clinician-Administered PTSD Scale. *J Trauma Stress* 1995; 8:1:75–90.
31. Brewin CR, Rose S, Andrews B, et al. Brief Screening Instrument for Post-Traumatic Stress Disorder. *Br J Psychiatry* 2002; 181:158–162.
32. Brewin CR. Systematic Review of Screening Instruments for Adults at Risk of PTSD. *J Traumatic Stress* 2005; 18:1: 53–62.

33. Felitti VJ, Jakstis K, Pepper V, et al. Obesity: Problem, Solution, or Both? *Perm J* 2010; 14:1:24–31.
34. Felitti VJ, Williams SA. Long-Term Follow-Up and Analysis of More Than 100 Patients Who Each Lost More Than 100 Pounds. *Perm J* 1998; 2:3:17–21.
35. Felitti VJ, Anda RF. The Relationship of Adverse Childhood Experiences to Adult Medical Disease, Psychiatric Disorders and Sexual Behavior: Implications for Health-care. The Hidden Epidemic: The Impact of Early Life Trauma on Health and Disease, Lanius R & Vermetten E (eds); 2009:2–18.
36. Lee KA, Vaillant GE, Torrey WC, et al. A 50-Year Prospective Study of the Psychological Sequelae of World War II Combat. *Am J Psychiatry* 1995;152:4:516–522.
37. Constantian MB. What Motivates Secondary Rhinoplasty? A Study of 150 Consecutive Patients. *Plast Reconstr Surg* 2012; 130:667–678.
38. Deckersbach T, Savage CR, Phillips KA, et al. Characteristics of Memory Dysfunction in Body Dysmorphic Disorder. *J Int Neuropsychol Soc* 2000; 6:673–681.
39. van der Kolk B. Trauma and Memory. In: van der Kolk B, McFarlane AC, Weisaeth L, eds. *Traumatic Stress*. New York: The Guilford Press; 2007:3289–3296.
40. Saar-Ashkenazy R, Cohen JE, Guez J, et al. Reduced Corpus-Callosum Volume in Posttraumatic Stress Disorder Highlights the Importance of Inter-Hemispheric Connectivity for Associative Memory. *J Traumatic Stress* 2014; 27:1:18–26.
41. Levine PA. *Trauma and Memory: Brain And Body In A Search For The Living Past: A Practical Guide For Understanding And Working With Traumatic Memory*. Berkeley [CA]: North Atlantic Books; 2015.
42. Brown DW, Anda RF, Edwards VJ, et al. Adverse Childhood Experiences and Childhood Autobiographical Memory Disturbance. *Child Abuse Neglect* 2007; 31:9:961–969.
43. Bassham L. *With Winning In Mind: The Mental Management System: An Olympic Champion's Success System*. mentalmanagement.com; 2011.
44. Sarwer DB, Wadden TA, Pertschuk MJ, et al. The Psychology of Cosmetic Surgery: A Review and Reconceptualization. *Clin Psychol Rev* 1998; 18:1–22.
45. Sarwer DB, Pruzinsky T, Cash TF, et al. *Psychological Aspects Of Reconstructive And Cosmetic Plastic Surgery: Clinical, Empirical, And Ethical Perspectives*. Philadelphia: Lippincott Williams & Wilkins; 2006.
46. van der Kolk BA. *The Body Keeps The Score: Brain, Mind, And Body In The Healing Of Trauma*. New York: Viking (Penguin Group); 2014.
47. Franzoni E, Gualandi S, Caretti V, et al. The Relationship Between Alexithymia, Shame, Trauma, and Body Image Disorders: Investigation Over a Large Clinical Sample. *Neuropsychiatric Dis Treat* 2013; 9:185–193.
48. Troop NA, Sotrilli S, Serpell L, et al. Establishing a Useful Distinction between Current and Anticipated Bodily Shame in Eating Disorder. *Eat Weight Disord* 2006; 11:2:83–90.
49. Brewin CR, Andrews B, Valentine JD. Meta-Analysis of Risk Factors for Posttraumatic Stress Disorder in Trauma-Exposed Adults. *J Consul Clin Psychol* 2000; 68:5:748–766.
50. van der Kolk B. The Black Hole of Trauma. In: van der Kolk B, McFarlane AC, Weisaeth L, eds. *Traumatic Stress*. New York: The Guilford Press; 2007:3–23.
51. Ogden P, Minton K, Pain C. *Trauma And The Body: A Sensorimotor Approach To Psychotherapy*. New York: W W Norton & Company; 2006.
52. Ogden P, Minton K, Pain C. Attachment: The Role of the Body in Dyadic Regulation. In: *Trauma and the Body*. New York: W W Norton & Company; 2006:41–64.
53. Pain C. *Attachment: The Role of the Body in Dyadic Regulation. In: Trauma and the Body*. New York: W W Norton & Company; 2006:41–64.

54. Frank JD, Frank JB. *Persuasion & Healing: A Comparative Study Of Psychotherapy*. Baltimore: Johns Hopkins University Press; 1961.
55. Ledoux JE, Romanski L, Xagoraris A. Indelibility of Subcortical Emotional Memories. *J Cogn Neurosci* 1989; 1:238–243.
56. Olff M, Langeland W, Draijer N, et al. Gender Differences in Posttraumatic Stress Disorder. *Psychol Bull* 2007; 133:2:183–204.
57. Veale D, De Haro L, Lambrou C. Cosmetic Rhinoplasty in Body Dysmorphic Disorder. *Brit J Plast Surg* 2003; 56:6:546–551.
58. Cash TF. Body Image and Plastic Surgery. In: Sarwer DB, Pruzinsky T, Cash TF, Goldwyn RM, Persing JA, Whitaker LB, eds. *Psychological Aspects of Reconstructive and Cosmetic Plastic Surgery*. Philadelphia: Lippincott Williams & Wilkins; 2006:37–59.
59. Jerome L. Body Dysmorphic Disorder: A Controlled Study of patients Requesting Cosmetic Rhinoplasty. *Am J Psychiatry* 1992; 149:4:577–578.
60. Andrews B, Qian M, Valentine JD. Predicting Depressive Symptoms with a New Measure of Shame: The Experience of Shame Scale. *Br J Clin Psychol* 2002; 41:29–42.
61. Picavet VA, Hellings PW. Reply: Preoperative Symptoms of Body Dysmorphic Disorder Determine Postoperative Satisfaction and Quality of Life in Aesthetic Rhinoplasty. *Plast Reconstr Surg* 2014; 133:1:60e–62e.
62. Sheen JH, Sheen AP. *Aesthetic Rhinoplasty*. 2nd edition. St. Louis: Mosby; 1987:874–897.
63. Andrews B. Bodily Shame as a Mediator between Abusive Experiences and Depression. *J Abnorm Psychol* 1995; 104:2:277–285.
64. Tangney JP, Wagner P, Fletcher C, et al. Shamed Into Anger? The Relation of Shame and Guilt to Anger and Self-Reported Aggression. *J Personal Soc Psychol* 1992; 62:4:669–675.
65. McKinley NM, Hyde JS. The Objectified Body Consciousness Scale: Development and Validation. *Psychol Women Quar* 1996; 20:181–215.
66. Connell BF, Gunter J, Mayer T, et al. Roundtable: Discussion of "The Difficult Patient." *Facial Plast Surg Clin N Am* 2008; 16:2:249–258.
67. Kelly MM, Walters C, Phillips KA. Social Anxiety and Its Relationship to Functional Impairment in Body Dysmorphic Disorder. *Behav Ther* 2010; 41:143–153.
68. Wertheim EH, Paxton SJ. Body Image Development in Adolescent Girls. In: Cash TF, Smolak L, eds. *Body Image*. 2nd edition. New York: The Guilford Press; 2011:76–84.
69. Constantian MB. Dorsal Deformities. In: Constantian MB, ed. *Rhinoplasty: Craft and Magic*. St. Louis: Quality Medical Publishing; 2009:864–876.
70. Heller L, LaPierre A. The Beginning of Our Identity. In: *Healing Developmental Trauma*. Berkeley [CA]: North Atlantic Books; 2012:125–160.
71. Heller L, LaPierre A. The Beginning of Our Identity. In: *Healing Developmental Trauma*. Berkeley [CA]: North Atlantic Books; 2012:87.
72. McFarlane A, Yehuda R. Resistance, Vulnerability, and the Course of Posttraumatic Reactions. In: van der Kolk B, McFarlane AC, Weisaeth L, eds. *Traumatic Stress*. New York: The Guilford Press; 2007:170.
73. Kelley LP, Weathers FW, Mason EA, et al. Association of Life Threat and Betrayal with Posttraumatic Stress Disorder Symptom Severity. *J Trauma Stress* 2012; 25:408–415.
74. Kushner, HS. *Overcoming Life's Disappointments*. New York: Alfred A. Knopf; 2006.
75. McFarlane A, de Girolamo G. The Nature of Traumatic Stressors and the Epidemiology of Posttraumatic Reactions. In: van der Kolk B, McFarlane AC, Weisaeth L, eds. *Traumatic Stress*. New York: The Guilford Press; 2007:129–155.

76. Yehuda R, Hoge CW, McFarlane AC, et al. Post-Traumatic Stress Disorder. *Nat Rev Dis Primers* 2015; 1:15057.

77. Edgerton MT, Langman MW, Pruzinsky T. Plastic Surgery and Psychotherapy in the Treatment of 100 Psychologically Disturbed Patients. *Plast Reconstr Surg* 1991; 88:4:594–608.

78. Bienvenu OJ, Samuels JF, Riddle MA, et al. The Relationship of Obsessive-Compulsive Disorder to Possible Spectrum Disorders: Results from a Family Study. *Biol Psychiatry* 2000; 48:287–293.

79. Phillips KA. *The Broken Mirror: Understanding and Treating Body Dysmorphic Disorder*. Revised and expanded edition. New York: Oxford University Press; 2005.

80. Picavet VA, Gabriels L, Grietens J, et al. Preoperative Symptoms of Body Dysmorphic Disorder Determine Postoperative Satisfaction and Quality of Life in Aesthetic Rhinoplasty. *Plast Reconstr Surg* 2013; 131:4:861–868.

81. Knorr NJ, Edgerton MT, Hoopes JE. The "Insatiable" Cosmetic Surgery Patient. *Plast Reconstr Surg* 1967; 40:3:285–289.

82. Scaer RC. *The Body Bears the Burden: Trauma, Dissociation, and Disease*. 2nd edition. New York: Routledge; 2007:138–140.

83. Dyl J, Kittler J, Phillips KA, et al. Body Dysmorphic Disorder and Other Clinically Significant Body Image Concerns in Adolescent Psychiatric Inpatients: Prevalence and Clinical Characteristics. *Child Psychiatry Hum Dev* 2006; 36:369–382.

84. Grant JE, Kim SW, Eckert ED. Body Dysmorphic Disorder in Patients with Anorexia Nervosa: Prevalence, Clinical Features, and Delusionality of Body Image. *Int J Eat Disord* 2002; 32:291–300.

85. Phillips KA, Quinn G, Stout RL. Functional Impairment in Body Dysmorphic Disorder: Prospective, Follow-Up Study. *J Psychiatry Res* 2008; 42:701–707.

86. Osman S, Cooper M, Hackmann A, et al. Spontaneously Occurring Images and Early Memories in People with Body Dysmorphic Disorder. *Memory* 2004; 12:4:428–436.

87. Buhlmann U, McNally RJ, Wilhelm S, et al. Selective Processing of Emotional Information in Body Dysmorphic Disorder. *Anxiety Disord* 2002; 16:289–298.

88. Neziroglu F, Barile N. Environmental Factors in Body Dysmorphic Disorder. In: Phillips KA, ed. *Body Dysmorphic Disorder: Advances in Research and Clinical Practice*. New York: Oxford University; 2017:277–284.

89. Byram V, Wagner HL, Waller G. Sexual Abuse and Body Image Distortion. *Child Abuse Negl* 1995; 19:507–510.

90. Sack M, Boroske-Leiner K, Lahmann C. Association of Nonsexual and Sexual Traumatizations with Body Image and Psychosomatic Symptoms in Psychosomatic Outpatients. *Gen Hosp Psychiatry* 2010; 32:315–320.

91. Fenwick AS, Sullivan KA. Potential Link between Body Dysmorphic Disorder Symptoms and Alexithymia in an Eating-Disordered Treatment-Seeking Sample. *Psychiatry Res* 2011; 189:299–304.

92. Harth W, Hermes B. Psychosomatic Disturbances and Cosmetic Surgery. *JDDG: Journal der Deutschen Dermatologischen Gesellschaft* 2007; 5:9:736–744.

93. Albertini RS, Phillips KA. 33 Cases of Body Dysmorphic Disorder in Children and Adolescents. *J Am Acad Child Adolesc Psychiatry* 1999; 38:453–459.

94. Simmons RA, Phillips KA. Core Clinical Features of Body Dysmorphic Disorder: Appearance Preoccupations, Negative Emotions, Core Beliefs, and Repetitive and Avoidance Behaviors. In: Phillips KA, ed. *Body Dysmorphic Disorder: Advances in Research and Clinical Practice*. New York: Oxford University; 2017:61–80.

95. Maltz M. *Psycho-Cybernetics*. New York: Pocket Books; 1960.

96. Maltz M. *Psychocybernetics*. New York: Pocket Books; 1960:9–11.

97. Hertzler AE. *The Horse and Buggy Doctor*. New York: Harper & Brothers; 1938, pp. 155, 291.

98. Nuzzi LC, Cerrato FE, Webb ML, et al. Psychological Impact of Breast Asymmetry on Adolescents: A Prospective Cohort Study. *Plast Reconstr Surg* 2014; 134:6:1116–1123.

Toward the End of the Thread

Trauma, Body Image, Plastic Surgery, and Resilience

9

ADVERSE CHILDHOOD EVENTS IN MEDICAL AND PLASTIC SURGERY PATIENTS AND THEIR EFFECTS ON ADULT HEALTH, PERSONALITY, AND SURGICAL HAPPINESS

Problems seemed to follow her like the tail on a kite, but even in jeans and a white T-shirt she was elegantly pulled together, with just enough expression lines in her face to look like a grown-up. Her jewelry was large and looked real.

She gathered her hands in her lap and read hesitantly from a scrap of paper, pausing after each phrase to make sure that I was still paying attention.

"I need to have my nose fixed, see?" She pointed. "And my facelift has loosened and my lower lids need to be redone. Oh—and do you do breast lifts and tummy tucks?"

It was true that she'd had these surgeries at an early age, some repeated several times. All the results I could see were satisfactory, except it was obvious that her airway had collapsed and her eyelids were stretched too low.

"Let's paint one room at a time," I said. "Why did you have your first nasal surgery?"

"Here, look at this picture." She handed me a photograph.

"Who is this?" I said. "It's not you."

"That's my mother. She's very pretty. Don't you think she is?"

She stared at the photo and spoke to it the way you scold a misbehaving puppy. "She told me I looked like her father. She hated her father. Imagine

DOI: 10.4324/9781315657721-14

that. She thought I looked like an old man. So I wanted her whole face, but I was only 17. So I settled for her nose."

Every minute this was getting more complicated.

"How was your nasal shape different than hers?"

She gave me a mechanical smile.

"I don't remember," she said.

I'd never heard that before. Her first surgery had been only a few years earlier. She was clearly a bright woman.

"Not the details," I said. "For example, your surgeon's note says that he made your tip smaller. What didn't you like about your tip?"

Her face was expressionless. "I don't remember."

She turned her head in front of the mirror and squinted at shadows cast by the ceiling light. She ran her finger along her nose.

"Right here, see, there's a dent on my bridge, right at the edge, where it curves up."

She tipped her chin up.

"And this nostril is a little lower. Can you fix that?"

Her eyes narrowed.

"The last doctor did that to me."

"Really," I said.

"No, I'm sure."

"Maybe," I said. "Branches waving don't make the wind blow." I was trying not to lose my train of thought.

"OK, then you had a second surgery. What was wrong after that?"

She looked at me without expression. "I don't remember."

I had a brief internal struggle, which I lost. I moved on.

"Can you tell me why you wanted a third operation?"

She stood and began to pace around the office, stopping momentarily at each wall photograph and moving quickly and efficiently, like a bee in a bottle.

"It was a lousy result, and we both knew it. He de-faced me." She looked back at me, pleased with her pun.

"And then he wouldn't redo my nose, even after I threatened him with a lawsuit."

"Hard to imagine," I said.

"You're damn right it is. I want another surgery or I'll find someone else."

I finished taking her history. "Just lie on the table so I can examine you and see how I can help," I said.

She stared at me and hesitated, then slowly lay down. As I came closer, she clutched her collar with both hands, crowding her shoulders together. Her breathing became deep and halting, exhaling in long sighs. She looked like a castle under siege.

"Please," she said. Her voice rose and tightened. "It will hurt."

I backed away. "Let's move on."

She sighed, still breathing heavily. Then she sat up and hugged her knees.

"I see that you already had body contour operations after weight loss surgery," I said.

Her face brightened. "Yes, I lost almost 200 pounds. I weighed 340 six years ago."

She looked at me, waiting for a response.

I paused. I wasn't sure how much I wanted to uncover, but I knew that pathologies are sometimes still pathologies; they don't always go away when they are through bothering you. I also knew that her reaction on the examination table had nothing to do with me. She had become the age of some dark memory. Other people filled the room from her past, just like they did from mine. It's always like that.

"I've read a lot about morbid obesity," I said. "Weighing more than 300 pounds is almost a full-time job."

"So what," she said. She stared at me while she lifted a water bottle to her mouth, pausing at the opening as if she were savoring its bouquet.

I continued. "I also know that many people who are that overweight had difficult childhoods."

She gathered herself. I was pushing on a door that was meant to remain closed. Something, like neediness or anger or desperation, passed behind her eyes and then vanished. She settled on outrage.

"The implication is insulting," she said. I waited. A few moments of disapproving silence passed.

"I wasn't implying," I said. "I was just talking. I'm interested."

She looked, defocused, at the ceiling and then back at me. The stiff, contained snap that she had maintained earlier had faded slightly. Her voice remained soft, but now had rich undertones that made each word seem dramatic.

She began to bite her lower lip and murmured into her lap.

"My father abused me. I was 5. It didn't stop till I was 17. So I ate. I got fat so the bastard wouldn't touch me." She paused.

"You told your mother," I said.

"I tried. She said I was lying."

Suddenly she laughed. *"And when I told the nurse at school, she said I should 'improve my dietary habits.' That was a joke. She was bigger than me."*

Her voice became low and dreamy again, just above a whisper.

"So I saw these doctors for the weight loss surgery and more doctors for my back and my knees and my diabetes, and new ones for my plastic surgery."

I waited.

"And you know what," she said. *"I still hate myself."*

There was another dialogue going on that I couldn't hear. I waited. It seemed as if she was disappearing and coming back to me, like a whale surfacing and diving. She looked up and spoke clearly for the first time.

"I want surgery to make me someone different from the girl who was abused."

She watched the water bottle turn in her fingers.

"It's very funny, really. You're the first doctor who ever asked me these questions."

The Historical Kaiser Permanente Adverse Childhood Events Study

About 20 years ago physicians at Kaiser Permanente in San Diego, California, devised an ingenious and highly effective supplemented starvation weight-loss program that seemed to have infinite promise. Obesity, aside from its psychosocial and economic effects, is contributing or root causes of type 2 diabetes; heart disease; high blood pressure; nonalcoholic fatty liver disease; degenerative arthritis; breast, colon, kidney, and endometrial cancers; stroke, and probably other diseases that we have not figured out yet. A secure and effective treatment for obesity would be profoundly important. Without conquering obesity, we cannot control healthcare costs.

The program was metabolically sound, safe, and effective—yet (amazingly, it seemed at the time) a complete failure. Half of the patients dropped out. Instead of thin, happy people the program generated depression, divorce, suicide attempts, and anxiety attacks. Many patients, especially those for whom the program had been most successful, regained their lost weight. The researchers reluctantly concluded from this unexpected and counterintuitive result that obesity was not a problem for these patients, but rather a solution.[1, 2] They also uncovered the disturbing fact that behind the medicating effect of overeating were stories of childhood abuse and neglect.[3] These patients were overeating because it helped.[4]

Compelled to look further, Drs. Vincent Felitti from Kaiser Permanente and Robert Anda from the Centers for Disease Control designed a study to determine what types of childhood trauma they were seeing, and ultimately released their findings in more than 17,000 patients. Because of the computerized databank available at Kaiser Permanente, these researchers and subsequent authors were able to explore possible dose-response relationships between childhood trauma prevalences and many common, serious adult diseases.[1, 4–31]

Perhaps most provocative was their study group. Their patients were 50% men and 50% women, middle-class and employed, 80% white or Hispanic, 10% black, and 10% Asian. Seventy-four percent had attended college; average age 57 years. Theirs was not a disadvantaged population, so that the results cannot be dismissed as merely signs of socioeconomic failure.

Specifics of the Study Protocol

The Adverse Childhood Events (ACE) study contained 10 "Yes" or "No," one-point-each questions with subparts totaling 17 topics:

Prior to Your 18th Birthday:

1. Did a parent or other adult in the household **often or very often** . . .

    Swear at you, insult you, put you down, or humiliate you
    or call you things like "lazy," "stupid," or "ugly"?

    > **or**

    Act in a way that made you afraid that you might be physically hurt?

2. Did a parent or other adult in the household **often or very**

    often . . .
    Push, grab, slap, or throw something at you?

    > **or**

    Ever hit you so hard that you had marks or were injured?

3. Did an adult or person at least 5 years older than you **ever** . . .

    Touch or fondle you or have you touch their body in a sexual way?

    > **or**

    Attempt or actually have oral, anal, or vaginal
    intercourse with you?

4. Did you **often or very often** feel that . . .

   No one in your family loved you or thought you were important or special?

   > **or**

   Your family didn't look out for each other, feel close to each other, or support each other?

5. Did you **often or very often** feel that . . .

   You didn't have enough to eat, had to wear dirty clothes, and had no one to protect you?

   > **or**

   Your parents were too drunk or high to take care of you or take you to the doctor if you needed it?

6. Was a biological parent **ever** lost to you through divorce, abandonment, or other reason?

7. Was your mother or stepmother . . .

   Often or very often pushed, grabbed, slapped, or had something thrown at her?

   > **or**

   Sometimes, often, or very often kicked, bitten, hit with a fist or something hard?

   > **or**

   Ever repeatedly hit over at least a few minutes or threatened with a gun or knife?

8. Did you live with anyone who was a problem drinker or used street drugs?
9. Was a household member depressed, mentally ill, or attempted suicide?
10. Did a household member go to prison?

(Adapted from Felitti[9])

The number of positive answers determined the ACE Score.

The authors were careful to group their neglect or abuse question types so that the results would not be exaggerated (e.g., both alcoholism and drug abuse within one household were only scored once).

Results of the Adverse Childhood Events Study

Despite favorable demographics, *only one-third of the study population had an ACE score of zero*. Any patient who had one positive answer also had an 87% chance of having additional positive answers. One patient in 6 had a score of 4 or more. Women were 50% more likely than men to have scores of 5 or more.

By subtype, the prevalences of different adverse childhood event types were as follows: [5]

- Emotional Abuse (humiliating speech or threats): 11%
- Physical Abuse (beatings): 28%
- Contact Sexual Abuse (22% total; 28% women, 16% men)
- Violence toward Mother: 13%
- Alcohol or Drug Abuse in Household: 27%
- Depression, Suicidality, or Chronic Mental Illness in a Household Member: 17%
- Parental Divorce: 23%
- Physical Neglect (not having enough to eat, wear): 10%

Correlations of Trauma to Adult Health

The computerized health databases available for this population allowed correlation of ACE scores with adult health. Their findings should be common knowledge among all healthcare providers, which is regrettably not yet the case.

Straight line, dose-response relationships were found between the ACE score and chronic depression;[21] suicidality;[23] impaired childhood memory;[16, 32] amnesia, or hallucinations;[30] psychosis;[33] use of antidepressants or anti-anxiety medications;[19] unexplainable somatic disorders;[5, 34] smoking;[5] alcohol abuse or illicit drug use;[35] impaired work performance;[5] having 50 or more sexual partners or three or more marriages; risky sexual behavior (teen pregnancy and promiscuity),[5, 14, 36] liver disease;[8, 14] chronic obstructive pulmonary disease;[18] coronary artery disease;[5] fibromyalgia;[37] headaches;[17] autoimmune disease;[24] hypertension, hyperlipidemia, and cancer;[5, 8] and even illnesses for which a stress etiology may be harder to imagine, like multiple sclerosis or primary pulmonary fibrosis.[5, 8, 18]

Even after correcting for all conventional risk factors (hypertension, hyperlipidemia, smoking, family history), these trauma types increased the risk of coronary artery disease by 1.4–1.7 times, depending on the type of abuse.[5, 8, 12, 14, 22, 38–41]

Each point in a patient's total ACE score increased a patient's odds of having another health issue by 33%. Similar adult health consequences followed the inevitable emotional trauma and physical neglect after the 1944–1945 Dutch Winter Famine.[42, 43]

★★★★★

Evidence of the family/disease association is easy to find.[44] In his biography of Theodore Roosevelt, historian David McCullough writes, "Asthma is . . . the family affliction. . . . 'A preternaturally nervous . . . temperament . . . wonderfully favors the attack of asthma.' . . . The onset of an attack . . . was frequently preceded by a spell of depression or 'heaviness' *(what Teedie [Theodore Roosevelt] called feeling 'doleful.') . . . 'Don't scold me,' he would say, if he had incurred his father's displeasure, 'or I shall have the asthma.' And so he would. . . . The likeliest source of the child's anxieties, it has long been thought, is the mother. Asthma is repeatedly described as a 'suppressed cry for the mother'—a cry of rage as well is a cry for help. . . . Mama's love and attention were magic."[45]*

★★★★★

Trauma seizes the body and distorts the mind. Incoming data becomes metabolized and distorted. Facts that cannot be objectively or logically true seem totally real. Musician and composer Brian Wilson recalls this about his childhood:

"I was afraid of my dad. He yelled all the time. . . . He grabbed us. . . . He drank too much. . . . He had trouble with his moods. . . . And then he was gone. . . . I know [my mother] loved me. . . . I know she would've told me so."

Yet later in life and now internationally acclaimed, he still processes his experience through his father's lens.

"Passing the Hollywood Bowl sign that says, 'Tonight, Brian Wilson, Pet Sounds . . . Sold Out' . . . my routine starts. . . . What if the audience doesn't like the show? What if they don't like my music? Suppose the goddamn voices start coming at me?"

". . . I gave myself the nickname . . . 'Brian Willpower Wilson.'. . . . It reminded me the only way to go was forward. . . ."[46]

Such is the power of toxic shame.

The Effect of Multiple ACE Scores

The cumulative effect of multiple ACE scores was impressive: Compared to patients with no ACEs, those with scores of 4 or more adverse childhood events (an intermediate score) had 3 times the likelihood of developing depression or using antidepressants;[47] twice the likelihood of hallucinations[30] or illicit drug use;[5] 5 times the prevalence of memory disturbance;[16] twice the likelihood of unexplained somatic symptoms;[1] twice the likelihood of smoking and 5 times the likelihood of alcohol abuse;[35,15] 4 times the likelihood of serious job problems;[1] 4–5 times the prevalence of early intercourse, teen pregnancy, or paternity;[14] 4 times the likelihood of teen promiscuity;[14] and 5 times the rate of prescription drug use.[5,19] Patients who scored 6 or more had a stunning 50 times greater chance of attempting suicide.[14]

A score of 6 or more predicted a 20-year decrease in life expectancy.[48] Appropriately, the oldest patients had the lowest scores. Consistent with that finding, when patients were stratified by birth year, abuse and neglect prevalences steadily increased over decades. However, among patients born from 1900 to 1931, the rela-tive odds for an ACE score of 6 or greater was lowest despite hardship, despite war.[23] Did older patients just forget more, or was hardship simply better accepted at a time when family ties were stronger and adverse events perhaps less prevalent? Hardship and deprivation during wartime or national poverty are often simply shouldered: "We just did what was necessary," one retired physician told me. *Hardship and trauma are different.* Traumatic experiences have specific meaning to the survivor and always contain the terrifying sense of powerlessness in the face of overwhelming stresses.

★★★★★

Though not fully elaborated, the connecting mechanisms between childhood trauma and adult health are likely to be self-medicating coping strategies (addic-tions or maladaptive behaviors); the effects of chronic, unrelieved stress disrupting neurological and neuroendocrine development and therefore social, emotional, and cognitive impairment; and the compensatory adoption of high-risk behavior, producing disease, disability, societal problems, and early death.[29, 49]

It is also not surprising that 87% of patients who had one answer also had other positive answers (80% in our study; see below). Abuse or neglect does not occur in otherwise perfect, supportive and nurturing families. In the household where the father is molesting his daughter, the ACE score is already 4, regardless of what patients indicate, because emotional abuse, emotional neglect, and physical abuse also co-exist. Mothers too depressed or drug-dependent to take children to the doctor are also likely to neglect their children's emotional and physical needs. A single answer may also reflect denial and memory loss for toxic experiences.[50] ACEs are interrelated, as we have confirmed below.[8, 11, 12]

Felitti also makes the point that patients benefit from being able to tell these dark secrets to someone else.[51] This story-telling is the human connection, missed by health professionals who do not engage and patients who cannot trust. Twenty-five years ago, Moeller and Bachman documented that only 9% of 668 women, 53% of whom recounted at least one type of childhood abuse, had ever been asked about their childhoods.[52] I am skeptical that these numbers have changed significantly since.[36, 53–76]

★★★★★

"It doesn't matter that I'm late. I'm a special case."
I had just entered the room and the atmosphere was already tight.
"And don't ask for my address or Social Security number."
Perhaps she was 50. She wore a black jacket and skirt, a black, broad brimmed hat with a wide ribbon, and black, knee-high boots. The hat was tilted on her head. Her hair was slanted to one side, sprayed and tucked behind an ear. I thought of a 1930's movie poster of Marlene Dietrich.

"Or my age," she added, and settled into the chair.

"I can tell you what's wrong," she added. "It's my nose. My keystone and scroll areas are disgusting."

I waited. She stared at me, hoping for a response. Evidently she liked drama. There was no reason not to be accommodating. It would be dark soon. Besides, I was curious.

"You'll have to show me what you mean," I said. "That's not a diagnosis, I know. But why won't you tell me your age?"

"Because you will hold it against me. You're all quislings." She tipped her head and scanned me, proud of her historical metaphor, and waited to see if I was paying attention.

"You studied more than rhinoplasty," I said.

"You're making fun of me."

I shook my head. "I was just listening."

"You can assume that I'm 40." She had a hard, narrow face with hollow cheeks and thin eyebrows that she had plucked and redrawn at an exotic angle. Her perfume was strong. Maybe she'd never been a child. But she wasn't 40.

"I see that you already had four rhinoplasties," I said. "Who operated on you?"

"I'm not going to tell you. They're your friends so you will lie and tell me they did great work. But my result is dreadful and you know it."

I took in some air. "Let's start with your surgical history."

"I was 12."

"What was wrong with your nose?" I said.

"It was broken." She paused.

"I broke it myself." She laughed as if she had said something witty.

"It was at school. I wanted to get away from my parents, so I got on the swing and crashed into the beam so my nose would break. But they sent me back home. So after I ran away I had surgery."

I was right: she had never been a child. There was no use pushing on that door today.

"What happened then?" I said.

"After the first operation my nose was no better so I went back to have it made smaller. But he made it wider. I looked like a colored woman."

"Black," I said.

She shrugged.

"Same thing," she said.

"No, it isn't," I said.

*She shook her head as if she were already exhausted from talking to me.
I looked more carefully. Her nose was too narrow. Surely she couldn't
breathe well.*

"What don't you like now? Show me."

*Her complexion had the sallow, scored patina of a long-time smoker,
which she tried hard to hide with pancake makeup*

*"I won't look at myself," she said, "but he put silicone in my nose.
I know it. He says he didn't, but he lied. All the other doctors say I should
get a lawyer."*

She looked absently around the room.

"I'll just kill myself if I can't get it right."

She shifted in her chair.

"And now I have fibromyalgia."

*She shook her head. "I didn't think you'd understand. It doesn't matter. I'm
obtaining consultations in New York. I have retained a private referral service.
This time I will have a good result. I won't tolerate any more skullduggery."*

I smiled.

*"I'll bet no one has ever used 'skullduggery' in this building," I said. "But
I can't feel any silicone. I think your surgeon is telling the truth. I don't see
how I can help you."*

Later I realized that there were demons that I would never have
uncovered. Standing in Logan Airport only one month later, my wife
and I saw her photograph on the front page of a Boston newspaper.
"Dominatrix Arraigned in Death of New Hampshire Man . . . Dominatrix accused of dismembering client's body after he died in bondage
session." Skullduggery indeed.

★★★★★

What many patients fear most is not being believed, or discovering that some
ailment only reflects another deficiency. From his experience in *Anatomy of an
Illness*, Cousins writes,

*"There was first of all the feeling of helplessness, a serious disease in
itself. . . . There was the reluctance to be thought the complainer. . . . There
was the conflict between the terror of loneliness and the desire to be left
alone. . . . There was the lack of self-esteem, the subconscious feeling perhaps that our illness was a manifestation of our inadequacy."[77]*

An Adverse Childhood Events Study in Plastic Surgery Patients, with Nick Zaborek, MA

Our own ACE study has been in progress for the past 30 months. To my knowledge, this survey is the first duplication of the original study in a different patient population using precisely the same questions without modifications.

Unlike the original research, we did not administer the survey through mail or routine intake for two reasons. For plastic surgery patients, the questions would have seemed too irrelevant and jarringly intrusive. Also, only consecutive *postoperative* patients were tested, which allowed us to put patient results in context. How demanding had the patients been? Was their behavior depressed or disempowered? Were they accompanied by protective persons who dominated the patients' goals or treatment? How much pain medication did patients need? Did the patients mention shame? What were their current health problems? Most importantly, were the patients satisfied, dissatisfied, or did they request more surgery?

The ability to observe these patients in context over time also allowed an assessment of "resilience," which I defined according to five criteria that assessed how well the patients managed their lives: Did they have appropriate self-esteem, functioning boundaries, observe and react to their surroundings without distorting their sensory input, practice self-care, and live moderated lives? Based on these parameters, the core attributes of functional adults (Chapter 3), resilience was scored from 1 to 4.

Our Patient Demographics

Our study group consisted of 175 consecutive postoperative elective plastic surgery patients. Patients under age 21 were excluded. Participation was explicitly voluntary, but not one patient refused to be included.

One hundred seventy-five patients completed the survey; 133 were women and 42 were men. Ninety-four percent of the patients were Caucasian, 2% black, 2% Asian, and 2% Latino. Their mean age was 56 (youngest 22, oldest 81). Seventy-nine percent had completed college or graduate school. Seventy-five percent were employed, 11% unemployed, and 14% retired. Of the entire group, 85% were aesthetic surgery patients (77% rhinoplasty and 23% other facial surgery or breast surgery) and 15% were reconstructive patients (skin cancers, reconstructive facial surgery, or hand surgery). The great majority of the patients had health insurance and our 148 cosmetic patients (85% of the total group) also had disposable income that would cover the cost of surgery.

Thus our population demographics, though not all general medical patients, shared similarities to the Kaiser group: this was not a disadvantaged population. If we had tested patients known to be refugees, orphans, objects of racial or ethnic discrimination, or those raised in poverty high-crime areas, it is certainly possible that the prevalences would be higher.

Among the 114 rhinoplasty patients, 33% never had nasal surgery; 67% had previous surgery ("revision rhinoplasty patients"). As we had found in our previous research (Chapter 8), 60 patients (77%) of the revision patients originally had normal noses. Because these patients had noses that they knew were normal but underwent surgery anyway they fulfilled the DSM-5 criteria for body dysmorphic disorder. This is the surgical BDD population: we shall consider their results in that context (See Table 9.1).

Results of the ACE Survey*

Table 9.1 compares each of our categories with the Kaiser group. Whereas 67% of the Kaiser patients had at least one positive answer, 80% of ours did ($p < 0.001$). Reconstructive patients had almost the same individual positive scores as the Kaiser patients (70% versus 64%, respectively) and lower ACE scores than all of the cosmetic patient groups, which scored 78%–91%. Not only were our overall prevalences higher than the Kaiser group, but 5 of the 10 individual trauma types were significantly higher than the Kaiser Permanente group (emotional abuse, emotional neglect, physical neglect, household substance abuse, and household mental illness, Table 9.2).

TABLE 9.1 ACE Component Analysis Comparing Kaiser Permanente and Nashua Prevalence

Patient Groups	Any Positive Answer	More Than 4 Positive Answers:	
Kaiser Permanente General Medical Patients:	67%	17%	
All Nashua Plastic Surgery Patients:	80%	34%	
A.C.E Question	Our Value	Kaiser Value	p-Value
1. Emotional Abuse	49	11	0.0001*
2. Physical Abuse	31	28	0.252
3. Sexual Abuse	24	21	0.163
4. Emotional Neglect	42	15	0.0001*
5. Physical Neglect	17	10	0.001*
6. Parental Separation or Divorce	26	23	0.253
7. Mother Treated Violently	15	13	0.223
8. Household Substance Abuse	37	27	0.002*
9. Household Mental Illness	25	19	0.034*
10. Incarcerated Household Member	7	5	0.121

* These values are significantly different between the groups.

We also separated the study groups according to their indications for surgery and found revealing differences:

> The mean ACE score for reconstructive patients was 1.9 but for BDD patients it was 3.1.($p < < 0.03$)

Similarly, whereas 17% of the Kaiser patients had a total of ACE of 5 or more, similar to our reconstructive patients (22%), the cosmetic patient groups had more than double the Kaiser rate at 36–41%. Twice as many women in the Kaiser study had scores of 5 or more; in our group, women also dominated men in scores of 5 or more by a factor of 2.9—all statistically significant differences.

Wherever we looked, our prevalences were worse than the Kaiser Permanente data. Though our reconstructive patients duplicated the Kaiser data closely, all cosmetic surgery patients had suffered noticeably more trauma—the BDD patients among the worst.

Clustering of ACEs

Adverse childhood events ought to occur in groups, and they do: e.g., a family unit can't be otherwise perfect if one of the children is being sexually abused or the mother is repeatedly beaten. Looking at conditional probabilities, emotional abuse, physical abuse, sexual abuse, and emotional neglect all clustered with other types of adverse events.

Among those, emotional abuse was associated with more other types of trauma than the others just mentioned, consistent with the prevalent view in the literature that it is most damaging type.[78–81] Children who were emotionally abused were also traumatized in the following ways with the accompanying percentages: physical abuse (89%), violence toward mother (81%), physical neglect (77%), family member in prison (75%), living with a mentally ill family member (70%), living with an alcohol or drug abuser (64%), sexual abuse (60%), and family divorce (49%).

The second trauma with the greatest associated clustering was emotional neglect, co-occurring with other trauma types in the following percentages: physical neglect (80%), family member in prison (75%), violence toward mother (73%), physical abuse (72%), living with a mentally ill family member (68%), emotional abuse (68%), sexual abuse (62%), and family divorce (56%). Childhood trauma not a discrete pathology in an otherwise perfect household; it is a destructive medium that suffuses the child's life and environment.

ACE Score and Patient Health

Like the Kaiser Permanente study, the number of positive ACE answers correlated with patient health. Even in our small population, dose related correlations existed with obesity, drug use, irritable bowel, asthma and chronic obstructive pulmonary disease, and arthritis. These are manifestations of autonomic dysregulation. Like the Kaiser study, the strongest correlation was with familial drug or alcohol abuse use.[5, 9] It is particularly disturbing to recognize that our patient population, with an average age of 56 (oldest 81), had health problems that correlated with their childhood trauma and—like the PTSD we documented in the last chapter—still manifested 35–50 years later. For many individuals, the effects of childhood do not dissipate: their minds, behaviors, lifestyles, and abilities to care for themselves each suffer.

ACE Score and Personality Characteristics

Furthermore, the number of positive ACE answers correlated strikingly with personality characteristics, specifically perfectionism, disempowered or demanding behavior, and patients who explicitly mentioned "shame" during their interactions with me. These personal traits also clustered: shame was particularly associated with positive ACE answers to emotional abuse, physical abuse, sexual abuse, emotional neglect, physical neglect, violence against the mother, and suicide in the family. Depression was associated with verbal abuse and emotional neglect. Even fibromyalgia correlated with emotional abuse. Disempowered behavior correlated with physical and emotional abuse, but more individual ACE types correlated with shame, childhood trauma's final common denominator: whereas shame was mentioned by 15% of reconstructive patients, it was mentioned by 70% of BDD patients.

Patient Characteristics Associated with Postoperative Satisfaction

Although total ACE score did not correlate with happiness after surgery, certain personality traits were characteristic of unhappy patients—nearly identical to our earlier data (Chapter 8): more than two previous cosmetic surgeries;[†] being unemployed; being disempowered, perfectionistic, demanding, depressed, and shame-filled. These associations should not be surprising: disempowerment and depression are characteristic of low self-esteem; demanding natures are characteristic of grandiosity; shame owns and generates them both.

ACE score did not predict happiness with the surgical outcome, presumably because of the confounding factor of resilience (See Chapter 10).

However,

- those patients who were not disempowered had a 76% chance of being happy after surgery;
- those patients who were not demanding (i.e., had functioning boundaries) had a 70% chance of being happy;

- those patients who were not shamed (i.e., had self-worth) had an 81% chance of being happy;
- those patients who were not perfectionistic (i.e., reality, moderation, self-care) had a 95% chance of being happy;
- and those patients who were resilient had 3.5 times greater chance of being happy than non-resilient patients.

★★★★★

Thus the following characteristics, in descending order of importance, are significantly associated with unqualified postoperative happiness—i.e., no dissatisfaction and no revision requested:

- Not being perfectionistic
- Being older
- Not being disempowered
- Not being shame-filled
- Having had fewer than two previous cosmetic surgeries
- Being resilient

How Our Data Construct a Portrait of Body Dysmorphic and Revision Rhinoplasty Patients

As we scanned our results, the patient data sorted into three distinguishing silos (Table 9.2).

1. *The Combined Cosmetic Non-Rhinoplasty Patients and the Reconstructive Patients.* Neither group had undergone many prior cosmetic surgeries, the majority were happy, most did not want revisions, only 20% mentioned shame, 20% or less were disempowered, 15% or less were demanding, no more than 25% were perfectionistic, and the majority had resilience scores of 4 (ACE > 1 = 70%).

2. *The Primary Rhinoplasty Patients.* Compared to the first group, these patients were still as happy and unlikely to request revision, but they were more likely to mention shame (35%), slightly more likely to be disempowered, and had higher ACE scores than the reconstructive patients (2.6 versus 1.9), though this difference was not statistically significant (ACE > 1 = 75%).

3. *The BDD patients (who originally had normal noses) and the Revision Rhinoplasty Patients (who originally had deformities).* Though unexpected, these patient groups were almost indistinguishable. They started having surgery earliest (in their 20's, rather than 40's or 50's); had the most rhinoplasties (average 3); the most other cosmetic surgeries (averaging 2 versus 0.5 for other patients); were half as likely to be happy and twice as likely to wish revisions than the other groups; expressed shame more commonly (65% to 70% versus 15% to 18%); were twice as likely to be accompanied by overbearing "protective" persons who

tried to dominate the patients' desires; twice as likely to be disempowered, demanding, or perfectionistic; and half as likely to have high resilience scores. The only measured difference between the groups was that the 60 BDD patients had undergone even more cosmetic surgeries (ACE > 1 = 91%).

★★★★★

Close similarities between the body dysmorphic and other revision patients seems counterintuitive: the BDD patients, who knew they never had nasal deformities but had surgery anyway, ought to score differently—i.e., worse-than patients who originally had deformed noses. But they don't. Why not?

There are at least two possibilities. Not everyone who can theoretically benefit from a rhinoplasty has one; the drivers to surgery are complex combinations of personal aesthetics, family values, ethnic identities, and the degree to which self-worth, shame, and body image are interrelated. Shame can compel patients to chase surgery even for minor or imaginary deformities: this incongruity is prominent in the body image literature.[82]

TABLE 9.2 Comparison of Body Dysmorphic and Revision Rhinoplasty Patients with Primary Rhinoplasty Patients, Cosmetic/Non-Rhinoplasty Patients, and Reconstructive Patients

	BDD and Other Revision Rhinoplasty Patients	*Primary Rhinoplasty, Cosmetic / non-Rhinoplasty, And Reconstructive Patients*
Adverse Childhood Events (Trauma) Score	3.1	2.3★
Age at First Cosmetic Surgery, years	25.6	47.5★
Number of Prior Cosmetic Surgeries	2.13	0.51★
Totally Happy with Result After One Operation	42%	82%★
Wanted Revision	53%	16%★
Unhappy	5%	2%
Expressed Shame	69%	24%★
Accompanying Disruptive/Protective Person	34%	16%★
Disempowered	44%	19%★
Demanding	30%	12%★
Perfectionistic	61%	31%★
Resilience Score of 4 (1–4)	34%	59%★

(★ indicates $p < 0.01$ or less)

Second, those personality characteristics exhibited by both groups—shame, perfectionism, demanding nature, disempowerment, and the pressing desire for revision—may not have manifested in the non-BDD revision patients until they had been through unsuccessful surgeries. Time, money, and emotion invested and then seemingly wasted when the results are repeatedly unfavorable can disequilibriate many of us. Recall the patients in Chapter 8 who screened positive for PTSD, some of them 30 years after their rhinoplasties. Surgery deemed unsuccessful by the patient can produce strong—and justifiable—emotions.

A Definition of Surgical Body Dysmorphic Disorder

Thus I believe that these 60 patients who had surgery for normal noses provide an empirical and useful portrait of *"surgical body dysmorphic disorder."* Although surgery is not listed as a compensatory behavior for BDD in the DSM-5, our patients satisfied each diagnostic criterion:

1. A deformity that was not observable: *The patients knew that their noses were normal*
2. Clinical distress: *The patients were driven to see surgeons*
3. Compensatory action: *The patients underwent surgery (an average of three times)*

Thus "surgical body dysmorphic disorder" is determined not by what happens after surgery, but what preceded it. Not every unhappy patient is body dysmorphic; some patients are justifiably unhappy. Postoperative distress is not the key. *The key to surgical body dysmorphic disorder is what drove the surgery: body shame and a desire for self-worth. BDD is a problem of emotions, not deformity.* Like the unhappy patients in many of our vignettes, these patients cite motives of self-esteem, self-perfection, or shame, not only deformity. Any addictive substance is never enough, never satisfies the patient's goal. That is why the size of the deformity—this weird, irreconcilable incongruity—may not justify the patient's level of distress. Why should it? It's not about the deformity.

★★★★★

In a very different patient population—a predominantly elective cosmetic surgery practice—80% of patients still documented histories of childhood trauma. Although there are established data indicating that being non-Caucasian, poor, raised by a single parent,[83] uneducated, or being male predispose to childhood trauma,[84] it does not necessarily follow that being Caucasian, educated, affluent, or female is protective. Interestingly, in both the Permanente study and in ours, the divorce prevalence was only 27% in our group and 23% in the Permanente group. The majority of patients had not even come from broken homes. Even in a largely elective aesthetic surgery population, the data indicate that what we think of as "privilege" sometimes means relatively little.

In many ways, our patient populations are the "lucky ones." The data therefore, like the original Kaiser/Permanente study, has significant societal implications. If we see these prevalences in patients who seem to have many of life's advantages and then were to include those who have withstood poverty, crime, or discrimination, the prevalences can only be imagined and are highly disturbing. How our early years go impacts personality, health, and happiness.

The ACE Study has considerably broadened what we define as "trauma."

The Societal and Public Health Implications of the ACE Data

The ramifications of the ACE data have percolated into the medical literature, though often with insufficient recognition of how much they mean. For example, patients with multiple chronic medical conditions have higher probabilities of substance use disorders or other mental health conditions than those not addicted.[85] Opioid abuse—highly related to the ACE score in our work and in the Kaiser study[5, 9]—is still regarded as a public awareness issue without adequate emphasis given to factors beyond simple availability—no different than the campaigns to reduce obesity that emphasize only nutritional guidance.[86–89] Some authors conclude that failures in substance abuse treatment suffer only from funding, psychiatric, social worker, police, ambulance, and juvenile judge shortages: we need better emergency department protocols, less opiate prescribing, better patient education, and better understanding of illicit fentanyl contamination in heroin.[87, 90] While each of those factors is relevant, other deficiencies—bigger and more common ones—lurk in the family of origin environment, rarely mentioned, even by the most caring researchers. If one one-third of individuals in the United States experience chronic pain—some of whom receive prescription opioids—it would be important to know what percentage of these patients get narcotics for trauma-generated somatic pain.[88] If we focus only on availability and not on motivation and other underlying driving forces, we will not solve the opioid crisis, obesity, alcohol abuse, or any of the dysregulated and self-destructive behaviors prevalent today.

★★★★★

The prevalence of childhood abuse and neglect means that physicians see these patients all day long, doggedly lugging the weight of their childhoods behind them.[91, 92] By recognizing only individual diseases, the physician has already passed the problem without fully appreciating the contributing sources beyond lifestyle or Mendelian genetics. Many adverse traits or "familial" diseases have been as influenced by early childhood environments, with or without their epigenetic impact, as by particularly unlucky coding sequences. Complex diseases are almost always multifactorial. While we search to isolate genetic causes, we cannot afford to overlook other obvious, treatable contributors.

The desire for plastic surgery adds the complex dimension of body image. The nature of attachment, attunement, and childhood environmental safety appears to influence body image and shame, the drive to plastic surgery, patient behavior, personality characteristics, surgical courses, and even patient satisfaction. When we see patients with addictions or BDD or eating disorders or anorexia or chronic pain or obesity, we are also seeing their childhoods.[93]

What This Information Means

All threads have two ends. So far ours has only one. What do we know so far?

From the cauldron of physical obsession and distress that we call body dysmorphic disorder, recurrent themes emerge: absent self-esteem, family disharmony, deliberate self-injury, childhood abuse, body shame, compulsive re-enactment, and dysregulated living seemingly without regard to personal safety. In many cases, body dysmorphic disorder can be traced to a punishing childhood environment.

If we begin with self-injurious, obsessive, intemperate, poor adult health, or addictive behaviors including body dysmorphic disorder and work backward, each began in dysfunctional family systems, shame, and childhood neglect or abuse, seemingly independent of favorable socioeconomic conditions.

If we begin with childhood, the effects of developmental trauma can produce body shame-based, self-injurious, obsessive, intemperate, or addictive behaviors, poor adult health, and BDD.

Thus the connection between family, childhood, body image, and body image disorders works in either direction—starting from childhood or starting from its adult sequelae.

Adding our observations to the existing literature, it is possible to trace a pathway in which childhood trauma is the seed; shame its core manifestation; and dysregulation, addiction, and disease are its poisonous blooms (Figure 9.1).

★★★★★

Consistent with the mental health and plastic surgery literature, it is not surprising that many elective plastic surgery patients have had traumatic childhoods that impact self-worth, boundaries, their views of the world, abilities to live in moderation, and self-care—and that can later manifest as body shame, perfectionism, an obsessive desire for plastic surgery, or postoperative anger, even with good surgical results. *Childhood must be a major component in the genesis of surgical body dysmorphic disorder.* The often inexplicable and sometimes irrational behavior that so taxes theses patients' families, friends, and caregivers is not their fault.

But something is still missing. The ACE score correlates with shame, depression, disempowerment, perfectionism, some diseases, and nasal appearance, but does not predict happiness with a surgical outcome. *The ACE score is not a preoperative screen.* More important seems to be the patient's clinical history, but even there inconsistencies remain.

Resilience makes a decisive impact on patient health, personality characteristics, and happiness with the surgical result, and in doing so disrupts what ought to be a simple connection from a chaotic and injurious childhood to self-harming

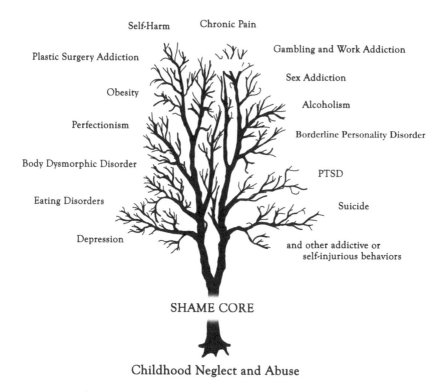

Self-Harm   Chronic Pain

Plastic Surgery Addiction

Gambling and Work Addiction

Sex Addiction

Obesity

Alcoholism

Perfectionism

Borderline Personality Disorder

Body Dysmorphic Disorder

PTSD

Eating Disorders

Suicide

Depression

and other addictive or
self-injurious behaviors

SHAME CORE

Childhood Neglect and Abuse

FIGURE 9.1   The Poisonous Fruits of Trauma and Shame

behaviors and addictions, including plastic surgery. But what is resilience and how does it affect a life? How do some patients pull the sword from the stone? That is where the thread leads next.

Notes

* Several patients whose behavior was immature had ACE scores of zero, which seemed doubtful. If those patients were counted, 87% of our population had at least one positive answer, $p < 0.0000001$—one in 1 million possibility of an erroneous result.
† Seventy-five percent of patients who had < 2 surgeries were satisfied, whereas only 37% of those who had two or more were satisfied ($p < 0.000007$).

References

1. Felitti VJ, Jakstis K, Pepper V, et al. Obesity: Problem, Solution, or Both? *Perm J* 2010; 14:1:24–31.
2. Maercker A, Hilpert P, Burri A. Childhood Trauma and Resilience in Old Age: Applying a Context Model of Resilience to a Sample of Former Indentured Child Laborers. *Aging Ment Health* 2016; 20:6:616–626.

3. Fantuzzo J, Fusco R. Children's Direct Exposure to Types of Domestic Violence Crime: A Population-Based Investigation. *J Fam Violence* 2007; 22:7:543–552.

4. Felitti VJ, Williams SA. Long-Term Follow-Up and Analysis of More Than 100 Patients Who Each Lost More Than 100 Pounds. *Perm J* 1998; 2:3:17–21.

5. Felitti VJ, Anda RF. The Lifelong Effects of Adverse Childhood Experiences, Chapter 10. In *Chadwick's Child Maltreatment: Sexual Abuse and Psychological Maltreatment*, 4th edition. Florissant, MO: STM Learning; 2014.

6. Zlotnick C, Mattia JI, Zimmerman M. The Relationship between Posttraumatic Stress Disorder, Childhood Trauma and Alexithymia in an Outpatient Sample. *J Traumatic Stress* 2001; 14:1:177–188.

7. Watkins LE, Han S, Harpaz-Rotem I, et al. FKBP5 Polymorphisms, Childhood Abuse, and PTSD Symptoms: Results from the National Health and Resilience in Veterans Study. *Psychoneuroendocrinol* 2016; 69:98–105.

8. Felitti VJ, Anda RF, Nordenberg D, et al. Relationship of Childhood Abuse and Household Dysfunction to Many of the Leading Causes of Death in Adults. *Am J Prev Med* 1998; 14:4:245–258.

9. Felitti VJ, Anda RF. The Lifelong Effects of Adverse Childhood Experiences. *Chadwick's Child Maltreat: Sex Abuse Psychol Maltreat* 2014; 2:203–215.

10. Briere J. The Long-Term Clinical Correlates of Childhood Sexual Victimization. *Ann NY Acad Sci* 1988; 528:1:327–334.

11. Felitti VJ. Reverse Alchemy in Childhood: Turning Gold into Lead. *Health Alert* 2001; 8:1:1–11.

12. Dong M, Anda RF, Felitti, VJ, et al. The Interrelatedness of Multiple Forms of Childhood Abuse, Neglect, and Household Dysfunction. *Child Abuse Neglect* 2004; 28:7:771–784.

13. Larsson S, Aas M, Klungsoyr O, et al. Patterns of Childhood Adverse Events Are Associated with Clinical Characteristics of Bipolar Disorder. *BMC Psychiatry* 2013; 13:97:1–9.

14. Felitti VJ, Anda RF. *The Relationship of Adverse Childhood Experiences to Adult Medical Disease, Psychiatric Disorders and Sexual Behavior: Implications for Healthcare. The Hidden Epidemic: The Impact of Early Life Trauma on Health and Disease.* Edited by Lanius R and Vermetten E. Cambridge, U.K.: Cambridge University Press; 2009:2–18.

15. Felitti VJ. Origins of Addictive Behavior: Evidence from a Study of Stressful Childhood Experiences. *Praxis der Kinderpsychologie und Kinderpsychiatrie* 2003; 52:8:1–13.

16. Brown DW, Anda RF, Edwards VJ, et al. Adverse Childhood Experiences and Childhood Autobiographical Memory Disturbance. *Child Abuse Neglect* 2007; 31:9:961–969.

17. Anda R, Tietjen G, Schulman E, et al. Adverse Childhood Experiences and Frequent Headaches in Adults. *Headache* 2010; 50:1473–1481.

18. Anda RF, Brown DW, Dube SR, Bremner JD, Felitti VJ, Giles WH. Adverse Childhood Experiences and Chronic Obstructive Pulmonary Diseases in Adults. *Am J Prev Med* 2008; 34:396–403.

19. Anda RF, Brown DW, Felitti VJ, et al. Adverse Childhood Experiences and Prescribed Psychotropic Medications in Adults. *Am J Prevent Med* 2007; 32:5:389–394.

20. Anda RF, Fleisher VI, Felitti VJ, et al. Childhood Abuse, Household Dysfunction, and Indicators of Impaired Worker Performance in Adulthood. *Perm J* 2004; 8:1:30–38.

21. Chapman DP, Whitfield CL, Felitti VJ, et al. Adverse Childhood Experiences and the Risk of Depressive Disorders in Adulthood. *J Affect Disord* 2004; 82:217–225.

22. Dong M, Giles WH, Felitti VJ, et al. Insights Into Causal Pathways for Ischemic Heart Disease: Adverse Childhood Experiences Study. *Circulation* 2004; 110:1761–1766.

23. Dube SR, Anda RF, Felitti VJ. Childhood Abuse, Household Dysfunction, and the Risk of Attempted Suicide Throughout the Life Span: Findings from the Adverse Childhood Experiences Study. *JAMA* 2001; 286:24:3089–3096.

24. Dube SR, Fairweather D, Pearson WS, et al. Cumulative Childhood Stress and Autoimmune Diseases in Adults. *Psychosom Med* 2009; 71:2:243–250.

25. Edwards VJ, Dube SR, Felitti VJ, et al. It's OK to Ask About Past Abuse. *Am Psychol* 2007; 62:327–328; discussion 330–332.

26. Lee C. Childhood Abuse and Elevated Markers of Inflammation in Adulthood: Do the Effects Differ Across Life Course Stages? *Psychosom Med* 2013; 75:3.

27. Meyer N, Richter H, Schreiber RS, et al. The Unexpected Effects of Beneficial and Adverse Social Experiences During Adolescence on Anxiety and Aggression and Their Modulation by Genotype. *Front Behav Neurosci* 2016; 10:97–124.

28. Nurius PS, Green S, Logan-Greene P, et al. Life Course Pathways of Adverse Childhood Experiences Toward Adult Psychological Well-Being: A Stress Process Analysis. *Child Abuse Neglect* 2015; 45:143–153.

29. Weiss JS, Wagner SH. What Explains the Negative Consequences of Adverse Childhood Experiences on Adult Health? Insights From Cognitive and Neuroscience Research (Editorial). *Am J Prev Med* 1998; 14:356–360.

30. Whitfield CL, Dube SR, Felitti VJ, et al. Adverse Childhood Experiences and Hallucinations. *Child Abuse Neglect* 2005; 29:7:797–810.

31. Winzeler K, Voellmin A, Hug E, et al. Adverse Childhood Experiences and Autonomic Regulation in Response to Acute Stress: The Role of the Sympathetic and Parasympathetic Nervous Systems. *Anxiety Stress Coping* 2016; 1:1–10.

32. Bottoms BL, Najdowski CJ, Epstein MA, et al. Trauma Severity and Defensive Emotion-Regulation Reactions as Predictors of Forgetting Childhood Trauma. *J Trauma Diss* 2012; 13:291–310.

33. Reininghaus U, Gayer-Anderson C, Valmaggia L, et al. Psychological Processes Underlying the Association between Childhood Trauma and Psychosis in Daily Life: An Experience Sampling Study. *Psychol Med* 2016; 46:13:2799–2813.

34. Simon NM, Herlands NN, Marks EH, et al. Childhood Maltreatment Linked to Greater Symptom Severity and Poorer Quality of Life and Function in Social Anxiety Disorder. *Depress Anxiety* 2009; 26:11:1027–1032.

35. Langeland W, Draijer N, van den Brink W. Psychiatric Comorbidity in Treatment-Seeking Alcoholics: The Role of Childhood Trauma and Perceived Parental Dysfunction. *Alcohol Clin Exp Res* 2004; 28:3:441–447.

36. SmithBattle L, Freed P. Teen Mothers' Mental Health. MCN *Am J Matern Child Nurs* 2016; 41:1:31–36.

37. Low LA, Schweinhardt P. Early Life Adversity as a Risk Factor for Fibromyalgia in Later Life. *Pain Res Treat* 2012; 1–15.

38. Lanius RA, Vermette E, Pain C, eds. *The Impact of Early Life Trauma On Health And Disease: The Hidden Epidemic.* Cambridge [UK]: Cambridge University Press; 2010.

39. Coughlin SS. Post-Traumatic Stress Disorder and Cardiovascular Disease. *Open Cardiovasc Med J* 2011; 5:164–170.

40. Cuijpers P, Smit F, Unger F, et al. The Disease Burden of Childhood Adversities in Adults: A Population-Based Study. *Child Abuse Neglect* 2011; 35:937–945.

41. Kaplow JB, Saxe GN, Putnam FW, et al. The Long-Term Consequences of Early Childhood Trauma: A Case Study and Discussion. *Psychiatry* 2006; 69:4:362–375.

42. Roseboom T, deRooij S, Painter R. The Dutch Famine and Its Long-Term Consequences for Adult Health. *Early Hum Develop* 2006; 82:485–491.
43. Schulz LC. The Dutch Hunger Winter and the Developmental Origins of Health and Disease. *Proc Natl Acad Sci* 2010; 107:39:16757–16758.
44. Hornor G. Childhood Trauma Exposure and Toxic Stress: What the PNP Needs to Know. *J Pediatric Health Care* 2015; 29:2:191–198.
45. McCullough D. *Mornings On Horseback: The Story Of An Extraordinary Family, A Vanished Way Of Life, And The Unique Child Who Became Theodore Roosevelt.* New York: Simon & Schuster; 1981:90–98.
46. Wilson, B. *I Am Brian Wilson.* Boston: DaCapo Press, 2016:136–138, 161, 270, 283–284.
47. Gaon A, Kaplan Z, Dwolatzky T, et al. Dissociative Symptoms as a Consequence of Traumatic Experiences: The Long-Term Effects of Childhood Sexual Abuse. *Isr J Psychiatry Relat Sci* 2013; 50:1:17–23.
48. Keller A, Litzelman K, Wisk LE, et al. Does the Perception That Stress Affects Health Matter? The Association with Health and Mortality. *Health Psychol* 2012; 31:5:677–684.
49. Russek LG, Schwartz GE. Feeling of Parental Caring Predict Health Status in Midlife: A 35-Year Follow-Up of the Harvard Mastery of Stress Study. *J Behavioral Med* 1997; 20:1:1–13.
50. MacDonald K, Thomas ML, MacDonald TM, et al. A Perfect Childhood? Clinical Correlates of Minimization and Denial on the Childhood Trauma Questionnaire. *J Interpers Violence* 2015; 30:6:988–1009.
51. Becker-Blease KA, Freyd JJ. Research Participants Telling the Truth about Their Lives: The Ethics of Asking and Not Asking About Abuse. *Am Psychol* 2006; 61:3:218–226.
52. Moeller TP, Bachmann GA, Moeller JR. The Combined Effects of Physical, Sexual, and Emotional Abuse During Childhood: Long-Term Health Consequences for Women. *Child Abuse Neglect* 1993; 17:623–640.
53. Davenport S, Goldberg D, Millar T. How Psychiatric Disorders Are Missed During Medical Consultations. *The Lancet* 1987 August; 439–440.
54. Epstein RM. Responding to Suffering. *JAMA* 2015; 314:24:2623–2624.
55. Adler HM. A Piece of My Mind—Actually. *JAMA* 2015; 314:16:1693–1694.
56. Berman SI. Gripers and Whiners. *JAMA* 2015; 313:16:1621–1622.
57. Bredlau A. Where Do You Put the Pain? *JAMA* 2016; 315:10:983.
58. Butow PN, Brown RF, Cogar S, et al. Oncologists' Reactions to Cancer Patients' Verbal Cues. *Psycho-Oncology* 2002; 11:47–58.
59. Colloca L, Finniss D. Nocebo Effects, Patient-Clinician Communication, and Therapeutic Outcomes. *JAMA* 2012; 307:6:567–568.
60. Del Piccolo L, Saltini A, Zimmermann C, et al. Differences in Verbal Behaviours of Patients with and without Emotional Distress During Primary Care Consultations. *Psychol Med* 2000; 30:629–643.
61. Del Piccolo L, Saltini A, Zimmermann C. Which Patients Talk about Stressful Life Events and Social Problems to the General Practitioner? *Psychol Med* 1998; 28:1289–1299.
62. Detsky AS. Reducing the Trauma of Hospitalization. *JAMA* 2014; 311:21:2169–2170.
63. Galint M. The Doctor, His Patient, and the Illness (revised). New York: International Universities Press; 1972, quoted in: Felitti VJ, Jakstis K, Pepper V, et al. Obesity: Problem, Solution, or Both? *Perm J* 2010; 14:1:24.
64. George DR, Greene MJ. Lessons Learned from Comics Produced by Medical Students. *JAMA* 2015; 314:22:2345–2346.
65. Goldberg DP, Jenkins L, Millar T, et al. The Ability of Trainee General Practitioners to Identify Psychological Distress among Their Patients. *Psychol Med* 1993; 23:185–193.

66. Gupta S. The Other Generation. *JAMA* 2015; 313:13:1319–1320.

67. Hall JA, Irish JT, Roter DL, et al. Gender in Medical Encounters: An Analysis of Physician and Patient Communication in a Primary Care Setting. *Health Psychol* 1994; 13:5:384–392.

68. Hall JA, Roter DL, Katz NR. Meta-Analysis of Correlates of Provider Behavior in Medical Encounters. *Medical Care* 1988; 26:7:657–675.

69. Kupfer JM. The Graying of US Physicians: Implications for Quality and the Future Supply of Physicians. *JAMA* 2016; 315:4:341–342.

70. Laskowski RJ. The Power of "My." *JAMA* 2016; 315:12:1235.

71. Maguire P, Faulkner A. Booth K, et al. Helping Cancer Patients Disclose Their Concerns. *Eur J Cancer* 1995; 32A:1:78–81.

72. Schneiderman H. Efficacy at the Bedside. *JAMA* 2015; 313:6:569–570.

73. Shaw WS, Pransky G, Winters T, et al. Does the Presence of Psychosocial "Yellow Flags" Alter Patient-Provider Communication for Work-Related, Acute Low Back Pain? *J Occup Environ Med* 2009; 51:9:1032–1040.

74. Smith RC, Hoppe RB. The Patient's Story: Integrating the Patient- and Physician-Centered Approaches to Interviewing. *Ann Inter Med* 1991; 115:6:470–477.

75. Stewart MA. What Is a Successful Doctor-Patient Interview? A Study of Interactions and Outcomes. *Soc Sci Med* 1984; 19:2:167–175.

76. Zimmermann C, Del Piccolo L. Cues and Concerns by Patients in Medical Consultation: A Literature Review. *Psychol Bull* 2007; 133:3:438–463.

77. Cousins N. *Anatomy of An Illness As Perceived By The Patient: Reflections On Healing And Regeneration.* New York: W W Norton & Company; 1979.

78. Mellody P, Freundlich LS. *The Intimacy Factor: The Ground Rules For Overcoming The Obstacles To Truth, Respect, And Lasting Love.* New York: Harper Collins; 2003.

79. Massie H, Szajnberg N. My Life Is a Longing: Child Abuse and Its Adult Sequelae: Result of the Brody Longitudinal Study from Birth to Age 30. *Int J Psychoanal* 2006; 87:471–496.

80. McFarlane A, Yehuda R. Resistance, Vulnerability, and the Course of Posttraumatic Reactions. In: van der Kolk B, McFarlane AC, Weisaeth L, eds. *Traumatic Stress.* New York: The Guilford Press; 2007:170.

81. Herman J, Russell D, Trocki K. Long-Term Effects of Incestuous Abuse in Childhood. *Am J Psychiatry* 1986; 143:10:1293–1296.

82. Cash TF, Smolak, eds. *Body Image: A Handbook Of Science, Practice, And Prevention.* New York: The Guilford Press; 2011.

83. Kendler KS, Neale MC, Kessler RC, et al. Childhood Parental Loss and Adult Psychopathology in Women. *Arch Gen Psychiatry* 1992; 49:109–116.

84. Koenen KC, Roberts AL, Stone DM, et al. The Epidemiology of Early Childhood Trauma. In: Lanius RA, Vermette E, Pain C, eds. *The Impact of Early Life Trauma On Health And Disease: The Hidden Epidemic.* Cambridge [UK]: Cambridge University Press; 2010:13–24.

85. Knickman J, Krishnan R, Pincus H. Improving Access to Effective Care for People with Mental Health and Substance Use Disorders. *JAMA* 2016; 316:16:1647–1648.

86. Schore AN. *The Science of the Art of Psychotherapy.* New York: W W Norton & Company; 2012:395.

87. Dowell D, Noonan RK, Houry D. Underlying Factors in Drug Overdose Deaths. *JAMA* 2017; 318:23:2295–2296.

88. Gostin LO, Hodge JG, Noe SA. Reframing the Opioid Epidemic as a National Emergency. *JAMA* 2017; 318:16:1539–1540.

89. Kolodny A, Frieden TR. Ten Steps the Federal Government Should Take Now to Reverse the Opioid Addition Epidemic. *JAMA* 2017; 318:16:1537–1538.

90. Rosland A. Assuming the Worst. *JAMA* 2015; 313:22:2229–2230.

91. Briggs-Gowan MJ, Ford, JD, Fraleigh L, et al. Prevalence of Exposure to Potentially Traumatic Events in a Healthy Birth Cohort of Very Young Children in the Northeastern United States. *J Traumatic Stress* 2010; 23:6:725–733.

92. Christoffersen MN, Armour C, Lasgaard M, et al. The Prevalence of Four Types of Childhood Maltreatment in Denmark. *Clin Pract Epidemiol Ment Health* 2013; 9:1:149–156.

93. Powers AD, Thomas KM, Ressler KJ, et al. The Differential Effects of Child Abuse and Posttraumatic Stress Disorder on Schizotypal Personality Disorder. *Compr Psychiatry* 2011; 52:4:438–445.

10

RESILIENCE

The Antidote and the Inspiration

Resilience is the great confounder. It empowers those whose lives have not begun well. It emboldens the fainthearted and strengthens the weak. In my own patient data, resilient patients are healthier and happier, even when their childhood environments have been dangerous, violent, tumultuous, and frightening and ought to have produced the types of brain and body damage, self-medicating behavior, addictions, and self-destruction that we can observe instead.[1] But that doesn't happen. Resilience is the antidote to trauma.

★★★★★

> "The most sacred thing in this universe is personality," says Fosdick, who might well have been describing resilience. "Powerful personality is never created simply by thought and work. Powerful personality has deep interior resources of inspiration and intake. . . . Great living is not all output in creative thought and work; it is also intake, the openness of the soul . . . those that can hear a still small voice. . . . Every time there are new branches, there must be stronger roots."[2]

And this from my friend Dee Steed, a wrangler in Wickenburg, AZ:
> Wet saddle blankets make good horses.

★★★★★

DOI: 10.4324/9781315657721-15

The Paradox of Happiness

Twenty-five years ago, Richard Bentall, a psychologist in Liverpool, England, wrote a cleverly provocative essay about happiness. He noted that truly happy people are seemingly rare, exhibit cognitive distortions (because who can really be optimistic?), try to force their moods on others, often behave in carefree, uninhibited manners, sometimes indulging in behaviors with life-threatening consequences (such as eating and drinking to excess), don't dwell on sad events (which shows impaired memory), and are *prima facie* irrational because happiness isn't grounded in reality. Bentall proposed therefore that happiness be classified in the DSM as a "Major Affective Disorder, Pleasant Type."[3]

While Bentall meant to be waggish, he accurately describes what we have noted repeatedly so far: Some people can be happy, optimistic, even triumphant despite life events that might, perhaps even should produce depression, addictions—substitutes for self-esteem[4]—or failure.[5, 6] We call these people "resilient." What does that mean, and how do they get that way?

★★★★★

"If you don't mind, my wife and I would like you to tell us what's wrong with her nose, before she tells you."

What an unusual request, I thought. Most patients cannot wait to flood me with the details of their own facial flaws.

"I don't prefer to do that," I said. "I think it's important for patients to define what is normal and what they wish were different, not me."

They both looked grim. Immaculately and conservatively dressed, she sat on the edge of my examination table with her hands folded in her lap, her ankles crossed, and her legs motionless. He leaned forward, elbows on his knees with his chin resting on his clasped fingers.

"We are an unusual case," he said, looking expectantly at his wife. It was her turn.

Her head remained down, but I could see her eyes slowly scanning the space in front of her. Doubt and melancholy played on her face.

"I have had BDD since I was in second grade," she said. Her voice was so soft I could barely hear it. "That's why the other plastic surgeon sent me to you."

I shook my head. "I am not a therapist," I said. "But I still may be able to direct you."

I thought about what she had told me.

"I've only met one other patient who knew that he had body dysmorphic disorder. Tell me your story."

Suddenly she looked directly at me. *"I can remember exactly when it started. In the playground this little girl came up to me . . ."* She dropped her chin and craned her head toward the ceiling to mimic the child's motion. Her face tightened.

"She looked at me and said, 'Your nose holes are too big.' That started it. Even in kindergarten the other children wouldn't play with me because of how I looked. It's been that way all my life."

She paused, and stared at the floor again, defocused. I didn't have anything to say yet, so I waited.

"Then I had rhinoplasty in my thirties. See. . . . The doctor cut me here. But my nose looked better before." She nodded to herself.

For an early spring afternoon, it seemed unusually dark. Rain slid down the window in little rivulets. Already people were hurrying across the parking lot to their cars.

I looked at her intake sheet.

"But you have worked all your life. That's uncharacteristic of many BDD patients."

"Yes, I know," she said.

"You teach."

"I do."

"I'll bet you are a very good teacher."

We were quiet. She looked at me for a while.

"Do you think you are a good teacher?" I said.

She lifted her shoulders in a small shrug. *"I had a good education."*

I smiled to myself at her deflection.

"The seeds still had to fall on fertile ground," I said.

She gave a small, solemn nod.

"I guess."

"So, are you a good teacher?"

She remained impassive. *"That's what they tell me."*

I did a quick calculation in my head.

"That means you've had BDD for sixty-five years."

Something unreadable passed across her face.

"There are a lot of ways to die."

I waited. Apparently she wasn't going to continue.

"You've had treatment for your BDD," I said softly.

She closed her eyes and let out a long sigh. "Oh, yes. Cognitive behavior therapy for thirty years."

She gave one of those little non-judgmental head gestures.

"They've done everything they can. It's just not helping me. Now I need another surgery." Her tone was still empty of inflection.

"BDD runs in families, you know," I said. "Twenty percent of patients have at least one affected first degree relative."

She brightened as if she'd heard something new. "I'm certain that's true. I know my aunt had it, and I'll bet my mother had it."

"And then they raised you," I said.

She nodded like a woman resigned to a consolation prize.

"But see. . ." she said, turning her head in front of the mirror. "From this profile it looks okay; when I turn my head like this, it's not so good. From the front, I'm not sure. But from this profile . . ."

She closed her eyes in a tiny shudder.

"I think people are disgusted when they see me from this side."

I was feeling something but didn't know exactly what it was. Perhaps empathy, perhaps just sadness.

Her husband raised his hand in benediction. "We're looking for your ideas. I love my wife." He sighed. "But I don't see what she sees."

I told her about my trauma research. As we spoke I had calculated an ACE score of 5: physical abuse and neglect, emotional abuse and neglect, alcoholism and mental illness in the family. There were probably others. There are often others.

"Your asymmetries are real, but I think you would be unhappy with surgery right now, even if I gave you what you asked. If CBT isn't helping you, let's try a different kind of trauma workshop. Then come back if you still want surgery."

There is no point in thinking about alternatives if you don't have any.

★★★★★

Resilience in the Literature

Just as it has been easier to find data about body dissatisfaction than about body satisfaction, it has always been easier to find studies cataloging the psychological and physical ravages of trauma than stories about the irrepressible survivors, the heroes. Now, however, there is an accumulating body of good research on resilience, which may encourage the sufferers.

Resilience has been studied for its biological, cognitive, and affective lifetime, social, and public policy ramifications. The major areas of agreement can be most efficiently captured in a series of bullet points.[7–10]

Generalizations

- Resilience is successful, flexible, *and sustainable* adaptation to adversity,[11–14]— the capacity to rebound.[15]
- Resilience is not only whether you recover, but how fast.
- Individual resilience is the amount of stress that someone can endure without losing the ability to pursue his or her meaningful life goals.
- Resilience is multifactorial and not just the opposite of vulnerability; different physiologic mechanisms are operative.[16]
- Resilience is characterized by empathy, optimism, humor, and social interconnectedness.[17, 18]
- Resilient, optimistic individuals have fewer physical symptoms and recover from surgery faster; their blood pressures are lower and their immune function is better.[19, 20]
- Our research confirms that resilient patients are not only healthier but have fewer aesthetic surgeries and are more likely to be happy with their outcomes (Chapter 9 and Table 9.2).
- Resilience, self-esteem, self-sufficiency, and lack of depression are more common among those who have had work stressors as young adults compared to individuals with little prior work stress: a graph of adversity (*x*-axis) versus life satisfaction (*y*-axis) forms a bell—shaped curve. Those who have overcome adversity report elevated capacities for enjoying life.[21–23] However, much data is self-reported, introducing a confounder.[24, 25]

*****

- A 24-year follow-up of 152 Harvard graduates exposed to combat in World War II indicated that those eager to join the military and despite stress symptoms when exposed to danger, later in life were well adjusted, not depressed or alcoholic, had good health, good psychosocial adjustment, and were more likely to be listed in *Who's Who in America*.[26]
- Resilience can be measured by a scale that measures "dispositional attributes" (self-esteem, hope, and realistic life orientation); "family cohesion and warmth" (family cooperation, loyalty, and stability); and "external support systems" from friends and relatives.[27] These criteria parallel the five core attributes of functional adults (self-worth, intact boundaries, accurate reality processing, living in moderation, and self-care[28]) detailed in Chapter 3.
- Resilient individuals display humor, "cognitive flexibility"—the ability to grow from disasters,[29] do not place blame, presume that any problem can be solved, assign positive meaning to events, redefine crises as challenges, and even look at disasters as positive and beneficial; this is "posttraumatic growth," shown to improve health in patients with colorectal or lung cancer.[30] Religious faith, spirituality, altruism, social support, mentors, role models,[31] and active, problem-solving attitudes seem to be critical resilience factors.[6, 29, 31–34, 36]

*****

In the fascinating *River of Doubt: Theodore Roosevelt's Darkest Journey*, author Candace Millard describes the power of unseen forces, our recurring theme:

> *"The most immediate problem was how to negotiate the river itself. . . . Even a seemingly benign ripple could be deadly. The danger was in the eddy line, the point at which the current, which is running downstream, collides with the eddy, which is heading upstream, causing a powerful and chaotic swirl of water just under the surface."*[35]

How Trauma Influences Resilience in Humans and Animals

- Unremitting verbal abuse and neglect are powerful stimuli for adult depression, anxiety disorders, and other aspects of the emerging adult personality.[11]
- In experimental animals, chronic unpredictable stress induces anxious behavior and anhedonia, decreased interest in novel foods, decreased grooming, and more aggressive physical and sexual behavior. Many of these stress-induced changes can be reversed by antidepressants.[36]
- Gender differences exist: female rodents succumb to chronic unpredictable stress in 6 days, whereas males are resilient until 20–28 days.[33]
- Behavioral changes influenced in rodents by chronic unpredictable stress, chronic social defeat stress, and learned helplessness are reflected in weight gain, insulin insensitivity, elevated corticosteroid levels and reductions in hippocampal synaptic spine number, all of which can be reversed by antidepressants.[33]
- Chronic, unpredictable stress, experienced by so many children in chaotic homes, produces a variety of depressive, anxious, and despairing behavior manifested as the inability to enjoy pleasurable foods, explore novel foods, impaired grooming, increased aggression, and abnormal sexual behavior.[37]
- In a long-term study of 76 abused and non-abused individuals followed till age 30, 53% of the non-abused were secure, whereas only 20% of the abused were secure.

  - Early in life, the abused children manifested somatic symptoms (predisposition to illness, injuries, insomnia, obesity, headaches, gastrointestinal symptoms) and personality problems (narcissism, schizoid or anhedonic personalities, or low self-esteem). Some symptoms appeared as early as age 1, many by age 7, and all by age 18.[11]
  - In this same study, the child of a neglectful mother who was preoccupied with her appearance became excessively concerned with her own body even as an infant, and by age 6 was significantly depressed.[11]
  - Ninety percent of the children in this study were resilient, measured by stable adult relationships in gainful employment. The resilient children's defenses were rationalization, intellectualization, humor, self-observation, sublimation through writing, addictions, and high-risk behavior.

- Hypertension, hypercholesterolemia, diabetes, obesity, chronic inflammation, a history of mental illness, depression, a history of childhood trauma, and being a victim of violent crime each threaten resilience.[38–40]
- Despite childhood trauma (Adverse Childhood Events) many children still become competent, well-adjusted adults because of "protective factors," "core resources,"[41] "pre-crisis resilience,"[42] early life experiences,[43, 44] and "adaptive capacity."[15, 23, 25, 29, 45–47]
- Resilience following childhood maltreatment often comes at the price of emotional vulnerability and compromise potential: e.g., as adults these individuals often choose work that is beneath their capacities, not work that they might have chosen if they had recognized their self-worth.[11]

Neurophysiologic Characteristics of Resilience

- Resilient individuals have healthy HPA-axis function,[33, 48] appropriate cortisol, norepinephrine, serotonin (attunement), dopamine (reward system [DRD4-exIII-VNTR genotype[49]]), (social caregiving) oxytocin,[50, 51] Neuropeptide Y, brain-derived neurotrophic factor and galanin levels,[8, 52] high DHEA-cortisol ratios, and absence of the short allele of the 5-HT transporter gene promoter polymorphism.[6]
- Neural circuits for reward, fear-conditioning and social behavior are well regulated in resilience but not in trauma and depression.[53, 54, 55]
- Research in Romanian orphans indicates that impairments from deprived environments do not persist when the child is adopted by the age of 6 months, but children institutionalized up to 12 months or beyond had impairments that lasted for many years, presumably from neural damage or biological reprogramming.[56]
- Adoption studies do not identify specific resilience genes, but environmental influences affect resilience.[8]
- Genetic and epigenetic influences,[57, 58] do not operate without environmental influences; thus parental resilience does not guarantee resilience in their children.[17]
- Epigenetic influences create synaptic changes and rewiring that affect resilience. Optimal early life experience appears to reduce stimulation of hypothalamic CRH (corticotropin releasing hormone)—producing neurons, whereas chronic, fragmented maternal care excites these same neurons. Synaptic plasticity probably initiates epigenetic expression programs that persist, perhaps even the subsequent generations. Thus resilience may be transgenerational.[44, 48]
- Animal models that simulate prenatal and early life stress manifest in adult outcomes as a U-shaped curve: moderate stress in early life allows better adaptation than minimal or severe stress.[33] Prolonged maternal separation or social isolation, however, increase stress and produce "despair-like" behavior.

- "Chronic social defeat stress," in which a test mouse is repeatedly subordinated by a larger, aggressive mouse, results in depressive behavior, social avoidance, anhedonia (i.e., inability to feel pleasure), learned helplessness, and weight gain. It is not hard to imagine the parallels to bullied teens.[44]

★★★★★

- These types of observable behavioral, neurochemical, and hormonal changes, as well as differences in brain micromorphology have been confirmed in rodents as well as humans. "Stress inoculation" in rodents—early life stress (including maternal separation and neonatal corticosteroid administration) alters HPA-axis function and is modified by maternal behavior in early life. Hippocampal glucocorticoid receptors become more responsive in resilient mice; and other mediators (increased thyroid hormone secretion, hippocampal serotonin turnover, and hippocampal expression of nerve growth factor inducible-protein A) reflect this maternal nurturing.[33] When these stress-inoculated animals mature, anxious behavior is harder to produce and cognitive tasks are performed better.
- Early life experiences and stress (the quality of maternal care and handling, maternal separation) create both cognitive and emotional vulnerabilities in rodents that can be measured by up-regulation of glucocorticoid receptors in the hippocampus and repression of corticotropin releasing hormone in the hypothalamus. Maternal nurturing (grooming and licking) induces synaptic rewiring, confirmed in murine pups, reduced hypothalamic stress sensitivity, and in turn affects intracellular programs. These synaptic changes induce genetic regulatory pathways and epigenetic mechanisms. Optimal early life experiences calm hypothalamic neurons, just like early stress and chaotic maternal care increase excitation in the same neurons.

★★★★★

- Gender-related changes are complex, so that women test superiorly to men in some resilience measurements and inferiorly in others. Women show greater cognitive and memory resilience, whereas men display better emotional resilience.[8, 32, 43, 59]
- A study of children with court-documented abuse and neglect before age 11 indicated that 30% were resilient at age 29 (women more resilient than men, as researchers have established).[8, 27]
- Genetic predisposition to neuroticism, extraversion, and openness influence stress sensitivity and resilience in older individuals.
- Behavioral changes induced by maternal behavior persist into adulthood.[51]
- Happiness, cognitive flexibility, active coping style, life meaning, social support, positive affect, humor,[60] mental toughness, psychological well-being, religiosity, and low catechol-0-methyltransferase (COMT) levels (which

permit higher brain dopamine) are beneficial to cognitive functioning and maintaining resilience.[8]

- Stress exposure reduces normal hippocampal neurogenesis, which can be reversed by some antidepressants, though it is not yet clear whether neurogenesis promotes resilience or stress susceptibility.[61]
- These stressors create measurable changes in the human autonomic nervous system, glucocorticoid response, serotonin levels, the locus coeruleus–norepinephrine system, and the HPA. Markers such as dehydroepiandrosterone (DHEA) and neuropeptide-Y have become measurable biomarkers for resilience and stress.
- Added to the mix are effects that reproductive hormones may have on stress susceptibility and resilience: because mood disorders and depression are twice as prevalent in women as men, sex hormone fluctuations may be significant factors. Conversely, testosterone appears to be protective in men for social connectedness, dominance, and stress tolerance; low testosterone levels are often found in patients with PTSD or major depressive disorder.

★★★★★

- Cortisol, DHEA, corticotropin releasing hormone (both CRA-1 and CRA-2), the locus ceruleus–norepinephrine system, Neuropeptide Y, dopamine, serotonin, benzodiazepine receptors, testosterone and estrogen each respond to stress; each is reflected in neurophysiologic brain changes, and each may affect resilience by reducing or augmenting environmental stress response in experimental animals.[5, 6, 58, 62]
- Cytokines, soluble proteins released by white blood cells at inflammatory or infectious sites, cross the blood-brain barrier and create the social withdrawal and anorexia that occur in illness and depression. Other details beyond our scope can be found in several excellent reviews.[6, 7, 32, 33] Clinicians often observe that uncontrolled patient stress impairs wound healing and increases the likelihood of complications.
- So-called reward circuitry in the mesiocorticolimbic system (medial pre-frontal cortex, hippocampus, nucleus accumbens, amygdala, ventral tegmental area, lateral hypothalamus, lateral habenula, and other regions) response to psychological and thinking processes are impacted by stress and compromised by depression or anxiety. Dopamine, GABA (gamma-aminobutyric acid), and other mediators modulate brain activity, respond to antidepressants, foster resilience appropriate circumstances, and are susceptible to epigenetic influences.[33]
- Increased amygdala activity is reflected in angry and sad faces.[48]

Thus early life stressors—physical, sexual, or emotional abuse or neglect—produce long-lasting and interrelated hormonal, neurotransmitter, and central nervous system changes that last into adulthood.[17, 63, 64]

Family Environment and Resilience

"Positive parenting" promotes resilience through mechanisms not fully understood:[65]

- Childhood family environment characteristics predict resilience even after controlling for demographics, trauma exposure, maltreatment, and PTSD symptoms. A warm, stable, nurturing, affectionate, loving atmosphere predicted resilience despite poverty, family discord, or environmental trauma outside the family.[50] These results emphasize the dominance of caring family settings in producing resilience, despite intrafamilial and community obstacles.
- Parental quality during childhood is the most potent predictor of resilience in adulthood.[66]
- Maternal warmth and nurturing childhood environments favor resilience.
- According to the 2011–2012 National Survey of Children's Health, 72% of children with no ACEs reported were resilient. Among children who reported one ACE, 63% were resilient; and among children with two or more ACEs 55% were resilient. Among individual ACEs, parental divorce yielded the highest percentage of resilient children; witnessing domestic violence produced the lowest. An average of 15% of children with two or more ACEs repeated a school grade; if a parent was imprisoned, 20% did. Among children with two or more ACEs, 37% were obese; 61% had behavior problems; 33% had asthma; 45% had attention deficit hyperactivity disorder; 52% had special healthcare needs or emotional, behavioral or developmental problems; and 55% were bullies. These physical and emotional challenges make the children's' resilience prevalences even more astonishing and hopeful.[67, 68]
- Resilient children who have been mistreated need supportive adults, clergy, or relatives to provide stable, adult, loving relationships.
- Childhood trauma, depression, obsessive-compulsive disorder, addictions, and other psychopathology impair self-regulation and therefore resilience.[8, 69]
- "Temperamentally balanced children" resist the damaging effects of discordant homes with depressed, irritable parents. Self-esteem plays a role.

★★★★★

- The Kauai Longitudinal study that followed 698 babies born in 1955 until age 40 identified high-risk children in one-third of the population (chronic poverty, parental mental illness, perinatal complications, and chronic family discord). Only one-third became competent, caring adults due to their sociability, intelligence, self-control, parental attachment, parental and peer emotional support, and religious,[70] school,[71] or work support.[72] Two-thirds did not become competent adults.
- Some children who seem resilient when they are young become vulnerable as adults, but 11% of abused or neglected children in one study who were

non-resilient as adolescents became resilient adults.[73] Thus resilience may change over the life span.

- Older adults are less susceptible to single-event (e.g., natural disaster) trauma than younger adults.[74]
- Close family relationships favor resilience.[8]
- Group identification and the ability to empathize favor resilience.
- Only 10% to 15% of bereaved people develop chronic depression; in one study of bereaved spouses, half of the sample did not even display mild depression. This is not cold, unfeeling attachment, but genuine resilience despite terrible loss. The differences in these buoyant people were belief in their abilities to adapt, belief in a just world, and social support.
- After the September 11, 2001, terrorist attacks in New York City, initial estimates projected 7.5% incidence of PTSD in Manhattan; at four months the prevalence was only 1.7% and 0.6% at six months.[75] The same was true after the Oklahoma City bombing.[5, 6] One determining factor in these low prevalences was the citizens' ability to run, to escape. They were not trapped.[76]
- Children cope better and are less likely to develop PTSD from isolated traumatic events ("Big T") than from multiple small, daily traumas ("small t").[1, 56, 77]
- Self-enhancing bias, the tendency to view the self favorably, even highly favorably, supports resilience.[78]
- Self-esteem, self-confidence, self-understanding, positive outlook, self-control of behavior and emotion, hardiness, good defense mechanisms, good interpersonal skills, sociability, and life coping favor resilience.[6, 79]
- Personal and emotional intelligence favor resilience.[80]
- Resilient individuals have life purposes and spiritual foundations.[32]
- Resilient individuals face fears and cope with adversity because of traits they possessed before the trauma occurred.[36, 81]
- Regular exercise, healthy immune response, optimism,[20, 45, 82, 83] high cognitive functioning, secure family ties,[7] close friendships, forgiveness,[84] active coping strategies,[16, 85] and satisfying work lives each foster resilience.

Notice, however, that each of these research and clinical findings are resilience *attributes*, not *origins*—branches, not roots. Let's look further for the source. What clues might our trauma study provide?

★★★★★

Actor Peter Falk was very young when he developed an eye malignancy (retinoblastoma) that required the eye be removed. His mother took him for surgery but suddenly realized that her wallet was in the car. She left her child at the elevator. "I was three and I remember getting out of the elevator [before surgery]. . . . I told them to wait for my mother. . . . That was the last thing I remember."

Youth, a hospital, understandable fear of the unknown with no protective parent—these are perfect ingredients for a deeply traumatic episode that would yield lifelong scars. Yet it didn't persist:

"As I was growing up, I recall dreading the moment when some kid would ask, 'Hey, what's the matter with your eye.'. . . . This sensitivity started decreasing in my early teens and was completely gone by high school. . . .—I never—but never—thought about it, and I was convinced that the eye would not be a problem."[86]

★★★★★

The Interconnections Among Resilience, ACE Score, Health, and Surgical Satisfaction, with Nick Zaborek, M.A.

In theory, at least, a higher trauma score ought to correlate with a lower resilience score—more difficulty as an adult ought to reflect more suffering as a child. Surprisingly this was not the case for our trauma study patients. The mean ACE score of those who had a resilience of 4 (the best) was 2.5, and the mean ACE score of those whose resilience was less than 4 was 2.9 ($p = 0.1$). Thus the most resilient patients did not necessarily have the easiest childhoods.

Among individual groups, however, these differences blurred except for the two most different: the reconstructive patients (who always had absolute medical indications for surgery) and the BDD patients (who never had absolute indications for surgery because their noses had always been normal). In these two groups, the resilience scores were 3.4 for the reconstructive patients but only 2.8 for the BDD patients ($p < 0.01$).

Our trauma study generated data that we did not expect: lower ACE scores—less trauma—did not predict greater postoperative happiness, though it seems like it should. In fact, as the study progressed, I found that I could not predict my patients' ACE scores by observing them through surgery and or noticing how they behaved and led their lives. Some of our most delightful, grateful patients had the highest ACE scores. Why? Can resilience soften or overcome some of the destructive effects of a difficult childhood?

It seems so, for the characteristics we measured;

Resilient patients were older at the time of their first surgeries, less likely to be depressed, demanding, or perfectionistic, and five and a half times more likely to be happy with their surgical results than non-resilient patients.

For each one point increase in a patient's total ACE score, his or her odds of having an additional health problem increased by 33 percent. However, the chance that a resilient patient (Resilience score 4) will have an additional health issue was 65 percent lower than a non-resilient patient.

Thus resilience, that magical human quality, is associated with different personality traits, better health, and surgical happiness but not with individual ACE scores. Resilience seems to intercept some of the damaging effects of childhood abuse and neglect.

★★★★★

Her Irish face was pretty and iridescent, with bright blue eyes, clear skin, wavy blond haircut to the nape of her neck, and just the right number of dimples. She smelled of good soap and looked blissfully healthy. Tiny hints of aging around her eyes only added mystery.

"These are nice exam chairs," she said, bouncing lightly. "Most doctors have school auditorium seats. I always liked your chairs."

She smiled. I smiled. Her face was open and soft.

"You helped me so much," she said.

"You had a difficult problem, but I don't surrender easily."

I paused. She was still giving me her full attention.

"When you were here last you took the childhood trauma test."

She thought about that. "I remember. It took me back."

"You had some positive answers."

"I did," she said.

"Yet you're always pleasant, you have a successful career and marriage, and you're charming to everyone here. Why aren't you bitter and depressed?" I said.

"It wasn't really so bad . . ." Her voice drifted. "I think my mother always tried to do her best for us. We went to good schools."

I looked at her test sheet.

"That may be true. But you checked emotional abuse, physical and emotional neglect, mental illness in the family, and divorce."

She wrinkled her nose. "It wasn't always fun."

She didn't say anything for a few moments. Her face had become expressionless. Then she spoke quietly, staring at nothing.

"Her screaming voice sounded like a tin can tied to a wedding car," she said. "I sure remember that."

She looked up and smiled. "Get this: She offered to buy me breast implants for my high school graduation."

"How thoughtful," I said.

"That's what I told her. I said they'd make great paperweights on my desk."

"Not easy," I said.

She pushed a lock of hair behind an ear. "I tried shrinks but most of them were crazier than me."

I waited. Apparently there wasn't any more.

"Then why are you so nice?" I said. "Some of my patients tell me that someone outside the family believed in them. I had a grandmother and a Latin teacher and a bishop I met when I was twelve."

She went somewhere else momentarily, then took a deep breath and sat up straighter.

"My college soccer coach. I was on an athletic scholarship but the week before my first practice I panicked and called him. I told him I was going home. He said, 'No, you aren't. You're not a quitter.' So I stayed."

"How did it work out," I said.

She smiled. "I was All-American for four years."

She stopped talking and looked past me through the window.

"I forgot to tell you, two of my brothers went to prison."

"It's easy to accept what we have as normal, no matter what it is," I said.

She laughed. "Like John Adams used to say of Jefferson, 'In Virginia, all geese are swans.'"

She got quiet again and nodded in agreement with a conversation that I couldn't hear.

"A thing is what it is, I guess," she said.

"And nothing more," I said.

The Gifts of Optimism

Notice that the same themes repeat: caregivers; acceptance, social support,[74] peer support, family support,[7] self-esteem, self-confidence, self-understanding, positive outlook, ego strength, defense mechanisms, sociability, emotional expressiveness, interpersonal understanding, empathy, optimism, friendships, spirituality.[87] These are the qualities of interpersonal connection.[88]

Optimism has its own curious salutary effects. Physicians know this from the "nocebo effect," the reverse of the placebo effect: Patients respond to negative messages like they respond to positive ones. Plant the idea of pain or side effects, and their prevalence triples.[89] A childhood that produces a default negative outlook makes it possible for any of us to self-impose our own nocebo effects and doom our own outcomes. The way we view the future affects both attitude and result, which is why optimism is such a critical component of resilience. Sometimes it is the ability to see purpose where there does not seem to be any. We call that faith. At her last imprisonment, 17-year-old Lady Jane Grey prayed, "Give me grace to await Thy leisure, and patiently to bear what Thou doest unto me.... Only arm me . . . that I may stand fast . . . comforting myself in those troubles which it shall please Thee to send me, seeing such troubles are profitable for me."[90]

★★★★★

Dietrich Bonhoeffer was a Christian theologian executed in 1945 for opposing the Nazis. While imprisoned, he wrote letters. Even after all clemency appeals were denied his letters remain suffused with optimism and gratitude. "Please don't ever get anxious or worried about me.... You must never doubt that I'm traveling with gratitude and cheerfulness along the road where I'm being led. . . . It is as though in solitude the soul develops senses which we hardly know in everyday life. Therefore I have not felt lonely or abandoned for one moment. . . . What is happiness and unhappiness? It depends so little on the circumstances; it depends really only on that which happens inside a person. I'm grateful every day that I have you, and that makes me happy."[91]

Bonhoeffer can be grateful because he feels connected. His life is a life of reciprocity. To get support, you have to be able to feel it. Impenetrable walls are not resilience.

"Nobody gets everything he or she yearns for," Harold Kushner writes. "I look at the world and see three sorts of people: those who dream boldly even as they realize that a lot of their dreams will not come true; those who dream more modestly and fear that even their modest dreams may not be realized; and those who are afraid to dream at all, lest they be disappointed."[92]

Viktor Frankl, a psychiatrist imprisoned at Auschwitz, Kaufering, and Türkheim during World War II, never lost the conviction that his life had purpose and that he would be able to write and teach again. But it was a struggle: "The majority of prisoners suffered from a kind of inferiority complex. We all had once been or had fancied ourselves to be 'somebody.' Now we were treated like complete nonentities."[93, 94]

"Then I spoke of the many opportunities of giving life and meaning. . . . Human life, under any circumstances, never ceases to have a meaning. . . . This infinite meaning of life includes suffering and dying, preservation and death.... I remember two cases of would-be suicide. . . . Both used the typical argument—they had nothing more to expect from life. *In both cases it was a question of getting them to realize that life was still expecting something from them* [italics mine]; something in the future.... Only creativeness and enjoyment are meaningful."[94]

The Gifts of Resilience

Thus resilience converts stress and adversity from insurmountable obstacles to events from which lessons can be learned and new meanings assigned. Early in childhood, our genes and their interaction with environmental factors shape our neural circuitry and neurochemical functioning in ways that are observable in behavior, measurable neurochemically, and that can be imaged. Studies in both humans and experimental animals indicate that the early environment alters gene expression and neurochemical transmitters. *Thus the biochemical characteristics found in resilience may be the result of resilience, rather than its cause.* In this regard, the family environment, proximity, support, loving caregivers, and especially exposure to stressors that the child can manage seem to be immutable requirements.[48, 95]

Fosdick describes it this way: "This inherent and ennobling capacity of ours to hope, to plan, to see possibilities, to entertain prophetic insights, necessarily involves the companion capacity to be disappointed. . . . Disappointment is the obverse side of one of the noblest attributes of human nature."[96]

★★★★★

The ability to be resilient contains the ability to see beyond suffering. Surgeon Paul Brand has noted that societies that gain the ability to limit suffering can lose the ability to cope with suffering that remains.[97] Self-worth makes it possible to set goals, to feel that it is "like me" to achieve, and to recognize that the lessons learned along the journey make the goal.[98] "Accomplishment is all about outcome and it is important. . . . What it does not measure is what you've learned. . . . It does not measure who you have become. . . . Attainment is the total of accomplishment and becoming."[98] We make the most of ourselves for the sakes of others. Eric Hoffer writes: "No matter what some anthropologists, sociologists, and geneticists may tell us, we shall go on believing that man, unlike other forms of life, is not a captive of his past—of his heredity and habits—but is possessed of infinite plasticity, and his potentials for good and evil are never wholly exhausted."[4] "The first pulse to take," Samuel Shem writes, "is your own."[99]

Late in life Robert E. Lee wrote, "All is bright if you will think it so. All is happy if you will make it so. . . . Live in the world you inhabit. Look upon things as they are. Take them as you find them. Make the best of them. Turn them to your advantage."[100]

How similar those words are to those of Elie Wiesel to his companions at Auschwitz: "Ahead of you lies a long road paved with suffering. Don't lose hope. You have already eluded the worst danger: the selection. Therefore muster your strength and keep your faith. . . . Hell does not last forever. . . . Let there be camaraderie among you. We are all brothers and share the same fate. The same smoke hovers over all our heads."

Happiness may not be the consequence of living well, but rather its source.[31]

★★★★★

Pete Huttlinger came from a large family where one brother became addicted to drugs and in which there were five suicides and one murder among close relatives. Yet he graduated from the Berkeley School of Music, played lead guitar for John Denver, performed three times at Carnegie Hall and at Eric Clapton's Crossroads festivals, composed and recorded many albums of his own compositions and in 2000 won the National Finger Style Guitar Championship.

But his story is infinitely more complicated. Born with a severe congenital heart defect and *situs inversus*, in which the internal organs are reversed to mirror-image position, Huttlinger had undergone cardiac surgery at a young age. "I felt like a loser but I knew there was nothing I could do to change the situation," he remembered of his childhood.[101] Despite incipient heart failure Huttlinger composed and performed brilliantly, but in 2010 had a stroke that paralyzed his right side. Following surgery he regained his speech and labored to compose, play, and perform again till congestive heart failure became so severe that he required an external ventricular pump and long months of hospitalization. For the third time Huttlinger taught himself to play and perform.

The autobiography that he wrote with his wife, Erin, fairly jumps with resilience.[102] Huttlinger had not played guitar for five months and had lost all desire. Then a hospital nurse asked him to play. "I used to be a player but not anymore," he told another patient. "Off I went to another room, IV pole in one hand and guitar in the other to play a few tunes for someone else. The next thing I knew I was on the circuit . . . playing for the patients. This was the best gig of my life. . . . I had been transformed from someone who was a sick patient to someone who was helping others heal. . . . This was when my attitude changed. . . . I was finally able to give something back to others. . . . I could stop focusing on me for a little while each day and focus on another patient who was worse off." One year to the day after being life-flighted from Nashville to Houston, he and his wife completed a half marathon carrying his external ventricular pump in a shoulder bag. "Don't just live," he writes. "Live well."[102]

I corresponded with him in 2015. "I would be happy to speak with you [about resilience] when you are ready," he wrote. "I have not always been successful but I continue to get up when I'm knocked off the horse. I guess I'm a slow learner. Cheers, Pete." Sadly, we never had that conversation. He died of another stroke three months later at age 54.

Yet Pete Huttlinger's story remains one of unbounded resilience manifested as impish humor, perspective, a life philosophy, and devotion to his wife, family, and music. *Resilience was the result, the product of his connectedness, not the cause of it. Resilience ultimately depends on factors that individuals can control themselves, not just external supports.* It is another measure of self-sufficiency. Childhood isn't destiny.

What This Information Means

Shame constricts, isolates, and turns us inward. Disempowerment or grandiosity, porous boundaries or walls, distorted thinking, poor self-care, and living to excess or hardly living at all disconnect us from our worlds. Trauma is isolating. Depression; eating disorders; mental illness; obesity; cutting; addictions to alcohol, drugs, sex, gambling, work; suicidal ideation; and body dysmorphic disorder are not group behaviors: they are almost always solitary. Untreated trauma detaches, sequesters, and isolates; it reflects distorted thinking, information processing, and behavior biased by childhood. Trauma is lonely. Thus the first part of resilience is the capacity to look outward and care about others. Like being fully relational, resilience requires connection.

The door to freedom must be opened from the inside.

★★★★★

Resilience cannot only be inherited or neurochemical. It is at least partly, perhaps primarily, a result—of opening out, of being relational. When we are exposed, we are not walled; we are free to connect. From that expansion of personality and spirit comes life philosophy, perspective, humor, optimism, and the capacity to receive support—impossible personal characteristics for those turned in on themselves. Each of the unhappy patients we have discussed, dragging their body shame, obsessions, addictions, and self-injurious behaviors behind them, are inwardly directed, closed to full human contact. People living in their wounds are humorless malcontents: we see them as sad or hostile. They ruminate and panic and don't listen because they cannot absorb and process outside information without altering it unfavorably: we see them as argumentative, judgmental, and irrational. They live with intolerable emotional pain: we call them addicts. Toxic shame circulates within them: we see depression or self-injury. When this shame attaches to a physical feature, plastic surgeons and therapists see them as body dysmorphic patients. They cannot be resilient.

Unraveling trauma opens us toward each other. Living as functional adults creates the abilities to connect, receive support, have life perspective, and be optimistic, perseverant, and spiritual. These are the characteristics that we see, admire, and call "resilience."

★★★★★

And so I propose that resilience might not be a trait, something that some people are just lucky to have, like pretty eyes. Resilience might really be an *outcome*, the result of a controlled, self-respecting life lived in moderation and connection with others. That's when resilience appears—in fact, resilience seems inevitable for a life lived in abundance. "Self-understanding," "optimism," "control," "hardiness," "good defenses," "interpersonal skills," "sociability," "support," "life perspective," "spirituality," "self-confidence"—all the attributes of resilience are also the antidotes to trauma. Such lucky survivors feel autonomous: valuable, contained, protected, temperate, and clear-thinking. Life becomes reciprocal.[103]

★★★★★

Helen Keller, who lost her sight and hearing at 19 months from an illness that was probably scarlet fever, curable today, wrote a wonderful book at age 23 with the unexpected title of *Optimism*.

> "If I had regarded my life from the point of view of the pessimist, I should be undone," she wrote. "I should seek in vain for the light that does not visit my eyes and the music that does not ring in my ears. . . . I should sit apart in awful solitude. . . . But . . . I consider it a duty to myself and others to be happy. Thus, the optimist believes, attempts, achieves. He stands always in the sunlight."[104]

Where We Have Gone

Thus this chapter ends where it began; our book about body image-disturbed patients ends somewhere new, and I believe better. Happiness doesn't turn out to be a major affective disorder, and a shame-based life consumed with physical appearance and surgery doesn't have to be the predestined result of a painful or destructive childhood. Those of us who never had trauma and those of us who have broken out and become engaged, empowered, and relational—to each other, to our families, and to our communities—can all display resilience. Others may call it a remarkable trait, but it is really just the upshot of being fully human, an inspiring possibility for us all.

References

1. Wright KA, Turanovic JJ, O'Neal EN, et al. The Cycle of Violence Revisited: Childhood Victimization, Resilience, and Future Violence. *J Interpers Violence* 2016; May 25. pii: 0886260516651090.
2. Fosdick HE. *Riverside Sermons*. New York: Harper & Brothers; 1958:122, 224, 227.
3. Bentall RP. A Proposal to Classify Happiness as a Psychiatric Disorder. *J Med Ethics* 1992; 18:94–98.
4. Hoffer E. *The Ordeal of Change*. Titusville [NJ]: Hopewell Publications; 2006.
5. Solomon RL. The Opponent-process Theory of Acquired Motivation: The Costs of Pleasure and the Benefits of Pain. *Am Psychol* 1980; 35:8:691–712.
6. Southwick SM, Vythilingam M, Charney DS. The Psychobiology of Depression and Resilience to Stress: Implications for Prevention and Treatment. *Ann Rev Clin Psychol* 2005; 1:255–291.
7. Meyerson MD. Resiliency and Success in Adults with Moebius Syndrome. *Cleft Palate-Craniofac J* 2001; 38:3:231–235.
8. Reich JW, Zautra AJ, Hall JS, eds. *Handbook Of Adult Resilience*. New York: The Guilford Press; 2010.
9. Valentino R, Sheline Y, McEwen B. Editorial Introduction to the Special Issue on Stress Resilience. *Neurobiol Stress* 2015; 1:80.

10. Walsh WA, Dawson J, Mattingly MJ. How Are We Measuring Resilience Following Childhood Maltreatment? Is the Research Adequate and Consistent? What Is the Impact on Research, Practice, and Policy? *Trauma Violence Abuse* 2010; 11:1:27–41.

11. Massie H, Szajnberg N. My Life Is a Longing: Child Abuse and Its Adult Sequelae: Result of the Brody Longitudinal Study from Birth to Age 30. *Int J Psychoanal* 2006; 87:471–496.

12. Francis M. *Diary Of A Stage Mother's Daughter: A Memoir.* New York: Weinstein Books; 2012.

13. McEwen BS. Stress, Adaptation and Disease. *Ann NY Acad Sci* 1998; 840:1:33–44.

14. Rowling JK. *Very Good Lives: The Fringe Benefits of Failure and the Importance Of Imagination.* New York: Little Brown and Company; 2008.

15. Seery MD, Holman EA. Whatever Does Not Kill Us: Cumulative Lifetime Adversity, Vulnerability, and Resilience. *J Personal Soc Psychol* 2010; 99:6:1025–1041.

16. Wood SK, Bhatnagar S. Resilience to the Effects of Social Stress: Evidence from Clinical and Preclinical Studies on the Role of Coping Strategies. *Neurobiol Stress* 2015; 1:164–173.

17. Feder A, Nestler EJ, Charney DS. Psychobiology and Molecular Genetics of Resilience. *Nat Rev Neurosci* 2009; 10:6:446–457.

18. Hood SC, Beaudet MP, Catlin G. A Healthy Outlook. *Health Rep* 1996; 7:4:25–32, 27–35.

19. Kiecolt-Glaser JK, Page GG, Marucha PT, et al. Psychological Influences on Surgical Recovery. *Am Psychol* 1998; 53:11:1209–1218.

20. Scheier MF, Carver CS. Dispositional Optimism and Physical Well-Being: The Influence of Generalized Outcome Expectancies on Health. *J Personal* 1987; 55:2:169–210.

21. Anthony B. *Chaplin's Music Hall: The Chaplins and Their Circle in the Limelight.* New York: LB Taurus; 2012:46–47.

22. Boyette LL, van Dam D, Meijer C, et al. Personality Compensates for Impaired Quality of Life and Social Functioning in Patients with Psychotic Disorders Who Experienced Traumatic Events. *Schizophr Bull* 2014; 40:6:1356–1365.

23. Croft A, Dunn EW, Quoidbach J. From Tribulations to Appreciation: Experiencing Adversity in the Past Predicts Greater Savoring in the Present. *Soc Psychol Personality Sci* 2014; XX:X:1–6.

24. Bethell CD, Newacheck P, Hawes E, et al. Adverse Childhood Experiences: Assessing the Impact on Health and School Engagement and the Mitigating Role of Resilience. *Health Aff* 2014; 33:12:2106–2115.

25. Seery MD, Leo RJ, Holman EA, et al. Lifetime Exposure to Adversity Predicts Functional Impairment and Healthcare Utilization among Individuals with Chronic Back Pain. *Pain* 2010; 150:507–515.

26. Lee KA, Vaillant GE, Torrey WC, et al. A 50-Year Prospective Study of the Psychological Sequelae of World War II Combat. *Am J Psychiatry* 1995; 152:4:516–522.

27. Friborg O, Hjemdal O, Rosenvinge JH, et al. A New Rating Scale for Adult Resilience: What Are the Central Protective Resources Behind Healthy Adjustment? *Intl J Methods Psychiatric Res* 2003; 12:2:65–76.

28. Mellody P, Freundlich LS. *The Intimacy Factor: The Ground Rules For Overcoming The Obstacles To Truth, Respect, And Lasting Love.* New York: Harper Collins; 2003.

29. McGonigal K. *The Upside Of Stress: Why Stress Is Good For You, And How To Get Good At It.* New York: Avery [Penguin Random House]; 2015.

30. Tedeschi RG, Calhoun LG. The Posttraumatic Growth Inventory: Measuring the Positive Legacy of Trauma. *J Traumatic Stress* 1996; 9:3:455–471.

31. Duckworth A. *Grit: The Power of Passion and Perseverance*. New York: Scribner; 2016.
32. Bonanno GA. Loss, Trauma, and Human Resilience. *Am Psychol* 2004; 59:1:20–28.
33. Pfau ML, Russo SJ. Peripheral and Central Mechanisms of Stress Resilience. *Neurobiol Stress* 2015; 1:66–79.
34. Weisel E. *Night: New Translation By Marion Weisel*. New York: Hill and Wang; 1958.
35. Millard C. *The River Of Doubt: Theodore Roosevelt's Darkest Journey*. New York: Anchor Books; 2005.
36. Pearce ME, Jongbloed KA, Richardson CG, et al. The Cedar Project: Resilience in the Face of HIV Vulnerability Within a Cohort Study Involving Young Indigenous People Who Use Drugs in Three Canadian Cities. *BMC Public Health* 2015; 15:1:1095.
37. Larkin H, Beckos BA, Shields JJ. Mobilizing Resilience and Recovery in Response to Adverse Childhood Experiences (ACE): A Restorative Integral Support (RIS) Case Study. *J Prev Interv Community* 2012; 40:4:335–346.
38. Schaan VK, Vögele C. Resilience and Rejection Sensitivity Mediate Long-term Outcomes of Parental Divorce. *Eur Child Adolesc Psychiatry* 2016; Jul 26. [Epub ahead of print] PubMed PMID: 27460656.
39. Schulz A, Becker M, Van der Auwera S, et al. The Impact of Childhood Trauma on Depression: Does Resilience Matter? Population-Based Results from the Study of Health in Pomerania. *J Psychosom Res* 2014; 77:2:97–103.
40. Sexton MB, Hamilton L, McGinnis EW, et al. The Roles of Resilience and Childhood Trauma History: Main and Moderating Effects on Postpartum Maternal Mental Health and Functioning. *J Affect Disord* 2015; 174:562–568.
41. Lanius RA, Vermette E, Pain C, eds. *The Impact of Early Life Trauma On Health And Disease: The Hidden Epidemic*. Cambridge [UK]: Cambridge University Press; 2010.
42. Franzoni E, Gualandi S, Caretti V, et al. The Relationship between Alexithymia, Shame, Trauma, and Body Image Disorders: Investigation Over a Large Clinical Sample. *Neuropsychiatric Dis Treat* 2013; 9:185–193.
43. Harris MA, Brett CE, Starr JM, et al. Early-Life Predictors of Resilience and Related Outcomes Up to 66 Years Later in the 6-Day Sample of the 1947 Scottish Mental Survey. *Soc Psychiatry Psychiatr Epidemiol* 2016; 51:5:659–668.
44. Singh-Taylor A, Korosi A, Molet J, et al. Synaptic Rewiring of Stress-Sensitive Neurons of Early-Life Experience: A Mechanism for Resilience. *Neurobiol Stress* 2015; 1:109–115.
45. Segerstrom SC, Taylor SE, Kemeny ME, et al. Optimism Is Associated with Mood, Coping, and Immune Change in Response to Stress. *J Personality and Social Psychol* 1998; 74:6:1646–1655.
46. Walter KH, Horsey KJ, Palmieri PA, et al. The Role of Protective Self-Cognitions in the Relationship between Childhood Trauma and Later Resource Loss. *J Trauma Stress* 2010; 23:2:264–273.
47. Wessells MG. Commentary: A Social Environment Approach to Promotive and Protective Practice in Childhood Resilience—Reflections on Ungar (2014). *J Child Psychol Psychiatry* 2015; 56:1:18–20.
48. McEwen BS, Gray JD, Nasca C. Recognizing Resilience: Learning from the Effects of Stress on the Brain. *Neurobiol Stress* 2015; 1:1–11.
49. Das D, Cherbuin N, Tan X, et al. DRD4-exonIII-VNTR Moderates the Effect of Childhood Adversities on Emotional Resilience in Young-Adults. *PLoS One* 2011; 6:5:e20177.
50. Bradley B, Davis TA, Wingo AP, et al. Family Environment and Adult Resilience: Contributions of Positive Parenting and the Oxytocin Receptor Gene. *Eur J Psychotraumatol* 2013; 4:1–9.

51. Carli V, Mandelli L, Zaninotto L, et al. A Protective Genetic Variant for Adverse Environments? The Role of Childhood Traumas and Serotonin Transporter Gene on Resilience and Depressive Severity in a High-Risk Population. *Eur Psychiatry* 2011; 26:8:471–478.

52. Charney DS. Psychobiological Mechanisms of Resilience and Vulnerability: Implications for Successful Adaptation to Extreme Stress. *Am J Psychiatry* 2004; 161:2:195–216.

53. Fossion P, Leys C, Kempenaers C, et al. Depression, Anxiety and Loss of Resilience After Multiple Traumas: An Illustration of a Mediated Moderation Model of Sensitization in a Group of Children Who Survived the Nazi Holocaust. *J Affect Disord* 2013; 151:3:973–979.

54. Fossion P, Leys C, Kempenaers C, et al. Disentangling Sense of Coherence and Resilience in Case of Multiple Traumas. *J Affect Disord* 2014; 160:21–26.

55. Suzuki A, Poon L, Kumari V, et al. Fear Biases in Emotional Face Processing Following Childhood Trauma as a Marker of Resilience and Vulnerability to Depression. *Child Maltreat* 2015; 20:4:240–250.

56. Rutter M. Implications of Resilience Concepts for Scientific Understanding. *Ann NY Acad Sci* 2006; 1094:1:1–12.

57. Kim-Cohen J, Turkewitz R. Resilience and Measured Gene-Environment Interactions. *Dev Psychopathol* 2012; 24:4:1297–1306.

58. Reul J, Collins A, Saliba RS, et al. Glucocorticoids, Epigenetic Control and Stress Resilience. *Neurobiol Stress* 2015; 1:44–59.

59. Levine PA, Kline M. *Trauma-Proofing Your Kids: A Parents' Guide For Instilling Confidence, Joy And Resilience.* Berkeley [CA]: North Atlantic Books; 2008.

60. Meyer N, Richter H, Schreiber RS, et al. The Unexpected Effects of Beneficial and Adverse Social Experiences During Adolescence on Anxiety and Aggression and Their Modulation by Genotype. *Front Behav Neurosci* 2016; 10:97–124.

61. Levis DJ. A Review of Childhood Abuse Questionnaires and Suggested Treatment Approaches. In: Kalfoğlu EA, Faikoğlu R, eds. *Sexual Abuse: Breaking the Silence.* Intechopin.com, IntechOpen; 2012:1.

62. Felitti VJ, Jakstis K, Pepper V, et al. Obesity: Problem, Solution, or Both? *Perm J* 2010; 14:1:24–31.

63. Wilson JZ, Marin D, Maxwell K, et al. Association of Posttraumatic Growth and Illness-Related Burden with Psychosocial Factors of Patient, Family, and Provider in Pediatric Cancer Survivors. *J Trauma Stress* 2016; 29:5:448–456.

64. Yi J, Kim MA. Postcancer Experiences of Childhood Cancer Survivors: How Is Posttraumatic Stress Related to Posttraumatic Growth? *J Traum Stress* 2014; 27:461–467.

65. Luthar, SS, Sawyer, JA, Brown, PJ. (2006). Conceptual Issues in Studies of Resilience. *Ann NY Acad Sci* 1094; 105–115.

66. Kesebir S, Ünübol B, Tatlıdil Yaylacı E, et al. Impact of Childhood Trauma and Affective Temperament on Resilience in Bipolar Disorder. *Int J Bipolar Disord* 2015; 3:3.

67. Kilpatrick DG, Resnick HS, Milanak ME, et al. National Estimates of Exposure to Traumatic Events and PTSD Using DSM-IV and DSM-5 Criteria. *J Traumatic Stress* 2013; 26:5:537–547.

68. Kessler RC, Sonnega A, Bromet E, et al. Posttraumatic Stress Disorder in the National Comorbidity Survey. *Arch Gen Psychiatry* 1995; 52:12:1048–1060.

69. Kunseler FC, Oosterman M, de Moor MH, et al. Weakened Resilience in Parenting Self-Efficacy in Pregnant Women Who Were Abused in Childhood: An Experimental Test. *PLoS One* 2016; 11:2:e0141801.

70. Lowe SR, Rhodes JE, Waters MC. Understanding Resilience and Other Trajectories of Psychological Distress: A Mixed-Methods Study of Low-Income Mothers Who Survived Hurricane Katrina. *Curr Psychol* 2015; 34:3:537–550.

71. Bethell C, Gombojav N, Solloway M, et al. Adverse Childhood Experiences, Resilience and Mindfulness-Based Approaches: Common Denominator Issues for Children with Emotional, Mental, or Behavioral Problems. *Child Adolesc Psychiatr Clin N Am* 2016; 25:2:139–156.

72. Warner, EE, Smith, RS. 1992. *Overcoming the Odds: High Risk Children From Birth to Adulthood.* Ithaca, NY: Cornell University Press.

73. Dumont, KA, Widom, CS, Czaja, SJ. Predictors of Resilience in Abused and Neglected Children Grown Up: The Role of Individuals and Neighborhood Characteristics. *Child Abuse and Neglect* 2007; 31:255–274.

74. Maercker A, Hilpert P, Burri A. Childhood Trauma and Resilience in Old Age: Applying a Context Model of Resilience to a Sample of Former Indentured Child Laborers. *Aging Ment Health* 2016; 20:6:616–626.

75. Frederickson BL, Tugade MM, Waugh CE, et al. What Good Are Positive Emotions in Crises: A Prospective Study of Resilience and Emotions Following the Terrorist Attacks on the United States on September 11th, 2001. *J Pers Soc Psychol* 2003; 84:2:365–376.

76. van der Kolk B. The Body Keeps the Score. In: van der Kolk B, McFarlane AC, Weisaeth L, eds. *Traumatic Stress.* New York: The Guilford Press; 2007:233–234.

77. Wrenn GL, Wingo AP, Moore R, et al. The Effect of Resilience on Posttraumatic Stress Disorder in Trauma-Exposed Inner-City Primary Care Patients. *J Natl Med Assoc* 2011; 103:7:560–566.

78. Daniels JK, Hegadoren KM, Coupland NJ, et al. Neural Correlates and Predictive Power of Trait Resilience in An Acutely Traumatized Sample: A Pilot Investigation. *J Clin Psychiatry* 2012; 73:3:327–332.

79. Watson D, Clark LA, Tellegen A. Development and Validation of Brief Measures of Positive and Negative Affect: The PANAS Scales. *J Personal Soc Psychol* 1988; 54:6:1063–1070.

80. Simeon D, Yehuda R, Cunill R, et al. Factors Associated with Resilience in Healthy Adults. *Psychoneuroendocrinol* 2007; 32:8–10:1149–1152.

81. Noeker M. Survivors of Pediatric Cancer. Developmental Paths and Outcomes Between Trauma and Resilience. *Bundesgesundheitsblatt Gesundheitsforschung Gesundheitsschutz* 2012; 55:4:481–492.

82. Marini J. Frank Capra's America and Ours. *Imprimis Hillsdale.edu* 2015; 44:3:3–7.

83. Scheier MF, Carver CS, Bridges MW. Distinguishing Optimism from Neuroticism (and Trait Anxiety, Self-Mastery, and Self-Esteem): A Reevaluation of the Life Orientation Test. *J Personal Soc Psychol* 1994; 67:6:1063–1078.

84. Porterfield KA, Lindhout A. Healing in Forgiveness: A Discussion with Amanda Lindhout and Katherine Porterfield, PhD. *Eur J Psychotraumatol* 2014; 5.

85. Campbell-Sills L, Cohan SL, Stein MB. Relationship of Resilience to Personality, Coping, and Psychiatric Symptoms in Young Adults. *Behav Res Ther* 2006; 44:4:585–599.

86. Falk P. *Just One More Thing: Stories From My Life.* New York: Carroll & Graf; 2006.

87. Brewer-Smyth K, Koenig HG. Could Spirituality and Religion Promote Stress Resilience in Survivors of Childhood Trauma? *Issues Ment Health Nurs* 2014; 35:4:251–256.

88. Chandler GE, Roberts SJ, Chiodo L. Resilience Intervention for Young Adults with Adverse Childhood Experiences. *J Am Psychiatr Nurses Assoc* 2015; 21:6:406–416.

89. Colloca L, Finniss D. Nocebo Effects, Patient-Clinician Communication, and Therapeutic Outcomes. *JAMA* 2012; 307:6:567–568.

90. Fosdick HE. *What Is Vital In Religion: Sermons On Contemporary Christian Problems.* New York: Harper & Brothers; 1955, pp. 50, 113.

91. Bonhoeffer D. *Letters and Papers From Prison.* New York: Touchstone; 1997.

92. Kushner, HS. *Overcoming Life's Disappointments.* New York: Alfred A. Knopf; 2006.

93. Carli V, Roy A, Bevilacqua L, et al. Insomnia and Suicidal Behaviour in Prisoners. *Psychiatry Res* 2011; 185:1–2:141–144.

94. Frankl, VE. *Man's Search For Meaning.* Boston: Beacon Press; 1945.

95. Cash TF, Smolak, eds. *Body Image: A Handbook Of Science, Practice, And Prevention.* New York: The Guilford Press; 2011, 135.

96. Fosdick HE. *Living Under Tension: Sermons On Christianity Today.* New York: Harper & Brothers; 1941, 22.

97. Brand P, Yancey P. *The Gift Nobody Wants: The Inspiring Story of A Surgeon Who Discovers Why We Hurt and What We Can Do About It.* New York: Harper Collins; 1993.

98. Bassham L. *With Winning In Mind: The Mental Management System: An Olympic Champion's Success System,* mentalmanagement.com; 2011.

99. Shem S. *House of God.* New York, Dell; 1978.

100. Thomas EM. *Robert E. Lee: A Biography.* New York: W W Norton & Company; 1995.

101. Iancu I, Cohen E, Yehuda YB, et al. Treatment of Eating Disordered Improves Eating Symptoms but Not Alexithymia and Dissociation Proneness. *Comp Psychiatry* 2006; 47:189–193.

102. Huttlinger P, Huttlinger EM. *Joined At The Heart: A Story Of Love, Guitars, Resilience And Marigolds.* Nashville [TN]: Instar Publishing; 2015.

103. Keller H. *The Story of My Life.* Mineola [NY]: Dover Publications; 1996:51, 70.

104. Keller, H. *Optimism.* New York: T.Y. Cromwell and Co.; 1903.

AFTERWORD

*"It is true that there are many patients. So very many patients. Each day they come. . . . At the time they stand before you and tell their story you make the contact. . . . It comes with being a doctor. A person comes to you and describes his ailment. You observe him carefully. You watch closely for a little sign that will tell you what you must know. And the patient will not have confidence in you if he senses that the contact has not been made."**

The words that Cousins quotes from Dr. Margaret van der Kreek at the Schweitzer Hospital articulate the dominant theme of this book. Patients desire and need human contact most of all, the attentive touch of the doctor—which, until the advents of morphine, digitalis, sulfanilamide for infectious disease, B12 for pernicious anemia, and insulin for diabetes—most of them within the last century—was all physicians had to offer. Sometimes it still is.

★★★★★

Like other trauma-based, self-injurious behaviors, body dysmorphic disorder is a continuum. At one end are successful adults who nonetheless organize their lives around improving their appearances compulsively and addictively. At the other end are the delusional, housebound, sometimes suicidal patients described in the mental health literature. But the inciting ingredients common to both are just two: *shame* and *body*. All they need is lighter fluid.

If the long arm of childhood trauma is so terribly ubiquitous, storing and manifesting its toxicity as body shame, depression, distorted memory, and self-injurious behavior, perhaps we have modeled body dysmorphic disorder exactly backwards. We see so much less when we are sure of where we are going. Perhaps we need new eyes.

★★★★★

The current model of body dysmorphic disorder hypothesizes teens and adults who suddenly become obsessed with certain features until their lives are distorted and their self-esteem, family relationships, and abilities to function disappear. No one is positive why this obsession happens.

Suppose we reverse cause and effect. Suppose childhood abuse and neglect impair self-esteem and produce the body-shamed, obsessive, delusional, and addictive behaviors that we call body dysmorphic disorder. Can't almost all BDD beliefs and behaviors findings be explained by the results of adverse childhood events? Extensive published data indicate that they can—and support the concept that many unhealthy and intemperate behaviors have one unifying origin (Figure 9.1). In that case genetic abnormalities become epigenetic changes; the disrupted families and the significant first-degree prevalence make sense. PTSD-like MRI and neurotransmitter findings reflect childhood, not inherited, damage. *Childhood trauma is the seed; shame its core manifestation and fuel; and dysregulation, addiction, and disease are its poisonous blooms. Body dysmorphic disorder becomes just one of those blooms.* There is a unity among the somatic, addictive, and self-injurious behaviors we have discussed: They share many of the same preceding events and leave the same trails.

Viewed this way, body dysmorphic disorder reflects another body-shame-based, somatic expression of complex trauma, another kind of addiction, with its isolating walls, obsessions, compulsions, deceits, shame, secrecy, self-injury, and persistent behavior despite poor outcomes—another legacy of inescapable danger. This, then, is the explanation for the high family prevalence. These links are not my conjectures: they are each in the literature. Many of the questions raised by one research branch have already been answered by another. We might help these patients more by thinking sideways than only straight ahead.† The body dysmorphic mystery is seriously incomplete without the trauma story.

★★★★★

My own ace score is 3. That's not much compared to many patients, but it was enough to affect me. The upshot as a young surgeon was that I did not fully understand why I had any real effect on the lives of my patients. I couldn't even explain why they kept postoperative appointments. In a home where my ideas were often discounted, I had modeled the rest of my world like that. I thought that I was invisible to others like I was to myself. Now I know better.

Physicians are teachers and health ministers. Medicine is more than curing diseases and rescuing patients from the edge of catastrophe. Sometimes—oftentimes—the cure is the relationship. That is what makes it so hard to help patients walled by their defenses and sequestered in their addictions. They are unable to be relational or resilient. Treating physicians must set their own bounda-ries, manage their own energies, listen, find out what their patients need and help them make safe plans, and remember that all patient behavior is not about the physician.

Serving patients whose lives have been distorted by childhood and whose memories and behavior have been hijacked by deeply wounding events may require less concentration on anatomy and more on their driving tumult. The most direct path to the heart of the body dysmorphic mystery may be, "Tell me about your childhood."

Notes

* Cousins, N. *Dr Schweitzer of Lambaréné*, New York: Harper, 1960, p. 74.
† 139A. Coulehan K. Negative Capability and the Art of Medicine. *JAMA* 2017; 318:24:2429–2430.

INDEX

Note: Page numbers in *italics* denote references to figures and in **bold** indicate tables.

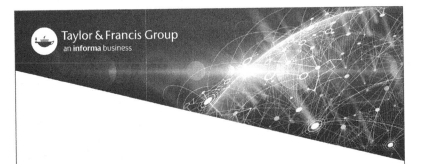

Printed in the United States
by Baker & Taylor Publisher Services